Lecture Notes in Bioengineering

Lecture Notes in Bioengineering (LNBE) publishes the latest developments in bioengineering. It covers a wide range of topics, including (but not limited to):

- Bio-inspired Technology & Biomimetics
- Biosensors
- Bionanomaterials
- Biomedical Instrumentation
- Biological Signal Processing
- Medical Robotics and Assistive Technology
- Computational Medicine, Computational Pharmacology and Computational Biology
- Personalized Medicine
- Data Analysis in Bioengineering
- Neuroengineering
- Bioengineering Ethics

Original research reported in proceedings and edited books are at the core of LNBE. Monographs presenting cutting-edge findings, new perspectives on classical fields or reviewing the state-of-the art in a certain subfield of bioengineering may exceptionally be considered for publication. Alternatively, they may be redirected to more specific book series. The series' target audience includes advanced level students, researchers, and industry professionals working at the forefront of their fields.

Indexed by SCOPUS, INSPEC, zbMATH, SCImago.

More information about this series at https://link.springer.com/bookseries/11564

José García-Alonso · César Fonseca
Editors

Gerontechnology IV

Contributions to the Fourth International Workshop on Gerontechnology, IWoG 2021, November 23–24, 2021, Évora, Portugal

Springer

Editors
José García-Alonso
University of Extremadura
Cáceres, Spain

César Fonseca
University of Évora
Évora, Portugal

ISSN 2195-271X ISSN 2195-2728 (electronic)
Lecture Notes in Bioengineering
ISBN 978-3-030-97523-4 ISBN 978-3-030-97524-1 (eBook)
https://doi.org/10.1007/978-3-030-97524-1

This Springer imprint is published by the registered company Springer Nature Switzerland AG
The registered company address is: Gewerbestrasse 11, 6330 Cham, Switzerland

Preface

The International Workshop on Gerontechnology (IWoG) aims to promote research and scientific exchange related to Gerontechnology and to bring together researchers and practitioners from various disciplines of the academia, public administrations and industry in order to tackle emerging challenges in the Gerontechnology applications and associated technologies, as well as to assess the impact of these technologies on society, media and culture.

This volume collects the full research papers (field, statistics, technical and vision works) and short research papers presented at the Fourth International Workshop on Gerontechnology (4th IWoG), held in Cáceres (University of Extremadura, Spain) and Évora (University of Évora, Portugal) during November 23–24, 2021.

The fourth edition of IWoG accepted contributions related to different dimensions of Gerontechnology: use of technology to improve functional ability and promote healthy aging; health interventions to support caregivers of elderly people; the effectiveness of public health initiatives and clinical interventions for prevent, reverse or mitigate decreases in physical and mental abilities; solutions for active aging, social integration and self-care; monitoring and management of chronic and non-chronic diseases in ambient assisted living; learning, training and coaching systems to promote healthy life in ambient assisted living environments; smart homes and sensor networks for ambient assisted living; context awareness in ambient assisted living environments; use of context and location information in user interfaces; elderly nutrition; health, wellness and disease monitoring; knowledge management for health (context, cognition, behavior and user modeling); health ecosystems (frameworks, models and methodologies); smarts technologies and algorithms for health.

This workshop was organized by the program committee (PC), with a senior PC composed of well-known experts from the field in charge of monitoring the work and animating the discussions of the broader regular PC. This made it easier to run the virtual PC meeting of the full research papers track and the discussion about each paper.

The program for IWoG 2021 was versatile and multifaceted. In this workshop, there were only full papers, and we selected 40 out of 135 submissions, resulting in an acceptance rate of 33 %.

This excellent and comprehensive program would not have been possible without the help of those who contributed to the success of the event. We would like to thank all the different chairs for their hard work. Our thanks also go to Helianthe Kort, Sumi Helal and David Mendes who imparted the main talks of the workshop.

We are grateful to our local organizers 4IE team of University of Extremadura and University of Évora for their logistical support and to Springer for publishing this volume. In addition, we want to thank the PC members, the additional reviewers and the student volunteers for their effort to make IWoG 2021 a very special event, both in terms of academic ambition and practical arrangements.

Finally, we want to thank you, authors and the IWoG community, for taking the time and effort to participate in IWog 2021.

January 2022

José García-Alonso
César Fonseca

Organization

Program Chairs

José García-Alonso	University of Extremadura, Spain
César Fonseca	University of Évora, Portugal
Manuel Lopes	University of Évora, Portugal

Proceeding Chair

Enrique Moguel	University of Extremadura, Spain

Program Committee

Juan Manuel Murillo	University of Extremadura, Spain
Javier Berrocal	University of Extremadura, Spain
Lorenzo Mariano Juárez	University of Extremadura, Spain
Sergio Cordovilla	University of Extremadura, Spain
Carlos Canal	University of Málaga, Spain
David Mendes	University of Évora, Portugal
Lara Guedes de Pinho	University of Évora, Portugal
Niko Mäkitalo	University of Helsinki, Finland
César Alberto Collazos	University of Cauca, Colombia
Julio Ariel Hurtado	University of Cauca, Colombia
Mohamed Mohamed	Ubiquitous Platforms Almaden Research Center, San Jose, California, USA
Luca Foschini	University of Bologna, Italy
Elena Navarro	University of Castilla-La Mancha, Spain
Javier Jaén	University of Valencia, Spain
Felismina Mendes	University of Évora, Portugal
Pedro Parreira	Nursing School of Coimbra, Portugal
Ana Paula Oliveira	Polytechnic Institute of Portalegre, Portugal
Adriano Pedro	Polytechnic Institute of Portalegre, Portugal

Rogério Ferreira	Polytechnic Institute of Beja, Portugal
Ana Canhestro	Polytechnic Institute of Beja, Portugal
Henrique Oliveira	Polytechnic Institute of Beja, Portugal
Maria Margarida Palma Goes	Polytechnic Institute of Beja, Portugal
Lucília Nunes	Polytechnic Institute of Setubal, Portugal
Lisete Mónico	University of Coimbra, Portugal
Laura Ruotsalainen	University of Helsinki, Finland
Ángela Barriga	Western Norway University of Applied Sciences, Norway
Alejandro Rodríguez	Western Norway University of Applied Sciences, Norway
Fabio Casati	University of Trento, Italy
Sergio Ochoa	University of Chile, Chile
Patricia Paderewski	University of Granada, Spain
Francisco Luis Gutiérrez	University of Granada, Spain
John Edison Muñoz	University of Waterloo, Canada
Jeferson Arango	University of Caldas
Francisco Chávez de la O.	University of Extremadura, Spain
Jaime Galán-Jiménez	University of Extremadura, Spain
Marino Linaje	University of Extremadura, Spain
Cristina Vicente-Chicote	University of Extremadura, Spain
David Conde-Caballero	University of Extremadura, Spain
Enrique Moguel	University of Extremadura, Spain

Sponsors

UEX UNIVERSIDAD DE EXTREMADURA

UNIVERSIDADE DE ÉVORA

SEPAD

Servicio Extremeño de Promoción de la Autonomía y Atención a la Dependencia

FS FundeSalud

IPP Instituto Politécnico Portalegre

IPBeja Instituto Politécnico de Beja

Unión Europea

Fondo Europeo
de Desarrollo Regional
"Una manera de hacer Europa"

Contents

Smarts Technologies and Algorithms for Health

Contigo: Monitoring People's Activity App for Anomalies Detection

Daniel Flores-Martin(✉), Sergio Laso, Javier Berrocal, and Juan M. Murillo

University of Extremadura, Badajoz, Spain
{dfloresm,slasom,jberolm,juanmamu}@unex.es

Abstract. The pandemic situation produced by COVID-19 has made access to medical services and personal treatment difficult. For the older adults, this has been a major problem because they often need assistance to facilitate their daily lives. Different types of solutions have been put into place very quickly to alleviate this problem, such as telemedicine or telecare. However, most of these solutions require people to perform some actions manually. This paper presents a solution to monitor people's activity in a way that is transparent to them. This solution is based on a mobile application that records their movements and estimates a certain amount of activity, and a web platform that allows authorized personnel to request this information by using different type of microservices. This application offers a simple and easy-to-access solution that allows the monitoring of the activity of the older adults to know their status and to be able to act accordingly in case of unusual situations.

Keywords: Older adults · Healthcare · Mobile devices · Monitoring · Microservices

1 Introduction and Motivations

Social isolation and loneliness have become increasingly relevant problems. This is of particular importance among older adults because the type of social relationships tend to be subject to close-knit groups of people and family members. This can lead to an increased risk of loneliness and isolation as these social relationships disappear or diminish [1].

Technology results useful for avoiding these situations and favoring the care of the older adults. Whether through smart devices, voice assistants, or robots, practically any technological development focused on the older adults can make their day-to-day life a little bit easier [2,3]. Some of the main benefits of technology in the lives of the older adults, such as reduction of social isolation, dependency or improved sense of security; and limitations such as physical impairments, cost of devices, or lack of interest in learning, were also indicated. The use of technology at the service of the older adults is also useful in nursing homes where, thanks to the use of different smart devices, their daily life becomes a

J. García-Alonso and C. Fonseca (Eds.): IWoG 2021, LNBE, pp. 3–14, 2022.
https://doi.org/10.1007/978-3-030-97524-1_1

little bit easier [4–6]. However, technology acceptance by older people is also the subject of study in [7], where the authors analyzed different theoretical models that provide the basis for building new applications and technologies targeted at older people. One of the factors that determine the perception that the older adults have about the use of technologies is influenced by the social factor. In a study conducted in [8], the authors observed that the older adults had been isolated and separated from their families during the pandemic in the COVID-19. In this sense, they realized the need and usefulness of new technologies and even appealed to the need to learn to use technological devices to help maintain the relationship with their loved ones without the need to resort to a person to facilitate this contact.

To mitigate these problems, different technological solutions have been developed that favor the recognition of people's activities to detect incidences related to the pandemic state [9,10]. However, there are also many barriers to these people coming into contact with new technologies, such as the difficulty of use, the need for supervision by third parties, or simply fear and mistrust.

In this paper we propose a solution based on the development of a mobile application called **Contigo**, which only by installing it on the mobile device of the older adults, can monitor their activity and detect possible anomalies in a completely passive way for the users.

The rest of this paper is structured as follows. After this introduction, Sect. 2 details the application structure. Then, Sect. 3 shows a real example of using the application. Next, in Sect. 4, some related work are detailed. Finally, in Sect. 5, the conclusions and future work are drawn.

2 Contigo App

The application, called Contigo, was developed during the initial phase of the COVID-19 pandemic to monitor older adults during this pandemic. Contigo is particularly aimed at older adults who live alone and therefore, in situations of isolation it is more difficult to know their state of health.

Contigo passively monitors whether a person has used their smartphone and what physical activities they performed over the last few hours via the mobile app. The activity and personal information (necessary for possible direct contact) is stored only on the mobile device and is provided through microservices. This information is aggregated and securely coordinated in the web application and is available for family members and healthcare personnel to be consulted.

2.1 Mobile Application

The mobile application is the main element of Contigo, which is responsible for the passive monitoring of the users' status. To quantify the status of the users, the application stores, on the one hand, the time with the screen active (the user is actively using the phone) and on the other hand, the time that the user is active without using the phone (sitting, standing up, walking, etc.). These activities are identified by means through the accelerometer and gyroscope sensor. The sum of the times is called activity time, which will be used to determine whether a person is active. Personal information is also stored in the mobile application in case it is necessary to contact the user directly.

Figure 1a shows the main interface of the application, where the user name and the activity time during the last 24 h are displayed. It is a very simple interface as the user does not have to interact with it, as explained above, the application automatically takes care of the monitoring.

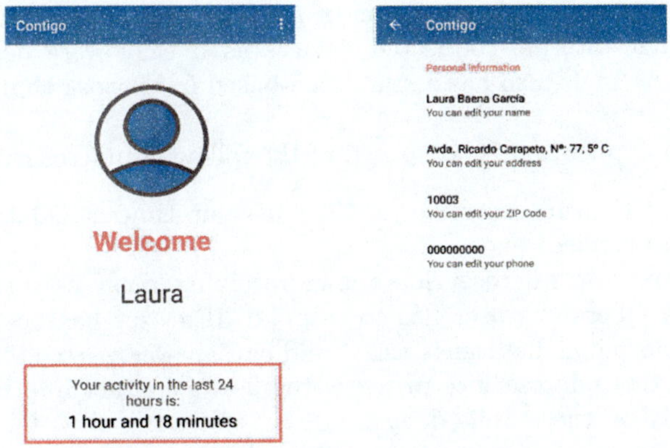

(a) Main screen (b) Preferences screen

Fig. 1. Contigo mobile app

To work properly, the application is composed of a set of permissions and requirements that must be fulfilled. These are detailed below:

- **Compatibility:** the application is developed for Android devices with operating OS version 6.0 (Marshmallow) or higher.
- **Location permission:** in order to obtain the location from the GPS sensor, it is necessary to accept the location permissions.
- **Background permission:** in order for the application to monitor and calculate the activity time correctly, it must run in the background. while the user has the phone locked or is using other apps, it has to monitor activity correctly. Therefore, it is essential to accept the background running permissions or in other cases, disable the device's power-saving limitations for the application.
- **Initial registration:** the phone stores personal information to be contacted by healthcare staff in case of low activity detection. This information is registered through a simple form when starting the application for the first time.

Figure 1b shows the settings section accessed from the main interface that allows editing the contact information once the initial registration is completed.

Microservices. To store and provide user data securely, the mobile application has been developed through Human Microservices [11,12]. These microservices provide accurate and up-to-date information about individuals (their owners) through embedded sensors or virtual profiles built and stored on their mobile devices. They allow greater control over data by not storing all this information in a remote environment, thus enhancing users' privacy. They can be consumed directly by other Internet-connected devices as if they were deployed in the cloud through APIs. It also has a standards-based framework that facilitates its development.

The mobile application is composed of the following microservices:

- **Get Status:** this microservice provides user up-time calculated and stored by the mobile device.
- **Post Status:** the microservice allows receiving push notifications for an active check where the user has to respond. If a user has been detected as having low activity, the user is asked and can answer yes/no.
- **Get User:** this microservice provides the user's contact information, which is stored only on the mobile device.
- **Get Location:** this microservice provides the user's current location. This is obtained directly from the GPS sensor of the mobile device, without having to store it beforehand.

For the implementation of these microservices, the development process of the Human Microservices has been followed. Firstly, the API has been defined with the microservices proposed above. For this, the OpenAPI standard [13], which is widely used in the industry for the design and implementation of APIs in the cloud, has been used. Secondly, with the design of the API, the skeleton of the mobile application has been automatically generated. The APIGEND tool[1] allows us to generate the API for Android mobile devices. Thirdly, before being able to deploy the API/mobile application, we had to finalize the implementation of the application. This includes the user interface, the business logic of each of the microservices, i.e. the behaviour of the different defined endpoints (obtaining the GPS location, the stored contact data, or the calculation of the activity), etc. For communication with the microservices, the MQTT protocol [14] is used, in this case, encrypted so that communication is secure. Finally, the application would be ready for deployment and installation on users' mobile devices.

2.2 Web Platform

For the development of the web platform, we followed a stack composed by Spring MVC, Spring Security, Spring Data JPA, JSP, and MySQL. These tech-

[1] https://openapi-generator-spilab.herokuapp.com/.

nologies allow the platform to be used in a secure and agile way while safeguarding user data. Currently, the platform is deployed for research purposes on a virtual machine with 2 cores and 4GB of Ram memory at the University of Extremadura[2].

This platform allows caregivers, healthcare staff, or management staff to keep track of the people who have installed the mobile application. In this way, it is possible to know in real-time if any person had little recent activity and, if necessary, send them a notification to find out their real status. For this purpose, it is possible to perform searches that return the status of different people, aggregating their data and displaying the information on an interactive map. Thanks to this, it is possible to detect which people were using their mobile devices with a certain degree of normality and which have been behaving unusually. In addition, the microservices used by the platform can also be consumed by authorized persons, such as neighbors or relatives of an older adult. The main features offered by the web platform are specified below:

Login. Caregivers, medical staff, or authorized people wishing to use the web platform must register. To do so, the access must be requested by justifying the reason for use (Fig. 2a). Since this is sensitive information about people, it has been decided that user registration will be supervised by a person and access will only be granted to those who really need it, whether to monitor a neighborhood, a nursing home, or a specific person. Once access is granted, the user can create a username and password to start using the platform (Fig. 2b).

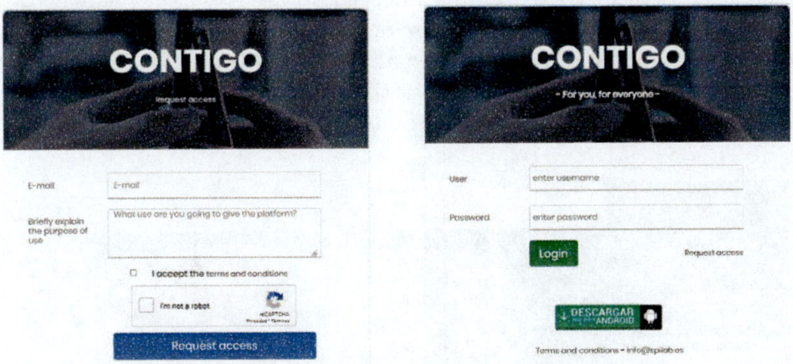

(a) Request access screen (b) Login screen

Fig. 2. Web platform register/access

[2] https://spilapps.unex.es/contigo.

Searching. Once the user has accessed the platform, he/she can perform different types of searching. To do so, the platform requests the user's location to position the map in the area where he/she is located, thus facilitating a possible search in the surrounding area. In this sense, several parameters were developed to allow the most precise searches possible. These parameters are:

- **Radius (meters):** this allows us to define the search radius on the map. In this way, only the data of people within this radius are received. For instance, 500 m.
- **Minimum activity (hours):** it sets the minimum time that people must have performed different activities for the results to return normal or anomalous behavior. For example, 3 h.
- **Activity in the last hours:** this parameter works as a complement to the previous one, defining the interval where the minimum activity performed must be fulfilled. It is possible to set 24 h, 12 h, and 8 h. Continuing with the previous example, it is possible to set the activity performed to be 3 h within the last 24 h.

Once the parameters have been set, the platform allows the user to configure the options for displaying the results. For this, it is possible to show only the answers that meet the configured parameters and therefore of the people who have performed the minimum recommended activity; the answers of those who do not meet the parameters and who, therefore, are likely to require attention in the event of a possible anomaly; or both answers. In addition, the results can be grouped for more convenient viewing. Finally, it is possible to create heat maps that allow users to see at a glance those areas where people are more likely to return anomalous answers, or on the other hand, the answers where the parameters are met. All these visualization options allow the user of the web platform to quickly and easily check the answers obtained. The figure below (Fig. 3) shows all this visualization options.

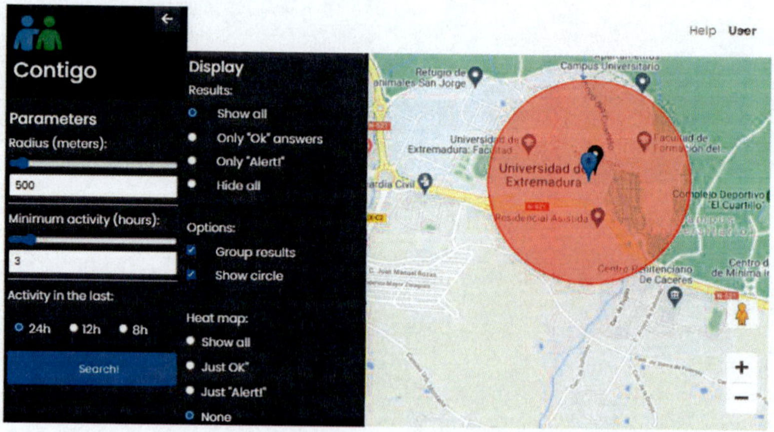

Fig. 3. Contigo web main searching screen

When a search is performed, a summary of the search is provided with the results obtained: number of responses, responses that meet the search parameters, and those that do not. In addition, an alert notification can be sent to all those who do not meet the search parameters entered.

Reports. The platform also allows different types of reports to be generated. These reports can be created in PDF and XML format and the information can be sorted by name, address, and postcode. In this way, the information obtained can be printed or analyzed easily.

In this section we detailed the main functionalities of both the mobile application and the web platform. The following section shows a complete example from when a user performs a search until a person receives a notification on their mobile device to inquire about their status.

3 Use-Case: Laura's Activity Time

In a real scenario, people downloaded the mobile application and installed it on their device. In addition, healthcare staff with access granted to the platform can perform different types of searches. In this example, the user *MedicalStaff1* set the following parameters to perform a search and check Laura's activity time:

- **Radius:** 500 m
- **Minimum activity:** 3 h
- **Performed in the last:** 24 h.

Once the parameters are set, the request return all the results (Fig. 4).

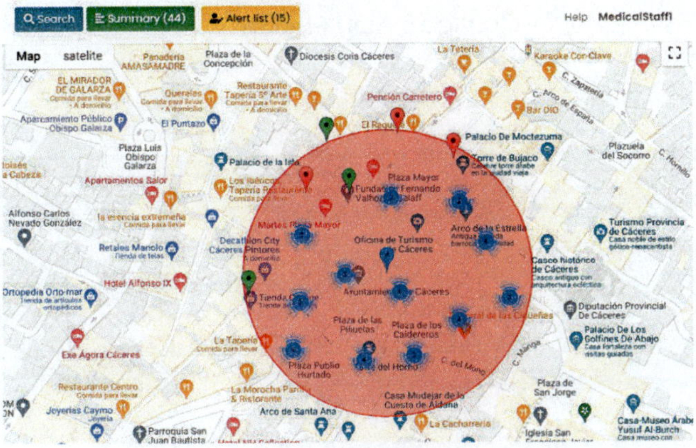

Fig. 4. Search results in the interactive map

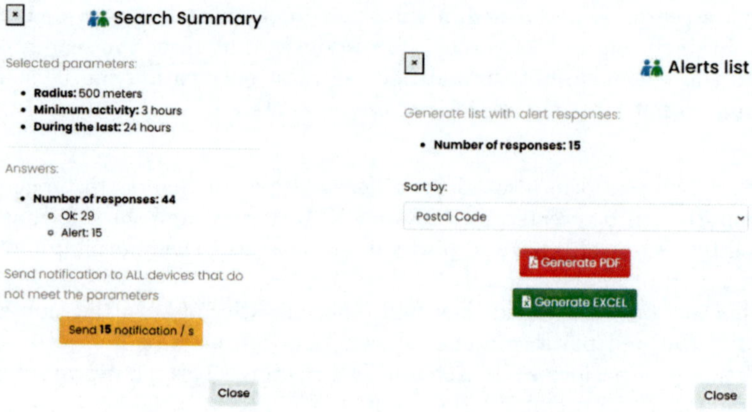

(a) Search summary (b) Alert list (reports)

Fig. 5. Search results

The platform allows the user to visualize the information on the interactive map, offering a summary (Fig. 5a) and allowing reports to be generated (Fig. 5b).

In this way, *MedicalStaff1* can check the status of the people who are within the parameters of the search he has performed. For this example, *MedicalStaff1* performs a search within the environment of the city of Cáceres to check the status of a specific person, *Laura*, who due to the pandemic situation can not go regularly to the health center for her check-ups, and therefore the healthcare staff must check if she is performing the minimum recommended activity. Thanks to the reports generated, *MedicalStaff1* can check Laura's condition (Fig. 6)[3].

Contigo's Alert Report

Date: Fri Oct 22 10:19:28 UTC 2021 - **User:** MedicalStaff1

Search location: 39.476900002187705,-6.373897270080559
Radius: 500 meters - **Minimum activity (hours):** 3.0 hours - **In the last:** 24 hours

Contigo

#	Name	Address	ZIP Code	Phone	Activity time
1	Laura Baena García	Avda. Ricardo Carapeto, Nº: 77, 5º C	10003	000000000	1 hour and 18 minutes
2	Antonio Chacón Pérez	C/ Alazán, Nº: 50, 2º A	10003	000000000	1 hour and 3 minutes
3	África Olmeda Suarez	Avda. Ricardo Carapeto, Nº: 165, 4º C	10003	000000000	1 hour and 21 minutes
4	Luis Manuel Nuñez Rivero	Ctra. de la Corte, Nº: 22, 3º E	10003	000000000	1 hour and 35 minutes
5	Esther Fernández Galván	Avda. Sabas Arias, Nº: 151, 2º F	10003	000000000	1 hour and 55 minutes
6	Luis Manuel Díez Ayuso	Calle Salvador Dalí, Nº: 2, 4º E	10003	000000000	1 hour and 46 minutes
7	Mari Luz Pérez Fernández	Avda. Ricardo Carapeto, Nº: 119, 1º F	10003	000000000	20 minutes
8	Beatriz Flores Martinez	Ctra. de la Corte, Nº: 86, 4º D	10003	000000000	2 hours y 50 minutes
9	Ángela Galván Fernández	Ctra. de la Corte, Nº: 31, 2º A	10003	000000000	42 minutes
10	Esther Rodríguez Díez	Plaza Francisco Bosh, Nº: 142, 5º B	10003	000000000	1 minute

Fig. 6. Search report with Laura's information

[3] The data generated in the report are simulated.

In view of the results, *MedicalStaff1* sets out to locate *Laura* in the area where she has her usual residence. Once located, her information can be checked and the activity performed analyzed. By clicking on Laura's marker, all her data are displayed on the interactive map (Fig. 7).

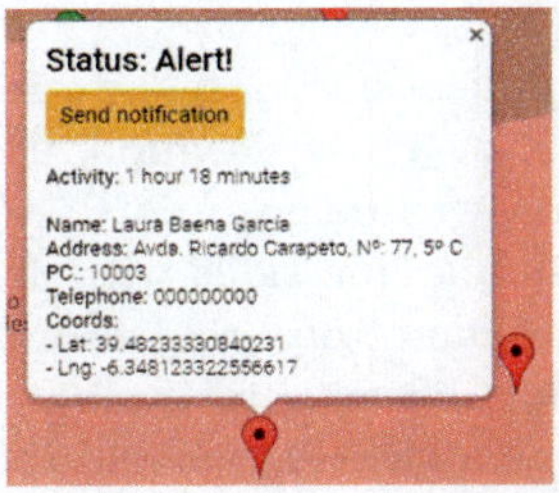

Fig. 7. Laura's information

In this case, *Laura* did not met the target requested in the search, so *MedicalStaff1* can send her a push notification to check her status (Fig. 8). In addition, Laura can reply to this notification to indicate that she is indeed well and that it may have been a specific anomaly of that day or, on the contrary, if she does not reply, *MedicalStaff1* can take the necessary actions for specialized staff to contact her personally at home.

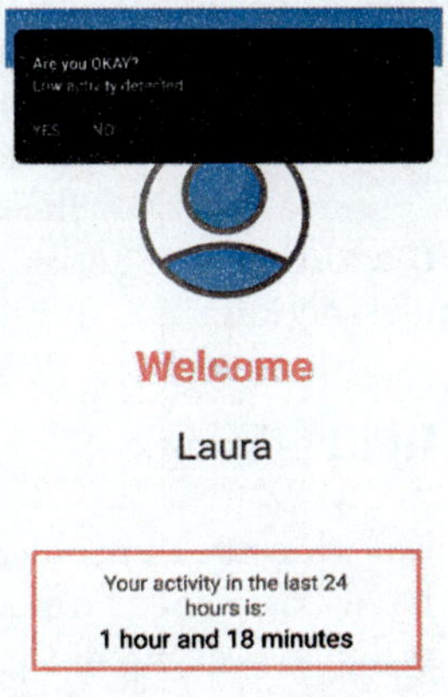

Fig. 8. Laura's Contigo app notification

This example demonstrates the usefulness of Contigo in detecting possible anomalies caused by the lack of activity of older adults, thanks to the combination of the mobile application and the platform.

4 Related Work

There are different mobile applications for monitoring different aspects of health. For example, Moodflow [15] is a mobile application that captures emotions, moods, thoughts, and general well-being, Ada [16] allows us to perform a small medical check-up through simple questions with an AI or Wave [17], an application to facilitate the maintenance of a record of physical and emotional well-being in patients with chronic diseases to track symptoms, medications, steps and other activities. All of them have in common the need to interact with them constantly, manually recording different information, answering questions, and so on. Therefore, those who are not familiar with and skilled in the use of mobile applications are not suitable for them. They need apps that monitor different aspects of their health with as little interaction as possible.

Some applications record different aspects of health passively without the user having to interact with them. For example, Google Fit [18] or Health Monitor [19] allows us to monitor different health parameters such as steps, heart rate, blood pressure, etc. However, for most of the parameters, it needs the help of other external devices. Moreover, these data are not reviewed by medical staff, so good use depends on the knowledge and interpretation of the users themselves.

A good example is Radar COVID [20], an application that uses the bluetooth sensor of the device itself to identify possible close contacts with people who have been diagnosed positive for COVID-19, alerting us when we have been near a COVID-positive person. In our case, we use the accelerometer and gyroscope sensors and the active screen detection of the devices themselves to detect the activity time of a person in a passive way, in which the user has minimal interaction with the application. In addition, the activity information is reviewed by healthcare professionals for quick action.

5 Conclusions and Future Work

Loneliness in the older adults is a widespread problem in our society. This, added to the pandemic situation we have experienced due to COVID-19, has generated truly alarming situations that have prevented the verification of the welfare status of our older adults. To counteract this, different types of solutions have been developed, such as those centered on telecare or telemedicine. However, the use of these solutions in most cases depends on people having to perform some action manually. This can be a barrier for people who are dependent on technology or do not have sufficient knowledge to use it.

In this paper, a mobile application has been presented that allows the monitoring of people's activity. This application uses different sensors of the mobile device to estimate the person's activity. All this is done in a transparent way for people and does not require any manual action. The security of the data has also been prioritized since, as it is personal and sensitive information, it is only stored in the person's device. In addition, as a complement to this mobile application, a web platform has been developed that allows customized searches to detect those people who have not performed a specific activity time and, therefore, could be considered as an alarm situation. In this case, a notification can be sent to the person's mobile device and, if necessary, a family member or the responsible medical staff can be contacted. As future work is intended to support other mobile operating systems such as IOs, since the mobile application is currently only available for Android. The application is also working on creating a history of people's activity to create statistics and schedule tasks and activities to encourage activity among the older adults, if necessary. Work is also being done to produce periodic queries of a specific person's activity, so that a family member or healthcare staff will have a record of the activity without having to perform a specific search.

Acknowledgments. This work was partially supported by the DIN2020-011586 grant, funded by MCIN/AEI/10.13039/501100011033 and by the European Union "NextGenerationEU/PRTR", by the Spanish Ministry of Science, Innovation and Universities (RTI2018-094591-B-I00 and RTI2018-101204-B-C21 projects, and FPU17/02251 grant), the 4IE+ Project (0499-4IE-PLUS-4-E) funded by Interreg V-A España-Portugal (POCTEP) 2014-2020 program, by the RCIS network (TIN2016-81978-REDT), by the Department of Economy, Science and Digital Agenda of the Government of Extremadura (GR18112, IB18030) and by the European Regional Development Fund.

References

1. Rivero Jiménez, B., Conde-Caballero, D., Juárez, L.M.: Loneliness among the elderly in rural contexts: a mixed-method study protocol. Int. J. Qual. Methods **20**, 1609406921996861 (2021)
2. López-Lago Ortiz, L., Arroyo Chacón, S., Cipriano Crespo, C., Luengo Polo, J., Muñoz González, B.: Technology in the face of the challenges of the long-term care system for the elderly in Spain. In: García-Alonso, J., Fonseca, C. (eds.) IWoG 2020. LNB, pp. 371–379. Springer, Cham (2021). https://doi.org/10.1007/978-3-030-72567-9_34
3. Mäkitalo, N., et al.: The internet of bodies needs a human data model. IEEE Internet Comput. **24**(5), 28–37 (2020)
4. Flores-Martin, D., Rojo, J., Moguel, E., Berrocal, J., Murillo, J.M.: Smart nursing homes: self-management architecture based on IoT and machine learning for rural areas. Wirel. Commun. Mob. Comput. **2021** (2021)
5. Flores-Martin, D., Laso, S., Berrocal, J., Canal, C., Murillo, J.M.: Allowing IoT devices collaboration to help elderly in their daily lives. In: García-Alonso, J., Fonseca, C. (eds.) IWoG 2019. CCIS, vol. 1185, pp. 111–122. Springer, Cham (2020). https://doi.org/10.1007/978-3-030-41494-8_11
6. Jesús-Azabal, M., Herrera, J.L., Laso, S., Galán-Jiménez, J.: OPPNets and rural areas: an opportunistic solution for remote communications. Wirel. Commun. Mob. Comput. **2021** (2021)

7. Klimova, B., Poulova, P.: Older people and technology acceptance. In: Zhou, J., Salvendy, G. (eds.) ITAP 2018. LNCS, vol. 10926, pp. 85–94. Springer, Cham (2018). https://doi.org/10.1007/978-3-319-92034-4_7
8. Chimento-Díaz, S., Sánchez-García, P., Franco-Antonio, C., Santano-Mogena, E., Cordovilla-Guardia, S.: Have people over 64 used technological devices during COVID-19? In: García-Alonso, J., Fonseca, C. (eds.) IWoG 2020. LNB, pp. 168–176. Springer, Cham (2021). https://doi.org/10.1007/978-3-030-72567-9_17
9. Ting, D.S.W., Carin, L., Dzau, V., Wong, T.Y.: Digital technology and COVID-19. Nat. Med. **26**(4), 459–461 (2020)
10. Marston, H.R., et al.: COVID-19: technology, social connections, loneliness, and leisure activities: an international study protocol. Front. Sociol. **5**, 89 (2020)
11. Laso, S., Berrocal, J., García-Alonso, J., Canal, C., Manuel Murillo, J.: Human microservices: a framework for turning humans into service providers. Softw. Pract. Exp. **51**, 1910–1935 (2021)
12. Laso, S., Linaje, M., Garcia-Alonso, J., Murillo, J.M., Berrocal, J.: Artifact abstract: deployment of APIs on android mobile devices and microcontrollers. In: 2020 IEEE International Conference on Pervasive Computing and Communications (PerCom), pp. 1–2. IEEE (2020)
13. Initiative, O.: The OpenAPI specification repository. Contribute to OAI/OpenAPI-Specification development by creating an account on GitHub. https://github.com/OAI/OpenAPI-Specification, https://github.com/OAI/OpenAPI-Specification. Accessed 3 Mar 2020
14. MQTT: MQTT. http://mqtt.org/, http://mqtt.org/. Accessed 20 Jan 2020
15. Monecke: Moodflow. https://play.google.com/store/apps/details?id=com.moodpixel. Accessed 20 Oct 2021
16. Ada, H.: Ada. https://play.google.com/store/apps/details?id=com.ada.app. Accessed 20 Oct 2021
17. Treatment Technologies & Insights: Wave. https://play.google.com/store/apps/details?id=com.waveapp.android. Accessed 20 Oct 2021
18. Google: Google Fit. https://play.google.com/store/apps/details?id=com.google.android.apps.fitness. Accessed 20 Oct 2021
19. Extrawest: Health Monitor. https://play.google.com/store/apps/details?id=com.extrawest.healthcare_flutter_app. Accessed 20 Oct 2021
20. Spain, G.: Radar COVID. https://play.google.com/store/apps/details?id=es.gob.radarcovid. Accessed 20 Oct 2021

SAMoA: A Self-adaptive Mobility Monitoring Framework for MCI Elderly People and Their Caregivers

José R. Lozano-Pinilla and Cristina Vicente-Chicote(✉)

Quercus Software Engineering Group, Universidad de Extremadura, Badajoz, Spain
{joserralp,cristinav}@unex.es

Abstract. People with Mild Cognitive Impairment (MCI) often experience a slight -but noticeable- decrease in their mental abilities, greater than other people of the same age, but not so severe as to interfere with their normal daily life and activities. MCI currently affects between 8 and 37% of people over 65 and, according to the latest findings, people with MCI are more likely to develop dementia. This paper introduces *SAMoA*: a self-adaptive framework aimed at helping elderly people suffering from MCI and their caregivers. *SAMoA* includes two self-adaptive mobile applications allowing to monitor the mobility of MCI elderly people, warning their caregivers when they leave their (previously defined) safe zones or change their daily mobility routines.

Keywords: Self-adaptive systems · Mobility monitoring · Mild Cognitive Impairment (MCI)

1 Introduction

Nowadays, more and more elderly people have a smartphone and use it in their day-to-day tasks, such as reading the news, talking with family and friends, or annotating reminders not to forget relevant information such as the pills they have to take or the appointments with their doctors.

Research shows that elderly people are more at risk of accidents, such as falling to the floor or getting lost or confused in certain situations. However, having a mobile phone with them would allow their relatives or caregivers to monitor their location at any time (of course, with their prior consent), for example when they go shopping or when they have to travel.

Monitoring the mobility of elderly people in order to identify potentially risky situations, may require using different sensors (e.g., GPS, accelerometer, etc.), communication networks and infrastructure (e.g., based on mobile data, WiFi or Bluetooth) and, eventually, external services (e.g., regarding weather forecast). The energy consumption associated with these devices and services may vary depending on their configuration (sample rate, precision, frequency and amount of data to communicate, etc.). Thus, in order to adequately manage the limited

J. García-Alonso and C. Fonseca (Eds.): IWoG 2021, LNBE, pp. 15–21, 2022.
https://doi.org/10.1007/978-3-030-97524-1_2

battery and computational resources available on smartphones, it is essential to adapt the mobility monitoring process so that it can work for as long as possible and, in particular, in the most risky situations.

The use of Information and Communication Technologies (ICT) has demonstrated to be very useful both for getting data from the elderly [1] and for making information more accessible to them [2]. In this vein, this paper presents *SAMoA* (Self-Adaptive Mobility Monitoring App): a monitoring framework based on *MoRES* [3], which aims at identifying unusual mobility behaviours to help the elderly prevent risky situations, while keeping their relatives and caregivers informed about them. This goal can be divided, in turn, into the following sub-goals:

- Provide elderly people in general, and those affected by MCI in particular, with an easy-to-use mobile app allowing them:
  - to receive relevant news based on their profile;
  - to send an SOS message to their relatives or caregivers in case they get lost or feel in trouble.
- Provide the elderly relatives and caregivers with a mobile app allowing them:
  - to define the elderly profile and mobility patterns (e.g., times when he/she usually gets out or should be at home);
  - to define different mobility zones according to their risk;
  - to define their notification preferences (e.g., according to their availability); and
  - to watch out the current location of the elderly person and his/her last movements when he/she sends an SOS message, gets into a risky area or exhibits a strange behavior (e.g., getting out late at night or under bad weather conditions);

The rest of the paper is organised as follows. Section 2 overviews related works; Sect. 3 outlines the architecture of the *SAMoA* framework and describes the behavior of each of its components; and, finally, Sect. 4 draws some conclusions and future works.

2 Related Works

The widely spread use of smartphones allows, among other increasingly complex tasks, to monitor people's mobility. Nowadays, it is possible to find many different applications that make use of this information in an aggregated (anonymous) way, for instance, for traffic estimation or crowded places identification. A good example of this kind of applications is Google Maps [5], which not only provides information about the best routes possible to reach any given destination, but also instant information about traffic jams, accidents or sections under construction. Google Maps also allows their users to share their instant location with a given person (or group of persons), for instance while traveling, and to register their mobile devices so that, if they get lost, it is possible to retrieve their current (and historical) location. Similarly, Find my iPhone [7] allows users to locate their iOS mobile devices just by logging in their Apple Account.

Among the personal mobility monitoring apps, it is possible to find SOS/rescue applications frequently used by hikers who want to be located in case they get lost. A good example of this kind of applications is Alpify [6], which allows hikers in trouble to send an SOS message to the local rescue services, indicating their location and personal information so that they can help them.

It is also possible to find tracking devices such as collars, bracelets or tags, which allow finding lost objects or persons (e.g., children). These devices are typically placed inadvertently and they allow tracking people location without their prior consent. Furthermore, some applications like Spyzie [4], also allow to instantly access, not only the current location of a device, but also additional personal information such as contacts, calls, messages or photos. Installing this kind of software on a mobile device without the consent of its owner is, of course, not only reproachable but illegal.

All the applications mentioned above allow to monitor the location of mobile devices (and thus the location of their owners) but, not being oriented to elderly people, they lack some valuable features such as enabling the definition of safe/risky areas or take into account their personal routines and potential visual or hearing impairments. Among the mobile apps specifically oriented to elderly people, it is worth mentioning the following ones:

- ***LoPe*** [8] is a service developed by Cruz Roja aimed at monitoring elderly people. *LoPE* is based on two main components: (1) a smartwatch application intended for elderly people, that sends the user location every 10 minutes and allows notifying emergency situations to caregivers; and (2) a mobile application intended for the caregivers allowing them to define secure/danger zones, setting alert preferences, and monitoring the current person location and distance covered;
- ***Safe365*** [9] is a mobile app for elderly monitoring. *Safe365* notifies the caregivers whenever the user enters or leaves a given area, or when a deviation in the daily routines (learnt using artificial intelligence techniques) is identified.

Although these two applications allow to monitor elderly people they are more oriented to caregivers than to end-users, and they are not self-adaptive in any sense. SAMoA aims at coping with these limitations by (1) offering added-value features specifically targeted to the elderly users, e.g., offering them relevant information according to their profile and routines, allowing them to easily manage reminders, and providing them with an interface adapted to their specific needs or impairments; and (2) supporting transparent, smart adaptation mechanisms the make the best out of the limited resources available in nowadays smartphones, in particular, to guarantee that they are available when really needed (e.g., in an emergency situation).

3 The *SAMoA* Framework

Before detailing the architecture of *SAMoA*, it is worth mentioning that it is based on the *MoRES* framework [3], aimed at helping elderly people to understand and comply with the mobility restrictions associated to the COVID-19 pandemic.

MoRES includes three applications: (1) a mobile app allowing end-users to identify allowed and forbidden places in their area (according to applicable restrictions) and crowded areas to be avoided; and (2) two web apps, one for politicians (allowing them to set up restrictions in a hierarchical way) and another one for the public security forces (allowing them to identify strange or forbidden mobility patters). *MoRES* builds on several software components, two of which have been fully reused in *SAMoA*: (1) a RoQME component [12,13], aimed at gathering real-time information from the smartphone sensors (e.g., GPS, accelerometer, etc.) and from some external APIs (e.g., a weather forecast service) and identifying relevant context patterns (situations) in it; and (2) an information storage and visualization component. Both the *MoRES* and the *SAMoA* frameworks rely on a loosely coupled architecture in which components are connected using a publish-subscribe middleware.

The *SAMoA* framework includes two apps aimed at covering the different needs of each kind of user in the system: a mobile app for the elderly people, and another mobile app supporting their caregivers. These apps provide customised functionalities and views, targeted to each user profile, and share data with each other. Figure 1 outlines the main components of the *SAMoA* framework and how they relate to each other. Each of these components are briefly described next.

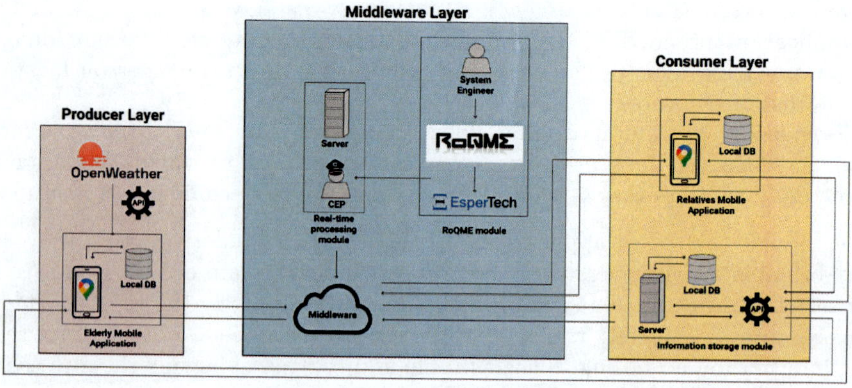

Fig. 1. Architecture of the *SAMoA* framework.

- **Elderly mobile app.** The main purpose of this application is, on the one hand, to provide the current location of the elderly person to the caregivers application and, on the other hand, to monitor the elderly mobility, checking how safe/risky is the area that person is in. High-safety areas are typically defined around the elderly person's home; medium-safety areas include the zones where they typically move through on a daily basis (e.g., for shopping,

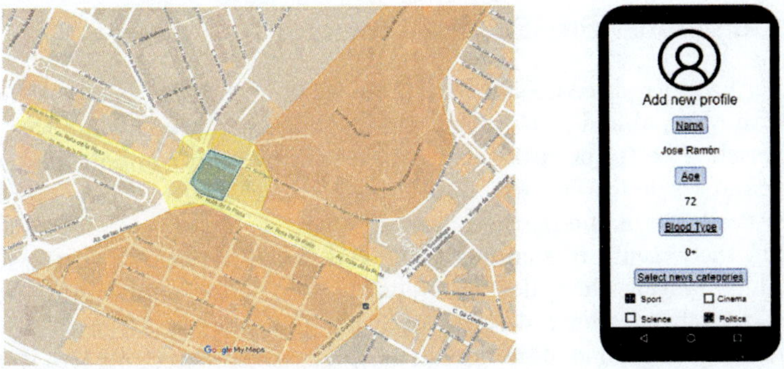

Fig. 2. *Left.* SAMoA zone range definition map, where green zones are associated to high-safety and orange zones to medium-safety. All other zones are considered unsafe. *Right.* Elderly person profile definition.

attending medical centers, or visiting close relatives and friends); and risky zones, which include unusual places or zones far away from their home. Note that these areas might be defined either by end-users themselves or by their caregivers (when end-user suffers from some cognitive impairment). Similarly, end-users (or their caregivers) may define (1) their personal profile (name, age, gender, blood type, preferred news categories, etc.); (2) the time intervals when they typically stay at home or go out; and (3) punctual or regular reminders (e.g., for taking their medicines, visiting their doctor, etc.). Finally, the application provides end-users with an SOS button they can press in case they feel lost or at risk, shows them relevant news based on their profile and location and displays how safe is the area in which they are (using a simple traffic-light color convention). It is worth mentioning that the risk level is not only based on the person location, but also on deviations from predefined behaviors and on the weather conditions (e.g., it is considered a risk if the person goes out late at night or under a heavy rain). It is also worth mentioning that the mobility monitoring process is zone and battery level dependent, that is, the safer the zone and the lowest the battery, the less frequently the location is sent to the caregivers application. However, if the user gets into a risky zone or if he/she presses the SOS button, the location is sent at the highest supported rate (every 2 min), regardless of the battery level.

- **Caregiver mobile app:** this application provides elderly caregivers with the following main features: (1) profile definition, including the time intervals when they are available for attending notifications; (2) when needed, definition of the elderly behavior routines and mobility zones (indicating their risk level); (3) setting up notification preferences (e.g., notifying all the caregivers or only those closest to his/her current position); (4) receiving notifications in a clear way; (4) visualizing the current location of the elderly person on a map; and (5) reviewing his/her routes and locations during the last 24 h.

Some of the functionalities supported by *SAMoA* are illustrated in Fig. 2.

4 Conclusions and Future Works

This paper has introduced *SAMoA*: a mobility monitoring framework for elderly people with MCI, aimed at helping them and their caregivers when they get lost or feel at risk. The framework architecture and its main components have been outlined, and its main features have been compared with similar applications currently available in the marketplace.

Among the extensions planned to be supported in *SAMoA* in the future, it is worth highlighting the following ones: (1) monitoring additional information obtained, e.g., from smart watches or other IoT devices, in order to provide end-users with additional functionalities (e.g., stress detection based on pulse alteration); (2) adding some "intelligent" features, e.g., allowing the mobile apps to adapt their behaviour according to the perceived situation, in line with some of our previous works on model-driven self-adaptive system development [10,11]; (3) supporting the integration with external services provided by some hospitals or by the Red Cross, and (4) using *artificial intelligence* techniques to learning elderly behavior patterns and detect deviations from their regular routines.

References

1. Flores-Martin, D., Laso, S., Berrocal, J., Canal, C., Murillo, J.M.: Allowing IoT devices collaboration to help elderly in their daily lives. In: García-Alonso, J., Fonseca, C. (eds.) IWoG 2019. CCIS, vol. 1185, pp. 111–122. Springer, Cham (2020). https://doi.org/10.1007/978-3-030-41494-8_11
2. Jesús-Azabal, M., et al.: Voice assistant to remind pharmacologic treatment in elders. In: García-Alonso, J., Fonseca, C. (eds.) IWoG 2019. CCIS, vol. 1185, pp. 123–133. Springer, Cham (2020). https://doi.org/10.1007/978-3-030-41494-8_12
3. Lozano-Pinilla, J.R., García-Pérez, D., Vicente-Chicote, C.: *MoRES*: a mobile app to help elderly people grasp and comply with COVID-19 restrictions. In: García-Alonso, J., Fonseca, C. (eds.) IWoG 2020. LNB, pp. 35–42. Springer, Cham (2021). https://doi.org/10.1007/978-3-030-72567-9_4
4. Spy Phone Application. https://spyzie.io/
5. Google Maps Platform. https://mapsplatform.google.com/
6. Alpify. http://www.alpify.com/
7. Apple Find my iPhone. https://www.icloud.com/find
8. People service locator developed by Cruz Roja. https://www.cruzroja.es/principal/web/teleasistencia/localizador-de-personas
9. Safe365 free monitoring mobile application for the elderly. https://www.diarioabierto.es/459872/safe365-una-app-gratuita-para-la-localizacion-y-seguimiento-de-personas-mayores
10. Inglés-Romero, J.F., Vicente-Chicote, C.: Towards a formal approach for prototyping and verifying self-adaptive systems. In: Franch, X., Soffer, P. (eds.) CAiSE 2013. LNBIP, vol. 148, pp. 432–446. Springer, Heidelberg (2013). https://doi.org/10.1007/978-3-642-38490-5_39
11. Rodríguez-Gracia, D., Criado, J., Iribarne, L., Padilla, N., Vicente-Chicote, C.: Runtime adaptation of architectural models: an approach for adapting user interfaces. In: Abelló, A., Bellatreche, L., Benatallah, B. (eds.) MEDI 2012. LNCS, vol. 7602, pp. 16–30. Springer, Heidelberg (2012). https://doi.org/10.1007/978-3-642-33609-6_4

12. Vicente-Chicote, C., et al.: A component-based and model-driven approach to deal with non-functional properties through global QoS metrics. In: 5th International Workshop on Interplay of Model-Driven and Component-Based Software Engineering (ModComp 2018), Held in Conjunction with MODELS 2018, Copenhagen, Denmark, pp. 40–45 (2018)
13. Vicente-Chicote, C., García-Pérez, D., García-Ojeda, P., Inglés-Romero, J.F., Romero-Garcés, A., Martínez, J.: Modeling and estimation of non-functional properties: leveraging the power of QoS metrics. In: Ferrández Vicente, J.M., Álvarez-Sánchez, J.R., de la Paz López, F., Toledo Moreo, J., Adeli, H. (eds.) IWINAC 2019. LNCS, vol. 11487, pp. 380–388. Springer, Cham (2019). https://doi.org/10.1007/978-3-030-19651-6_37

Blockchain-Supported Health Registry: The Claim for a Personal Health Trajectory Traceability and How It Can Be Achieved

Javier Rojo[1(✉)], Juan Hernández[1], Sumi Helal[2], Juan M. Murillo[1], and José García-Alonso[1]

[1] University of Extremadura, Cáceres, Spain
{javirojo,juanher,juanmamu,jgaralo}@unex.es
[2] University of Florida, Gainesville, FL, USA
helal@cise.ufl.edu

Abstract. The digitalization of health processes is a reality. Each time, there are more services and institutions generating and interacting with the health data of a patient. This put in manifest some deficiencies of actual health systems, such as the need for data no longer revolve around the institutions that generate them and start to revolve around the users or patients to whom they belong. Otherwise, patients will end up losing focus and control of their data, which is distributed among different information systems. To address this, many researchers around the world have proposed software solutions that integrate a patient's data into a global view, even though it is still stored in a distributed way in the systems that generate it. However, the mere integration of data does not allow a patient to have real knowledge of the entire life cycle of her different records. To this end, data integration solutions must go a step further and convert the structure that maintains the overall view of a patient's health, her Personal Health Trajectory, into a registry ensuring the traceability of the patient's health. As a result, patients will have a real understanding of everything that surrounds their health data and true patient-centered healthcare systems will be one step closer.

Keywords: Data integration · Data interoperability · eHealth · Blockchain · Health traceability

1 Introduction

Today's society is a digitalized one. All being susceptible of be digitalized is translated to electronic support that processes and store the attached information. In this context, health processes, as well as their input and output data, are being digitalized [8,21]. Concepts such as Electronic Health Records (EHRs) [11] and Personal Health Records (PHRs) [16] have arisen in the last few years. Particularly, the lasts have been widely employed recently to store any kind

J. García-Alonso and C. Fonseca (Eds.): IWoG 2021, LNBE, pp. 22–33, 2022.
https://doi.org/10.1007/978-3-030-97524-1_3

of health information about patients—including those generated by intelligent health devices such as Internet of Medical Things (IoMT) [4,6,19] or Web of Medical Things (WoMT) devices [15].

The broader capability of each new electronic support to store more diverse sources' health information highlights the need to offer mechanisms to patients in order to collect all their health information provided by different agents [9,18]—understanding by agents different types of healthcare entities or connected smart devices generating health data. Moreover, it can even arise *data-ownership*'s doubts in the patients, who are not confident about which systems store information about their health, as well as each of them does not have full knowledge about the interactions involving their data [22].

Due to all this, the advantages of digitalizing health processes are mitigated. Not having a way to access all her health data makes it difficult for a patient to manage it and apply its ownership's rights—since she is the real owner of her health data [18]. Health data can be generated, but they can also be modified in case there is an error in them and even deleted [12]—if requested by the patient to whom they belong. For any of these actions, the patient should have a way to keep track of and be aware of all the changes that occur in her health reality.

The first step to obtain empowers patients and allowing them to be aware of all concerning their data is to obtain a complete vision of their health trajectory [20]. In this sense, the most promising proposals in the literature are the ones using blockchain to obtain a data structure referencing where each health record of the user are stored [1,17]—due to its distributed nature, as well as its guarantees on data security and privacy [2,12]. Authors of this paper has contributed to it with previous works [18]. However, although these proposals offer unified access and the integration of each patient's health data, none of them take advantage of having a structure per patient to employ it as a registry of changes in the patient's health reality, rather than just as a directory to access their data.

It is clear that having this registry would help the patient to have greater control over their data, to validate the authenticity of the test data—detecting addictions, modifications or undue deletions of data—and to have complete traceability of the patient's health reality—as is done in other domains, such as food's traceability [3]. That is the reason why this paper makes efforts in the definition of this registry and proposes a theoretical implementation of it.

The obtainment of this registry contributes to the achievement of the *Personal Health Trajectory* of patients, proposed by the authors of this paper in previous works [20]. In addition, having a data structure such as the one proposed in this paper, new patient-centered health systems—instead of current institution-centered ones—come to a step closer [20].

The rest of the paper is structured as follows: Sect. 2 shows the motivations of this work and related work. Section 3 presents the concept of Personal Health Trajectory and its relationship to the health's registry presented in this paper. Then, Sect. 4 deeps on how to obtain this registry by means of their implementation with blockchain. Section 5 brings a brief discussion over the consequences and real applications of this registry. Finally, in Sect. 6 the conclusions of this work and some future lines of research are exposed.

2 Motivations and Related Works

In the current health systems, the data about its patients is stored in an isolated way. Data stored in the information system of a health system—or in cloud services from smart devices—for a patient is not aware of data stored in other health systems' information systems for the same patient [9]. Therefore, if a patient interacts with many of these health systems or uses smart devices to monitor her health, multiple, fragmented representations of her health reality are generated [18]. Further the duplicity and inconsistencies problems concerning these multiple, fragmented representations, this also makes difficult for patients to manage their health reality and be aware of all operations involving it.

As a first step to achieve it, each time more proposals try to integrate the patients' health data in a unique, global vision. On the one hand, proposals such as that of Spil et al. [23] or that of Kyazze et al. [13] advocate for the integration of health data physically integrating it on the same storage system. On the other hand, proposals such as that of Zhang et al. [24], advocate for the interoperability of data stored in a distributed way—reducing the intrusiveness of the first type of proposals—even using the same technology of the first ones. In this line, proposals using blockchain as support to enable this interoperability have arisen—being this one of the main suggested applications of this technology on health domain in last years[2,12]. Proposals such as that of Roehrs et al. [17] or that of Chen et al. [1] present the creation of a blockchain-supported data structure per patient that stores in their blocks references to where it is stored each of their health records. Jalali et al. [10] propose the Personicle concept, a chronicle of live events related with health of users. To generate it, they propose a framework integrate, store, and analyze data from heterogeneous data streams.

Moreover, the authors of this paper had been working on their own proposal defining the blockchains' federation concept [18], having a blockchain per patient with access to all their records and another upper blockchain that allows health professionals to locate the blockchains of patients sharing their data.

Although all these proposals achieve a solution to the problem of the multiple, fragmented visions of the health reality of a patient, all of them are only considering operations of the addition of new records. Some of them even affirm that health data does not need to be modified or deleted after their addition [1], so only the addition of data must be registered in the global vision. Despite this, as some studies on blockchain for eHealth affirm [12], these others operation can be necessary for some situations. This is solved by proposals that do not integrate physically records, but they make them interoperable through an additional data structure. Nevertheless, this has other implications, such as the global vision is not aware of what is happening in records—i.e., blockchain's security properties are applied to the global vision, but not to the records referenced by it.

Proposals generating this global vision could take advantage of having a data structure with all patient's health data to offer new mechanisms that empower patient with the control on her data—and even that improve the security of it [14]. This single, global view, in which the all health data of a patient are integrated, could offer users greater control over what is happening at any given moment in their medical history: the traceability of their health data.

Achieving this traceability, beyond the simple integration of health data, can be useful for the patient for multiple reasons. It will give the user complete control over what happens to his health data: when it is added, when it is modified, or when it is deleted—as well as where and by whom these actions are performed. In addition, it also allows verification of the authenticity of the records. For example, by saving a value computed with the content of a record at the time of adding or modifying it, it is possible to check whether its content has been maliciously altered at the time of accessing it. Likewise, it is possible to check whether a record has been deleted without the patient's consent or, at least, without the patient's knowledge. All this leads to greater empowerment of the data on the part of the patient and greater security for the records.

The fact of using a blockchain to perform traceability is not new. There are already many proposals in other fields where blockchain is used as a registry to ensure the traceability of elements such as food. In the case of alimentary traceability, public blockchains—where anyone can read—are employed to share the different stages by which a concrete aliment has passed since it was collected until it is on the hand of consumer [5]. Even within the health domain, no proposal talking about health traceability are found, in the field of smart health and eHealth there are already proposals that talk about the need to offer a certain grade of security in health data that could be achieved by means of health traceability [7,25]. Specifically, the works found claims for the need to ensure personal health data provenance, as well as right confirmation, by means of smart contracts, and the control of who is performing changes in health information to prevent malicious activity by means of the control of access keys' sharing.

Other proposals such as that of Li et al. [14] limit their application only to the insurance of health data security and not to the complete traceability of it. From the analysis of these works, it can be concluded that health traceability required a private approach where only patient to which health data belongs and their authorized users can access their health data traceability—in contrast to the public approach followed in alimentary traceability. This analysis reveals also that none of the proposals found trying to offer a full traceability solution such as this offered in other domains—e.g., the commented alimentary traceability. Each proposal faces only concrete parts of this traceability: data provenance, content validation, malicious accesses, among others.

The authors of this article believe that providing health data traceability and providing mechanisms for integrating distributed health data are intimately linked—as they have been trying to illustrate throughout this section. That is why they want to take advantage of the data structure already generated by many proposals—including their own—to integrate or make interoperable distributed data and enable it to perform the tasks of health data traceability. To this end, it is proposed to refocus the information to be stored, obtaining a solution that solves both problems. In this way, the aim is to bring closer the arrival of patient-centered health systems that are more complete without complicating their integration into current information systems.

3 Extending Personal Health Trajectory for Traceability

Personal Health Trajectory is a concept that arises in the minds of this paper's authors in previous researches [20], when they try to offer a solution to the problems of actual institution-centered health systems from the patient perspective. Among others, this concept implies the creation of new patient-centered health systems, where the information revolves around and in virtue of this, and not of the institutions—as it has up to now. In order to make this possible, the need to the creation of a data structure where all the patient's distributed data are aggregated into a complete view of the patient's health throughout her life arises—see Fig. 1.

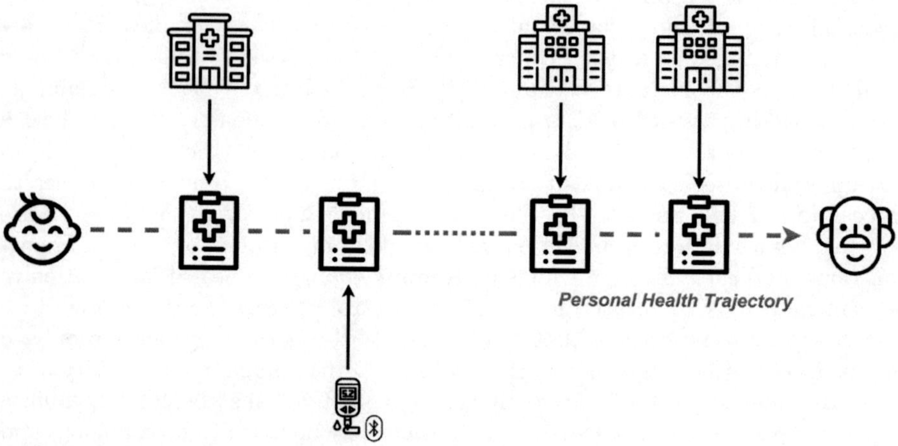

Fig. 1. Personal Health Trajectory concept

However, as motivated in the previous section, this structure does not have to remain just a system of links to patient records. It can take advantage of them to record all the changes that occur in the patient's health reality. Following the scheme of CRUD operations (create, read, update, and delete) that can be performed on the data, these would be: read (GET), add (POST), modify (PUT), and delete (DELETE).

Moreover, next to each operation associated with a health record, a value can even be stored to reflect the status of that record at the time a written operation—the creation or updating of the record—is recorded in its Personal Health Trajectory. In this way, it can be guaranteed that, if the state of the record is not the same as the one saved the last time this record was referenced in the Personal Health Trajectory, someone has spoiled it.

On the other hand, all this leads to empowerment of their health data by the patient. By belonging to the Personal Health Trajectory, the patient can control who has access to it and who does not. Thanks to traceability mechanisms, such as the one mentioned above, all those who interact with or generate patient health records without going through their Personal Health Trajectory can be considered unidentified users. Therefore, the authenticity and purpose of this data cannot be verified. Thus, this data may be treated with a different level of caution than data written by recognized agents—those to whom the patient has allowed access to the Personal Health Trajectory to write their changes.

4 Blockchain as Physical Support for Personal Health Trajectory Traceability

One of the most widely used technologies for the creation of the data structure that integrates patient health data is blockchain. Specifically, this is the main technology used in the proposal of the authors of this paper to create their Personal Health Trajectory [18].

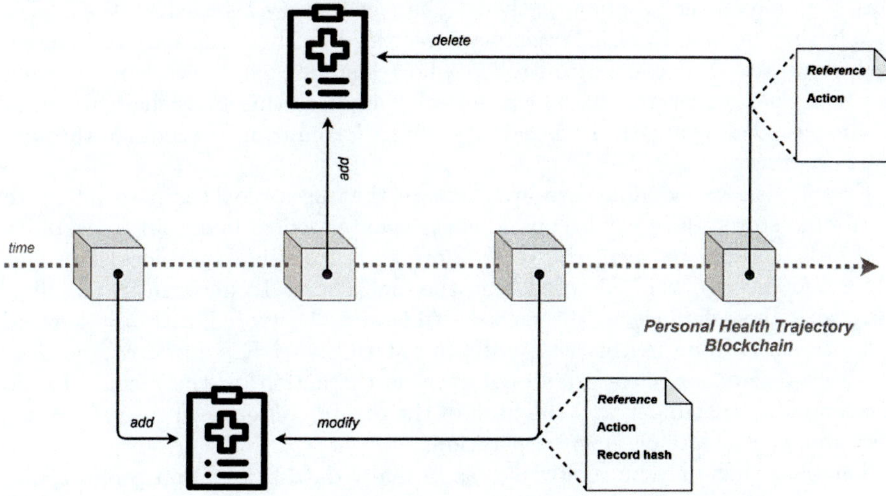

Fig. 2. Blockchain-based registry for Personal Health Trajectory

Blockchain as a technology to perform traceability on the Personal Health Trajectory allows the generation of a blockchain with the changes in the patient's health records. In this way, each block is associated with a CRUD operation on one of the patient's records—see Fig. 2. So, those records that do not have any associated block in the chain may be treated as data from untrusted sources, as discussed above. For records with blocks that store transactions on them, all the advantages discussed in the previous section can be applied.

In addition, the fact of using blockchain to obtain traceability over the Personal Health Trajectory allows not only to obtain the advantages already mentioned in the previous section, but also offers another series of extra advantages. For example, saving in the Personal Health Trajectory the status of a record when it is referenced from a block is more secure with blockchain. If the status of a record is obtained by calculating a hash associated with the content of the record, this hash should be stored in the block of the operation on the record. This block has the advantages of being stored in a blockchain, such as being part of an immutable chain, protected by a hash associated with the content of the block that does not allow anyone to change the content of the block without breaking and invalidating the chain—this is one of the security principles of blockchain. Therefore, it could be said that the integrity of the content of the record is guaranteed by the use of a double-hash. If someone were to maliciously attempt to alter the contents of the record, the hash associated with its contents, stored in the last block of a write operation on the blockchain record, would have to be rewritten. If someone tried to do this, it would invalidate the blockchain chain and the attack would be detected.

On the other hand, blockchain technology already offers advanced mechanisms to secure other aspects such as who accesses a blockchain and the permissions they have over it, among others. Therefore, every interaction that takes place in the Personal Health Trajectory is recorded by the blockchain technology itself. In this way, it can be controlled who registers each record—by knowing who and when generates the block—or who accesses this blockchain to register and visualize changes in traceability—even formalizing procedures through smart contracts.

Figure 3 shows what a base architecture that uses blockchain to integrate distributed stored data would look like if it is extended to maintain traceability of records. As can be seen, the records are stored outside the blockchain and only a reference to them is stored from the blockchain. To perform traceability, along with the reference to the record—which can be stored with any type of attribute, as is done in this case with the attributes *URL Resource* and *Key resource*—, new attributes are stored such as the action on the record that is represented by that block and the hash of the record content—in case of a write operation, as a *create* or *modify* operation.

The data that may be referenced, as in many data integration proposals, is data generated by healthcare institutions or data generated by IoMT or WoMT devices.

Similarly, it can be seen how the user's smartphone maintains a copy of the blockchain that it integrates and provides traceability over its Personal Health Trajectory. However, this blockchain can be shared with institutions for them to read or write to their Personal Health Trajectory, maintaining the integration and traceability of records at all times. How this sharing is done is more dependent on the data integration proposal than on this proposal on traceability.

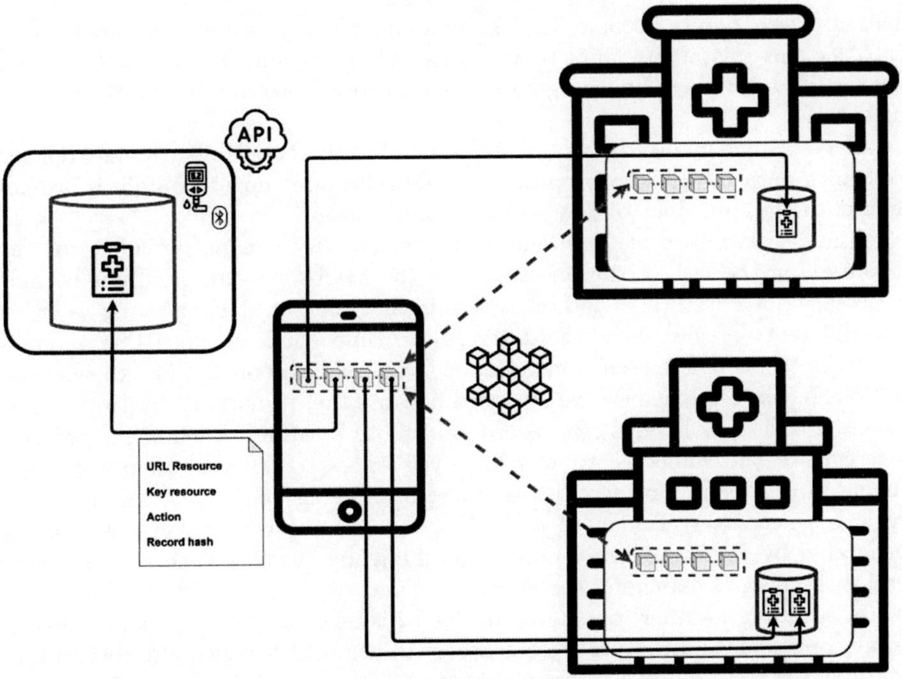

Fig. 3. Blockchain registry working on records from institutions and IoT services

Some proposals perform this step through the user, who shares a key for institutions to access their blockchain. Other proposals, such as that of the authors of this paper, seek more complex mechanisms, such as blockchains' federation [18], but which allow verified institutions associated with a data-sharing program to access the data of any of the verified institutions without the user's explicit consent for each access–something interesting for treating emergency patients, for example.

To finish, from the above it is intuited that creating such a proposal implies the use of private blockchains with permissions, where it is controlled who can read and generate new blocks in the blockchain of each user.

5 Discussion

As it has been manifested during all the manuscripts, the advantages of having a health registry that maintains the traceability of health records are clear. The achievement of this registry is closely linked to the existence of health data integration proposals. Despite this, the usage of other different structures to obtain this registry could be proposed, having a structure that maintains data integration and another one that maintains data traceability. However, to have real traceability of a patient's health, the need to having a global vision of all patient's health data becomes necessary. If no data integration structure is taken into account as starting point to access this global vision, the data integration's task must be replayed once again by new proposals to obtain the traceability structure.

Even being convinced that the obtaining of health traceability is an extension of health data integration proposals, the details about how to obtain it are not free of discussion, since different topics emerge around it.

The clearest example is about if real traceability can be provided only by maintaining the last version of records in the health system, or if it is become necessary to have stored—and referenced in the different blocks about a record—the different versions of a record across the time—at least until the record is solicited to be deleted—if done. In the proposal presented, it is known that various blocks reference the same record because their pointers refer to the same point. If different versions of a record become to be stored, each of the pointers referring to the same record will have references to different points. So, the inclusion of a common identifier to all records being versions of a unique real record is necessary. Taking as a premise that all the versions of a record are generated by the same institution—something that has so much sense—makes easier the task of managing the identifier of records.

In addition, another topic to be discussed is how the patient—being the real owner of this data structure—grant access to her health registry to institutions and IoT services to begin writing and/or read on it. In the case of IoT services, a possible solution is that patient's smartphone—having a copy of the registry—perform the writing tasks associated with records of IoT devices. However, in the case of health institutions, this is not so simple. The health professionals must access the registry not only for writing but also to read on it when the patient is under treatment. How to achieve this is discussed by several proposals on data integration, and their solutions can be applied in this case also—since on our approach architecture under data integration is the same under data traceability. Some issues arise around this, such as how access is granted in case of emergency if the user is the one granting it. In this sense, the authors of this paper are already working on solving problems of this type with other proposals such as the blockchain federation [18]. With all this, it is still up in the air that access to all patient health data traceability, and not only to their integrated data, will be given to them.

6 Conclusions and Future Work

This paper has discussed how distributed health data integration processes can be improved and taken into account to provide traceability of patient health data—as is already done in other fields. Specifically, the concept of Personal Health Trajectory—on which the authors of this paper have worked—has been presented and it has been shown how it can be extended to guarantee traceability.

Finally, efforts have been focused on showing a more pragmatic proposal—although without reaching its implementation—of how the traceability of the

Personal Health Trajectory could be achieved by implementing the latter as a registry of changes of the patient's health reality in blockchain. Different security mechanisms have been proposed around this registry, which takes advantage of the traceability offered to achieve levels of security that mere data integration does not achieve.

However, this proposal have already work to do. What is proposed here is to highlight the need for this traceability and its relationship with existing data integration proposals. There is still work ahead in terms of its implementation and the inclusion of new security techniques around the blockchain registry—some of which are already mentioned in the discussion, such as the use of smart contracts.

Acknowledgments. This work was supported by the projects 0499_4IE_PLUS_4_E (Interreg V-A España-Portugal 2014-2020) and RTI2018-094591-B-I00 (MCIU/AEI/FEDER, UE), the FPU19/03965 grant, the Department of Economy and Infrastructure of the Government of Extremadura (GR18112, IB18030), and the European Regional Development Fund.

References

1. Chen, L., Lee, W.K., Chang, C.C., Choo, K.K.R., Zhang, N.: Blockchain based searchable encryption for electronic health record sharing. Future Gener. Comput. Syst. **95**, 420–429 (2019). https://doi.org/10.1016/J.FUTURE.2019.01.018
2. Dubovitskaya, A., et al.: Intelligent health care data management using blockchain: current limitation and future research agenda. In: Gadepally, V., et al. (eds.) DMAH/Poly - 2019. LNCS, vol. 11721, pp. 277–288. Springer, Cham (2019). https://doi.org/10.1007/978-3-030-33752-0_20
3. Feng, H., Wang, X., Duan, Y., Zhang, J., Zhang, X.: Applying blockchain technology to improve agri-food traceability: a review of development methods, benefits and challenges. J. Clean. Prod. **260**, 121031 (2020)
4. Flores-Martin, D., Rojo, J., Moguel, E., Berrocal, J., Murillo, J.M.: Smart nursing homes: self-management architecture based on iot and machine learning for rural areas. Wirel. Communi. Mob. Comput. **2021** (2021)
5. Galvez, J.F., Mejuto, J.C., Simal-Gandara, J.: Future challenges on the use of blockchain for food traceability analysis. TrAC Trends Anal. Chem. **107**, 222–232 (2018)
6. Gatouillat, A., Badr, Y., Massot, B., Sejdic, E.: Internet of medical things: a review of recent contributions dealing with cyber-physical systems in medicine. IEEE Internet Things J. **5**(5), 3810–3822 (2018). https://doi.org/10.1109/JIOT.2018.2849014
7. Gong, J., Lin, S., Li, J.: Research on personal health data provenance and right confirmation with smart contract. In: 2019 IEEE 4th Advanced Information Technology, Electronic and Automation Control Conference (IAEAC), vol. 1, pp. 1211–1216. IEEE (2019)
8. Helal, S., Jain, R.: Digital health-active and healthy living. Computer **52**(11), 14–17 (2019)
9. Henly, S.J., Wyman, J.F., Gaugler, J.E.: Health trajectory research: a call to action for nursing science. Nurs. Res. **60**(3 SUPPL.) (2011). https://doi.org/10.1097/NNR.0b013e31821cc240

10. Jalali, L., Huo, D., Oh, H., Tang, M., Pongpaichet, S., Jain, R.: Personicle: personal chronicle of life events. In: Workshop on Personal Data Analytics in the Internet of Things (PDA@ IOT) at the 40th International Conference on Very Large Databases (VLDB), Hangzhou, China (2014)
11. Kalra, D.: Electronic health record standards (2006)
12. Kassab, M., Defranco, J., Malas, T., Graciano Neto, V.V., Destefanis, G.: Blockchain: a panacea for electronic health records? In: Proceedings - 2019 IEEE/ACM 1st International Workshop on Software Engineering for Healthcare, SEH 2019, pp. 21–24. Institute of Electrical and Electronics Engineers Inc., May 2019
13. Kyazze, M., Wesson, J., Naude, K.: The design and implementation of a ubiquitous personal health record system for South Africa. Stud. Health Technol. Inform. **206**, 29 (2014)
14. Li, H., Zhu, L., Shen, M., Gao, F., Tao, X., Liu, S.: Blockchain-based data preservation system for medical data. J. Med. Syst. **42**(8), 1–13 (2018). https://doi.org/10.1007/S10916-018-0997-3
15. Philip, N., et al.: Design of a restful middleware to enable a web of medical things. In: 2014 MOBIHEALTH, pp. 361–364, November 2014. https://doi.org/10.1109/MOBIHEALTH.2014.7015986
16. Roehrs, A., Da Costa, C.A., da Rosa Righi, R., De Oliveira, K.S.F.: Personal health records: a systematic literature review. J. Med. Internet Res. **19**(1), e13 (2017). https://doi.org/10.2196/jmir.5876, http://www.jmir.org/2017/1/e13/
17. Roehrs, A., da Costa, C.A., da Rosa Righi, R.: OmniPHR: a distributed architecture model to integrate personal health records. J. Biomed. Inform. **71**, 70–81 (2017). https://doi.org/10.1016/j.jbi.2017.05.012
18. Rojo, J., Hernandez, J., Murillo, J.M., Garcia-Alonso, J.: Blockchains' federation for integrating distributed health data using a patient-centered approach. In: 2021 IEEE/ACM 3rd International Workshop on Software Engineering for Healthcare (SEH), vol. 1, pp. 52–59. IEEE Computer Society, Los Alamitos, June 2021. https://doi.org/10.1109/SEH52539.2021.00016, https://doi.ieeecomputersociety.org/10.1109/SEH52539.2021.00016
19. Rojo, J., Flores-Martin, D., Garcia-Alonso, J., Murillo, J.M., Berrocal, J.: Automating the interactions among IoT devices using neural networks. In: 2020 IEEE International Conference on Pervasive Computing and Communications Workshops (PerCom Workshops), pp. 1–6. IEEE (2020)
20. Rojo, J., Hernandez, J., Murillo, J.M.: A personal health trajectory API: addressing problems in health institution-oriented systems. In: Bielikova, M., Mikkonen, T., Pautasso, C. (eds.) ICWE 2020. LNCS, vol. 12128, pp. 519–524. Springer, Cham (2020). https://doi.org/10.1007/978-3-030-50578-3_37
21. Rojo, J., Moguel, E., Fonseca, C., Lopes, M., Garcia-Alonso, J., Hernandez, J.: Time series forecasting to predict the evolution of the functional profile of the elderly persons. In: García-Alonso, J., Fonseca, C. (eds.) IWoG 2020. LNB, pp. 11–22. Springer, Cham (2021). https://doi.org/10.1007/978-3-030-72567-9_2
22. Helou, S., Abou-Khalil, V., El Helou, E., Kiyono, K.: Factors related to personal health data sharing: data usefulness, sensitivity and anonymity. Stud. Health Technol. Inform. **281**, 1051–1055 (2021). https://doi.org/10.3233/SHTI210345, https://pubmed.ncbi.nlm.nih.gov/34042839/
23. Spil, T., Klein, R.: Personal health records success; why google health failed and what does that mean for Microsoft HealthVault? In: Proceedings of the Annual Hawaii International Conference on System Sciences, pp. 2818–2827. IEEE Computer Society (2014). https://doi.org/10.1109/HICSS.2014.353

24. Zhang, Y., Qiu, M., Tsai, C.W., Hassan, M., Alamri, A.: Health-CPS: healthcare cyber-physical system assisted by cloud and big data. IEEE Syst. J. **11**, 1–8 (2015). https://doi.org/10.1109/JSYST.2015.2460747
25. Zhang, Y., Li, J., Zheng, D., Chen, X., Li, H.: Towards privacy protection and malicious behavior traceability in smart health. Pers. Ubiquit. Comput. **21**(5), 815–830 (2017). https://doi.org/10.1007/s00779-017-1047-8

A Graph-Based Healthcare System for Quantum Simulation of Medication Administration in the Aging People

Javier Romero-Álvarez(✉), Jaime Alvarado-Valiente, Jose Garcia-Alonso, Enrique Moguel, and Juan M. Murillo

University of Extremadura, Cáceres, Spain
{jromero,jaimeav,jgaralo,enrique,juanmamu}@unex.es

Abstract. Drug treatment is necessary to treat most illnesses, maintain health or prevent further deterioration. Above all, medication in the ageing population is a very important aspect because a large number of hospital admissions in this age group are due to adverse reactions caused by the misadministration and misprescription of medicines. So it is an area where medical experts need to take special care. However, inappropriate prescribing is a major and constant problem for this sector of the population. This is one of the principals reasons that both the relationships between genetic determinants and variables in the health trajectory of the aging people throughout their lives are involved. In this paper propose a graph-based system that, using a quantum simulation, will allow medical experts to predict the possible adverse effects that a particular drug may have on the health of an aging person, based on their history of taking drugs, the described effects of these drugs and the physiological and genetic determinants of the patient. In this way, with the use of this system, health professionals will be able to prescribe in a personalized way for each patient, avoiding, as far as possible, the inappropriate prescription of drugs.

Keywords: Aging · Quantum computing · Pharmacogenetics · Drug treatment · Architecture

1 Introduction

In recent times the concept of health is changing and adapting to multidimensional approaches, one of the factors being the transition from infectious to chronic diseases and the prescription of drugs to treat them [1,2].

Currently in Spain, one of the largest expenditures in healthcare budgets is pharmaceutical costs. 65% of people over 65 take at least one drug per week, more than 40% take at least 5 drugs per week, and 12% take more than 10. Adverse effects of these drugs account accounts for 7% of emergency hospitalizations for these patients. In studies of hospitalized patients, between 12% and 58.5% receive an inappropriate drug [3]. This is why, in order to solve these problems,

J. García-Alonso and C. Fonseca (Eds.): IWoG 2021, LNBE, pp. 34–41, 2022.
https://doi.org/10.1007/978-3-030-97524-1_4

ICT tools could be used to support healthcare professionals, and also eHealth applications for treatment have been advocated for many years as a promising tool to improve treatment prescriptions.

The current software is useful in identifying potential problems and facilitating the individualization of the administration of certain drugs [4]. However, providing safe and effective drug therapy with this software is a rather complex problem due to several reasons. Reasons such as the data to be considered, which is of such magnitude that with current tools it is unmanageable [5]. This is why, unfortunately, the adjustment of medication in the aging people is a complex and still unresolved challenge, and is currently done on a trial and error basis [6,7].

The possibility of having models that can handle a large amount of data, variables, and relationships between them could allow healthcare experts to choose the most optimal combination of drugs for each patient, the most appropriate prescribing regimen, and to model scenarios over time, thus allowing them to establish a strategy appropriate to the context [5]. In this way, therapeutic optimization would improve the health of patients and their evolution, avoiding the development of diseases and preventing potential adverse reactions. Thus improving the quality of life and the dependency of the aging people [8].

Therefore, prescribing medicines for the aging people is a challenge, which requires adaptation to their genetic and environmental characteristics, and to the pathophysiological changes that occur as a consequence of these and of aging [9,10].

To solve the problems mentioned above, we propose a system that will serve as a technological support for health experts for the preparation of data sets and the extraction of the relationships between the different variables. Providing a dashboard that will allow complex queries and facilitate the visualization of the information in a useful way. They will thus be able to predict the possible adverse effects that a given drug may have on a person's health based on their drug-taking history and genetic condition.

In order to present our proposal, the rest of the paper is structured as follows: Sect. 2 presents the motivations of this work. Section 3 describes our proposal in which we will highlight the architecture. And finally, Sect. 4 shows the conclusion and future works.

2 Motivations

Software engineering is making great progress in almost every field, and in every aspect of life. But with the increasing number and complexity of problems, software engineering requires more and more computing power, greater speed, and better results. To overcome these computational barriers, one of the most promising options is Quantum Computing [11,12].

The arrival of Quantum Computing has brought about a new paradigm in computing and software engineering, opening the door to new horizons in the applications of computing to solve problems [13]. Quantum computing not only allows problems to be solved in much less time than classical computers, but it also enables the use of its computational power to tackle problems beyond the scope of classical computing as we know it. In this way, the Theory of Computation is generating new categories of problems to classify those that cannot be reasonably solved with classical computing, and which can be solved with quantum computing [14]. In particular, the power of quantum computers makes it possible to segregate a new category within the class of P-SPACE problems called BQP [15]. The existence of this class of problems is very important because although we know that the benefit of quantum computing will not come from doing faster what classical computers can already solve efficiently, they will offer better and more efficient solutions [16].

The interaction of a new molecule with existing molecules in a person's organism, which in itself determines its own rules of behavior according to its genetic markers, is a quantum process in which a series of scenarios coexist, each with its own probability, recognized as a BQP-COMPLETE problem [15], one of the most complexes within the BQP class [17]. Given the characteristics of the problems in the BQP-COMPLETE class, some research work is already pointing to the usefulness and necessity of quantum computing in the life sciences and in particular in the health sector [18].

3 Graph-Based Healthcare System for Quantum Simulation of Medication Administration

We propose an architecture of a graph-based system with which we intend that health experts can analyze the relationships between genetic conditioning factors and other variables in the health trajectory of aging people throughout their lives, including the reaction that drugs can cause them. In this way, with this system, which uses quantum computing techniques, we intend to be able to predict the possible adverse effects that a particular drug may have on the health of an aging people person based on their history of taking drugs, the effects of these drugs and their physiological and genetic factors.

The proposed architecture is divided into two layers: front-end and back-end [19]. The front-end is the layer that is responsible for receiving user requests, invoking the business logic, and returning the results to the user. It controls the navigation of screens, opening, and closing of the web session, etc.

On the other hand, the back-end is where the business logic itself resides and consists of various modules or components, as will be discussed below. This division of the architecture has been established following the principles defined for the development of architectures based on microservices, where the need to decouple these two layers for a better design and development of the systems is established.

The components for the architecture detailed in Fig. 1 are as follows:

Microservices
Set of microservices that will contain the back-end of the system. Microservices are an architectural and organizational approach to software development

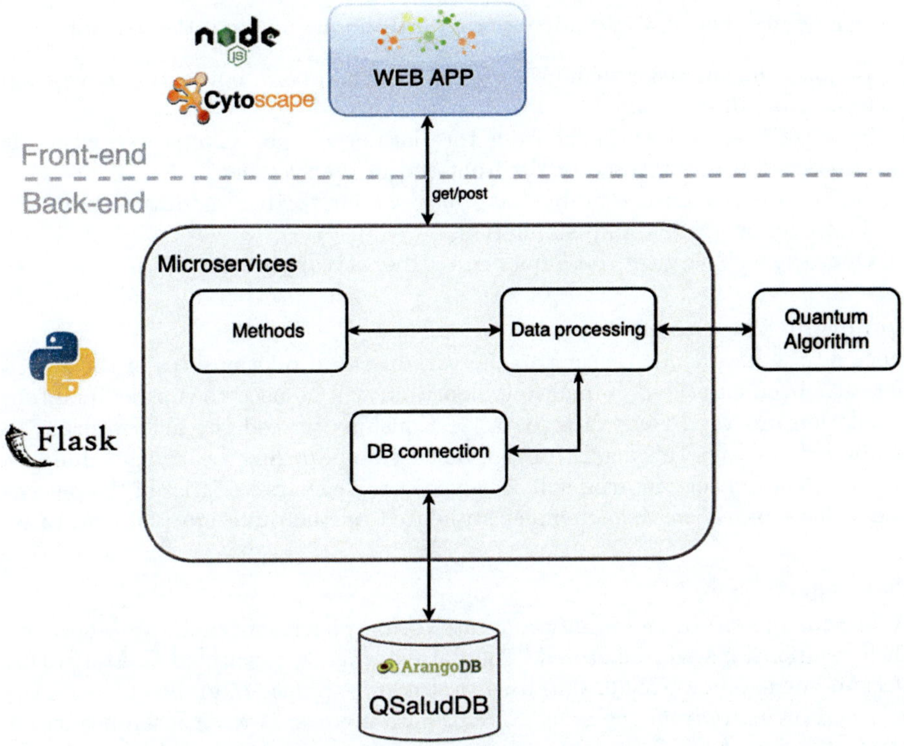

Fig. 1. General architecture of the proposed system

where the software is composed of small independent services that communicate through a well-defined application programming interface (REST API) [20,21]. By designing our architecture with this approach, it will allow it to be easier to scale, faster to develop, and, being composed of independent modules, it will be simpler to deploy and operate. Thus, the proposed *back-end* is composed of several modules, where its functions will be to make the necessary connections to the database, process the data to display them in the graphical interface, provide a REST API to invoke the services, and the transformation of the data represented in the graph so that they can be used by the quantum algorithm.

They will be implemented in the Python programming language, using an OpenAPI specification. OpenAPI is a standard for the description of programming interfaces, which will be used, therefore, for the description and documentation of the microservices. With this, the visual documentation is created and facilitates the implementation of the back-end.

Finally, they will be published through a REST API using the Flask framework. Flask is a Python library that provides useful tools and functions that allow you to create Python web applications in a simple way. Its use will facilitate collaboration between developers because it adapts to each project by installing project-specific extensions and includes its own web server for testing.

Therefore, this *back-end* microservices will be in charge of the following:

- Perform the operations/connections with the database, both reading, writing, modifying, or deleting.
- Serialize the data obtained from the database to be compatible with the visualization library used in the front-end of the system.
- Deserialize the data sent by the *front-end* for further modification in the database, or for quantum simulation.
- Offer the web services to be queried by the web application.

Quantum Algorithm
Once all the knowledge relating to the variables and relationships of the stored data has been extracted, a quantum algorithm will be used to run the quantum simulation process (using these data relationships to feed the algorithm). The study and design of this algorithm will be based on Machine Learning techniques to predict how a certain drug will act given specific characteristics of the patient and will be based on the principles stipulated by the quantum platform to be used.

Database
A database where the information of interest on pharmacogenetic variables and their relationships will be stored. The data storage tool selected is ArangoDB. It is an open-source NoSQL database that allows the use of graphs to store the information apart from the other NoSQL data models. It was chosen because it allows the use of graphs to store the information, thus offering the best model design that considers the relationships between the data.

On the other hand, to determine the typology and structure of the data to be stored in ArangoDB, the variables considered being determinant in the response to a drug by a patient, in this case, an aging people patient, were defined. The variables considered to be determinants of variability in drug response were as follows:

- **Pharmacogenetics** (dependent on the individual genetic endowment)
- **Pharmacogenetic interactions** (dependent on the treatment set)
- **Clinical and physiological conditioners** (physiology and pathophysiology dependent)

Once the variables that will be part of the data model were selected, the design of the data model was carried out in the selected data storage technology, taking into account the different fields in each of the variables presented in the previous enumeration. It was decided that the data model will be based on the use of the ArangoDB document graph.

Web APP. Web module developed with NodeJs that will act as the system's front-end. This framework supports the development of dynamic websites, web services, and web applications, as is the case of our system, providing libraries for accessing databases, template structures, session management, etc. NodeJs has been selected because it is the Javascript-based runtime environment that best allows applications to have scalability, excellent performance, optimized costs, and because it is one of the most widely used tools for web development today, such as Netflix or PayPal [22].

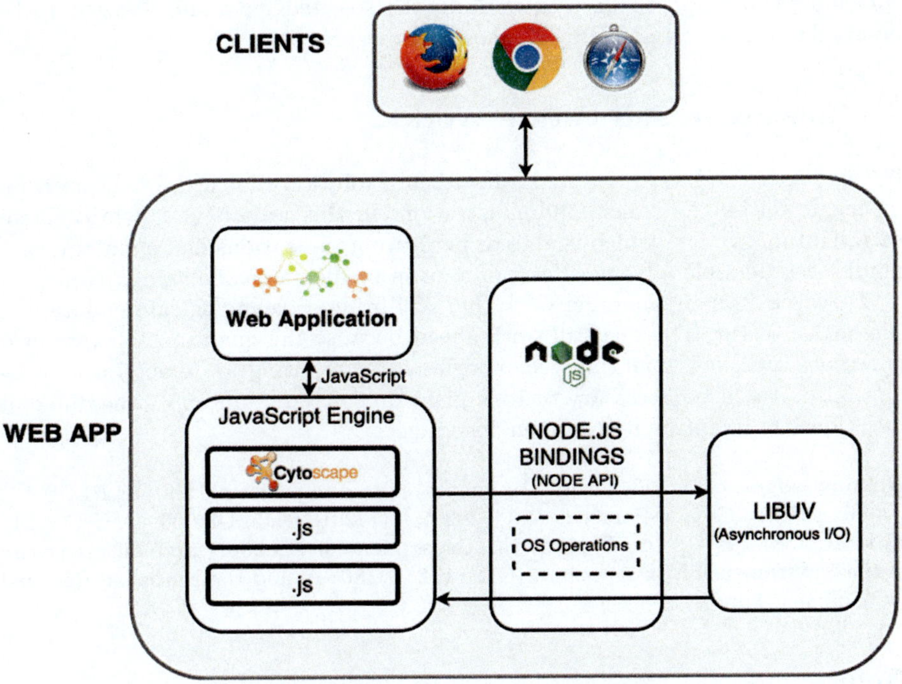

Fig. 2. Web APP module of the system

So, the function of this module will be to provide to the user a graphical interface with which to manipulate the graph with the pharmacogenomic variables of a patient, add new variables, and invoke the quantum simulation with the data represented.

A visualization tool will be used to manipulate and visualize the graph. This visualization technology has been selected after analysis and evaluation of different Hypergraph technologies that allow visualization of the information and relationships between the variables involved. By this way, the visualization tool that has been selected is the JavaScript library CystoscapeJS, as it has been the best value from a quantitative scale. In addition, this library is capable of natively offering events on the canvas where the data is represented and will allow operations to be performed on the nodes or arcs, which is essential in this work.

As can be seen in Fig. 2, the development of the Web APP module using Node.js allows the use of a non-blocking, asynchronous I/O model that is event-driven. This makes the adaptation of Javascript easier, providing a much higher code execution. Thanks to Javascript and Node.js, code runs faster in the server-to-client direction. This will improve the performance of the application. Another important dependency is *libuv*, a C library used by Node to abstract non-blocking I/O operations to a consistent interface on all supported clients.

As discussed above, being event-driven and using the CytoscapeJS library will allow the graph to be created from the selected data and allow it to be manipulated and visualized by the health experts.

4 Conclusion and Future Work

In this paper, we have presented a healthcare solution that uses quantum computing to optimize medicine administration. In this way, it is a hybrid classical/quantum system, which is able to perform optimizations and simulations to predict the possible adverse effects of a given medicine on the aging people.

However, it is an emerging work that will bring a technological revolution in the health sector. There is still work ahead because the quantum software field is recent, with new quantum technologies for computing are emerging day by day. Also, it will be necessary to test quantum software and apply the different techniques of quantum software engineering.

Acknowledgements. This work was supported by the projects 0499_4IE_PLUS_4_E (Interreg V-A España-Portugal 2014–2020), RTI2018-094591-B-I00 (MCIU/AEI/FEDER, UE) the QSalud Project, the Department of Economy and Infrastructure of the Government of Extremadura (GR18112, IB18030), and the European Regional Development Fund.

References

1. Bygbjerg, I.C.: Double burden of noncommunicable and infectious diseases in developing countries. Science **337**(6101), 1499–1501 (2012). https://doi.org/10.1126/SCIENCE.1223466
2. Mueller, C., Schur, C., O'Connell, J.: Prescription drug spending: the impact of age and chronic disease status. Am. J. Public Health **87**(10), 1626–1629 (2011). https://doi.org/10.2105/AJPH.87.10.1626
3. Merle, L., Laroche, M.L., Dantoine, T., Charmes, J.P.: Predicting and preventing adverse drug reactions in the very old. Drugs Aging **22**(5), 375–392 (2005). https://doi.org/10.2165/00002512-200522050-00003/FIGURES/TAB2
4. Cao, Y., Romero, J., Aspuru-Guzik, A.: Potential of quantum computing for drug discovery. IBM J. Res. Dev. **62**(6), 6-1 (2018)
5. Dash, S., Shakyawar, S.K., Sharma, M., Kaushik, S.: Big data in healthcare: management, analysis and future prospects. J. Big Data **6**(1), 1–25 (2019). https://doi.org/10.1186/S40537-019-0217-0/FIGURES/
6. Barry, P.J., O'Keefe, N., O'Connor, K.A., O'Mahony, D.: Inappropriate prescribing in the aging people: a comparison of the Beers criteria and the improved prescribing in the elderly tool (IPET) in acutely ill aging people hospitalized patients. J. Clin. Pharm. Ther. **2006**(31), 617–626 (2006)

7. Gallagher, P., Barry, P., O'Mahony, D.: Inappropriate prescribing in the aging people. J. Clin. Pharm. Ther. **32**, 113–121 (2007)
8. Mohseni, M., et al.: Commercialize quantum technologies in five years. Nature **543**(7644), 171–174 (2017). https://doi.org/10.1038/543171a
9. Spinewine, A., et al.: Appropriate prescribing in elderly people: how well can it be measured and optimised? Lancet (London Engl.) **370**(9582), 173–184 (2007). https://doi.org/10.1016/S0140-6736(07)61091-5
10. Feinstein, A.R., Horwitz, R.I.: Problems in the "evidence" of "evidence-based medicine". Am. J. Med. **103**(6), 529–535 (1997). https://doi.org/10.1016/S0002-9343(97)00244-1
11. Shubham, Sajwan, P., Jayapandian, N.: Challenges and opportunities: quantum computing in machine learning. In: Proceedings of the 3rd International Conference on I-SMAC IoT in Social, Mobile, Analytics and Cloud, I-SMAC 2019, pp. 598–602 (2019). https://doi.org/10.1109/I-SMAC47947.2019.9032461
12. MacQuarrie, E.R., Simon, C., Simmons, S., Maine, E.: The emerging commercial landscape of quantum computing. Nat. Rev. Phys. **2**(11), 596–598 (2020)
13. Zhao, J.: Quantum software engineering: landscapes and horizons (2020). https://arxiv.org/abs/2007.07047v1
14. Bernstein, E., Vazirani, U., Comput, S.J.: Quantum complexity theory *. Soc. Ind. Appl. Math. **26**(5), 7 (1997). http://www.siam.org/journals/sicomp/26-5/30092.html
15. Aaronson, S.: BQP and the polynomial hierarchy. In: Proceedings of the Annual ACM Symposium on Theory of Computing, pp. 141–150 (2009). https://doi.org/10.1145/1806689.1806711
16. Ozhigov, Y.: Quantum computers speed up classical with probability zero. Chaos Solitons Fractals **10**(10), 1707–1714 (1998). https://doi.org/10.1016/S0960-0779(98)00226-4
17. Zhang, S.: BQP-complete problems. Handb. Nat. Comput. **3–4**, 1545–1571 (2012). https://doi.org/10.1007/978-3-540-92910-9_46
18. Shaikh, T.A., Ali, R.: Quantum computing in big data analytics: a survey. In: 2016 IEEE International Conference on Computer and Information Technology (CIT), pp. 112–115 (2016). https://doi.org/10.1109/CIT.2016.79
19. Erickson, J., Siau, K.: Service oriented architecture: a research review from the software and applications perspective. Innov. Inf. Syst. Model. Methods Best Pract. 190–203 (2009)
20. Nadareishvili, I., Mitra, R., McLarty, M., Amundsen, M.: Microservice Architecture: Aligning Principles, Practices, and Culture. O'Reilly Media, Inc. (2016)
21. Taibi, D., Lenarduzzi, V., Pahl, C.: Processes, motivations, and issues for migrating to microservices architectures: an empirical investigation. IEEE Cloud Comput. **4**(5), 22–32 (2017)
22. Casciaro, M., Mammino, L.: Node.js Design Patterns: Design and Implement Production-Grade Node.js Applications Using Proven Patterns and Techniques. Packt Publishing Ltd. (2020)

Check for updates

Distributed Sustainable IoT Architecture for Detecting Loneliness in Isolated Rural Areas

Manuel Jesús-Azabal[1](✉), Lorenzo Mariano[2], José García-Alonso[1], and Jaime Galán-Jiménez[1]

[1] Department of Languages and Telematics, University of Extremadura, Avda. Universidad S/N, 10003 Cáceres, Spain
{manuel,jgaralo,jaime}@unex.es

[2] Department of Nursing, University of Extremadura, Avda. Universidad S/N, 10003 Cáceres, Spain
lorenmariano@unex.es

Abstract. Loneliness among ageing people has become a significant issue for society. Its impact on health can even be exacerbated in isolated rural areas. Furthermore, the lack of Internet connection is common for these areas, contributing to such isolation. Considering this, it is important to proactively detect ageing people who experience loneliness. In this work, we propose a distributed Internet of Things (IoT) architecture to detect loneliness among elderly population living in isolated villages. The solution is based on the identification of encounters of elderly people, tracing a graph of the recurrent contacts they have. Then, this graph reflects ageing people as nodes and the social encounters as links between the nodes. Hence, it is possible to identify nodes with few contacts, reveling potential candidates to suffer unwanted loneliness. For this, the architecture draws on the collaboration between smartwatches, smartphones and Bluetooth beacons. Then, ageing people are provided with smartwatches which may store all the encounters they experience with other ageing people and neighbours in the village. Once smartwatches registry this information, it is transmitted to Bluetooth beacons. The proposed architecture aims to address the lack of communication infrastructure with a sustainable solution, exploiting the autonomy of the devices. For this, a consumption model is estimated to study the viability of the proposal, achieving successful results at power sustainability.

Keywords: Loneliness · Distributed architecture · Internet of Things · Smartphones · Sustainable

1 Introduction

Loneliness have become a concern for society. In recent years, many works have addressed how social isolation and solitude impact on health and well-being [1]. In this context, loneliness among ageing people has been identified as a high

J. García-Alonso and C. Fonseca (Eds.): IWoG 2021, LNBE, pp. 42–54, 2022.
https://doi.org/10.1007/978-3-030-97524-1_5

priority problem, which is connected to other factors like their health but also with the place they live. Thus, rural areas become challenging contexts for ageing people who feel alone. In these cases, loneliness can be aggravated by the limited possibilities of interactions and the difficulties to relate with others. Many of these rural areas count with a very low population density and a significant proportion of ageing people. This is the case of the so-called "empty" Spain, where many small villages fit with these definitions. In this scenario, feelings of loneliness and social isolation have become normal. Then, it is necessary to tackle the problem and develop effective public policies.

However, obtaining loneliness information can become difficult. Many works are based on quantitative approaches which make use of scales and questionnaires to evaluate loneliness [2]. They provide reliable results, however, these approaches are not always able to reflect the reality and the whole context of solitude [3]. The problem of solitude, especially for ageing people, requires a more detailed qualitative perspective. Considering it, technology could notably enrich the way these works approach the problem.

Nevertheless, many of the existing technological approaches are not applicable for isolated rural areas where there are no communication infrastructures. Factors like the lack of interest of companies due to economic budget or the difficult geographical conditions derive in the absence of Internet coverage [4]. Then, these conditions motivates the application of alternative communication mechanisms.

In the present work, a distributed sustainable Internet of Things (IoT) architecture for studying loneliness is presented. The approach aims to provide a solution to identify potential candidates to suffer solitude among the elderly population in an isolated rural area. For this, the architecture draws on the collaboration of autonomous devices to detect the encounters of ageing people to recognise a contact map with the most recurrent contacts. Thus, a graph of relationships is provided, displaying ageing people as nodes and contacts as links between these nodes. Therefore, encounters among the population can be identified, including those nodes which are mostly isolated. As a result, it is possible to know potential candidates of suffering unwanted loneliness, propitiated by the lack of social contacts.

Our work proposes equipping ageing people with smartwatches which detect surrounding devices. Thus, storing social contacts is possible. For this, Bluetooth is used to perform the detection and the data transmissions. Therefore, Internet connection is not required to perform data sends, drawing on the physical movement and proximity to communications. Considering this collaboration between autonomous devices demands very concrete power needs, the energy consumption becomes a relevant factor in the technical viability [5,6]. For this, this work also details a consumption model to assess the sustainability of the approach.

The rest of the paper is organised as follows: Sect. 2 details the state of the art. Then, Sect. 3 describes the proposed algorithm and its implementation. In Sect. 4, a performance evaluation is provided. Finally, Sect. 5 draws the conclusion and details the future works.

2 State of Art

Loneliness has become a relevant field of study in the recent years. Multiple studies analyse how solitude affects people and their mood [7]. Then, this situation involves largely elderly population [7]. In many cases, ageing people experience how their social life is reduced as years pass. As a result, there is a large percentage of elderly people who live alone and use to spend their day-to-day with no companion. In this scenario, the identification of the situation is critical in order to provide a response. However, detecting loneliness can be difficult if there are not effective mechanisms to identify it [3].

Studies like [8] manifest how the traditional methods for identifying and recruiting ageing people at risk of isolation are hard to interpret. Furthermore, works like [9] also manifest how the lack of evidences question many experiments. As a response for some of these considerations, technology can become a suitable allied for loneliness detection.

Internet and social networks are a relevant domain to analyse loneliness. The work in [10] shows how approaches focused on communication technologies result to be positive on social support, social connectedness and social isolation. Works like [11] show how the use of technological devices and the inclusion of Internet in the routines of the elderly people become favourable for their well-being. In some cases, the interactions through social networks and the use of digital platforms can contribute to mitigate the feeling of loneliness. Thus, the communication between ageing people even though geographical or health obstacles become a strong incentive. However, these solutions raise two considerations: i) the lack of Internet in many isolated rural areas make these applications hard or impossible to use; and ii) the approaches are not centred on identifying loneliness since they are focused on providing mitigation and a response to it. In this way, our proposal adopts a different position in the loneliness topic and aims to detect solitude in rural areas. In fact, we propose a system based on Bluetooth and local communication for loneliness detection in rural areas with no Internet infrastructure. For this, physical encounters and movements in the village are used to perform communications. Next section details the insights of the proposal.

3 Detecting Loneliness with a Distributed IoT Architecture

In order to monitor and detect loneliness patterns, our approach is based on the collaboration between Internet of Things (IoT) devices and wearables, while exploiting social behaviour. The proposal is aligned with the works introduced in [12,13] and it is designed to be applied in specific rural areas such as small villages. In many of these contexts, Internet connection is not available or it is restricted to particular points. Considering the limitations of connectivity, the proposed solution makes use of Bluetooth to perform data transmissions in a local environment. Then, three main entities collaborate in the solution:

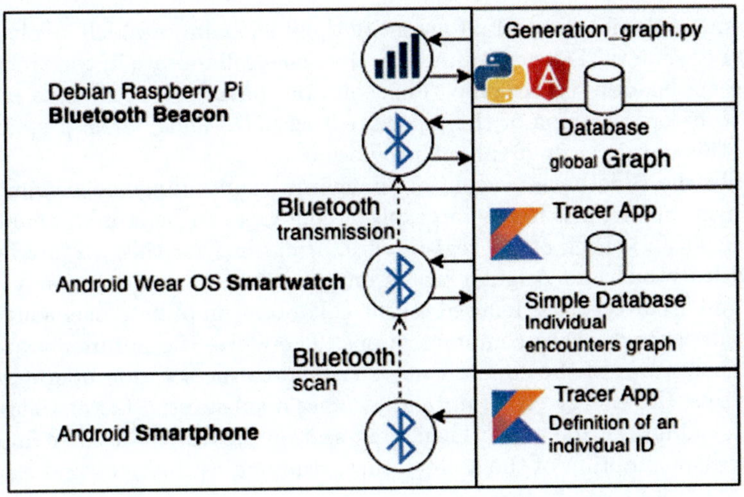

Fig. 1. Elements and relations in the proposed architecture.

ageing people, volunteer neighbours of the village, and the destination Bluetooth beacon.

1. **Ageing people** are equipped with smart bracelets which register all encounters they have with other ageing people and neighbours. Thus, the bracelets are able to constantly scan the context and detect other surrounding devices. The gathered information will be transmitted to a Bluetooth beacon which aims to build a contact graph of the inhabitants to detect potential candidates of suffering loneliness.
2. **Volunteer neighbours** are inhabitants of the same village who are recognised by the smartwatches. Thus, it is possible to identify encounters of the elderly with the rest of the population.
3. The **destination** node represents the entity which receives the information about the encounters and companion patterns of the elderly. The destination node, which is connected to the Internet, is able to transmit the data remotely or to process it locally. Finally, a graph of the encounters is obtained, providing a set of potential candidates of suffering loneliness.

As Fig. 1 represents, the system draws on an architecture based on the collaboration between three different devices: smartwatches, smartphone and Bluetooth beacon. In the case of the smartwatches, they make use of Wear OS [14] to execute Tracer App, a Kotlin [15] application which scan the context using BLE to detect and to registry surrounding devices. For this, the smartwatch requires the user ID of the entities and monitors the contact time. This way, the device stores internally the registered encounter, keeping the time it occurs and the user ID associated to the recognised device.

The smartphones are useful to identify those encounters which involve people who are not seniors. Thus, volunteers in the place collaborate in the architecture with the application Tracer App. This solution makes use of BLE to provide a service to listen petitions of the associated user ID. Thus, when a smartwatch requires this data, the smartphone provides it.

Finally, the Bluetooth beacons are in charge of obtaining the encounter data from the smartwatches. Hence, a graph of contacts can be stored, enabling the management and check of the registered information. For this, an interface provided with Python and Angular [15] is implemented.

The full architecture is focused on the collaboration of heterogeneous devices to perform context-aware communications. Therefore, the autonomy and independent behaviour of the components is critical to the solution operative. Considering this, the energy consumption becomes a substantial factor to study the technical viability of the work. Then, next section provides a detailed analysis of the power consumption of the architecture, studying estimations and extracting conclusions from these values.

4 Power Consumption Evaluation

The proposed architecture relies on the performance and autonomy of the devices to implements the encounters detection and the contacts graph. This way, the limitations at energy and power capabilities become critical factors for the potential implementation of the solution. As a response for this, this section details a theoretical power consumption model, analysing the potential threshold for the devices involved. Thus, it is possible to assess the technical viability of the work. This section introduces two parts: the energy consumption model and the estimation of energetic cost in hypothetical scenarios.

4.1 Energy Consumption Model

The devices in the architecture draw on BLE to perform the communications and data transmission. This way, depending of the operation executed, the power requirements vary. Following the states shown in Fig. 2a and the metrics defined in work [16], the stages involved in the BLE communication can be simplified into six: sleeping, waking-up, scanning, receiving and sending. These phases count with an estimated cost in battery which can be extracted from the work [16]. Next, these stages are explained:

1. Sleeping. This is the first state of the BLE communication. It refers to the period that the device is not available to perform operations such as scanning, receiving or sending. This interval is useful to save battery and to reduce the impact of BLE on the device operative. The energetic cost of sleeping, S_e, is insignificant, then it is estimated with $S_e = 0.001$ mA.
2. Waking-up. This stage is the previous step to scan the context. This way, this phase prepares the resources required to perform the scanning operation. The energetic cost associated to waking-up, Wu_e, is $Wu_e = 6.0$ mA.

3. Scanning (Pre-Rx-Tx). This step turns on in preparation to receive and to send data with BLE. For this, the device scans the context, becoming available for the other devices and recognising surrounding elements. The consumption of this operation, Prt_e, is $Prt_e = 7.4$ mA.
4. Receiving (Rx). The device listens for incoming packets from surrounding devices. This stage is fundamental to answer petitions and provide response. The energetic cost associated to receiving, Rx_e, is $Rx_e = 17.5$ mA.
5. Sending (Tx). This stage involves the transmission of data to another device. The cost of sending information, Tx_e, is $Tx_e = 17.5$ mA.

After the operations of sending or receiving, the device performs an intermediate task before sleeping in which a pre-processing is done. Considering the main objective of the study is assessing the viability of the proposed architecture, these stages are assumed as not critical and they are not considered in the analysis. This way, the average cost for each task is provided on Table 1, which also provides the average time of the actions: average time to sleep, Av_s; average time to wake-up, Av_w; average time to scanning, Av_{prt}; average time to receive, Av_{rx}; and average time to send, Av_{tx}. Considering the metrics associated to each task of the BLE operative, the estimation of energetic requirements of the devices in the architecture can be calculated. For this, the power consumption varies between a set of potential variables. These conditions involve the operations that the device performs and the defined connection interval, I. Also, the battery capacity is a significant factor, B.

Table 1. Operational cost with BLE

Operation	Cost (mA)	Average time (μs)
Sleeping	0.001	Connection interval (I)
Waking-up	6.00	400
Pre-Rx-Tx	7.4	160
Rx	17.5	190
Tx	17.5	115

The operations that devices performs are defined on Figs. 2a, 2b, 2c. Each of these tasks involve a concrete set of operations with BLE. For example, when a device does not recognise any surrounding element, Rx and Tx are not required, so consumption decrease. Considering this, the Eq. 1 defines the energy required for a single interval (E_i), i.e. an unique iteration with BLE,

$$E_i = \frac{(S_e \times Av_s) + (Wu_e \times Av_e) + (Prt_e \times Av_{\text{prt}}) + (r \times Rx_e \times Av_r) + (s \times Tx_e \times Av_e)}{Av_s + Av_e + Av_{\text{prt}} + Av_r + Av_e} \quad (1)$$

where r refers to the number of received messages and s refers to the number of sent messages. Considering the value in E_i, the absolute duration of a battery

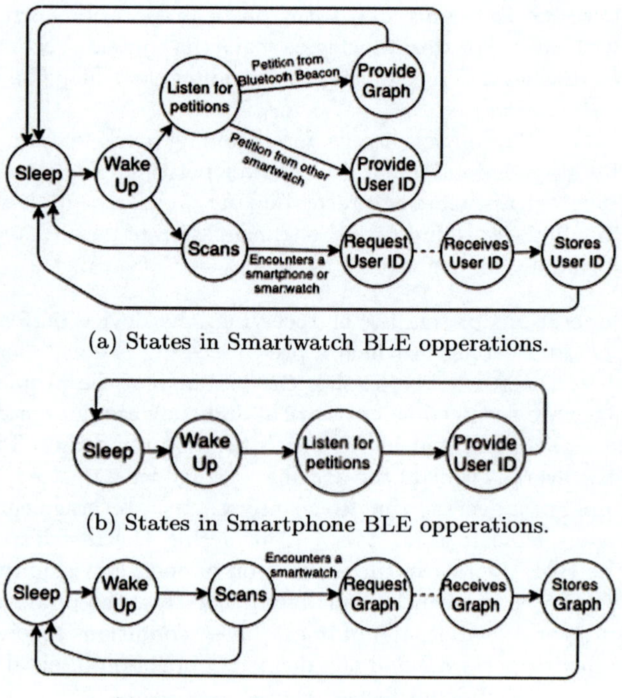

(a) States in Smartwatch BLE opperations.

(b) States in Smartphone BLE opperations.

(c) States in Beacon BLE opperations.

Fig. 2. BLE states of the different devices.

can be calculated. For this, the connection interval, I, has to be defined. This variable specifies the sleeping time of the device. This way, if $I = 1000$ ms, the device will wake-up, scan and communicate every 1000 ms. Hence, this is a critical factor to calculate the average consumption in a device, E_g. Equation 2 shows how this average is calculated, dividing the cost of an interval E_i between the length of an interval T.

$$E_g = \frac{E_i}{I} \tag{2}$$

As a result, the average current consumption is obtained. Thus, the length of the battery of the device, B can be calculated. For this, Eq. 3 reflects the length in hours of the battery,

$$B = \frac{L}{E_g} \tag{3}$$

where L is the capacity of the battery in mAh and E_g is the average consumption of BLE. As a result, B reflects the duration in hours of the battery that runs the BLE communication continuously. However, these numbers may not be applied to all devices in the proposed architecture since they perform different tasks in the scenario.

The devices in the architecture share three main context: 1) the device scans but none contact is detected; 2) the device scans, finds a contact and receives data; and 3) the device scans, finds a contact and provides data. Additionally, in the case of the smartwatch, scenario 3) and 4) may happen simultaneously. Considering this, the power requirements are not the same for every device. Then, it is necessary to detail the consumption for each one, so next subsections provide this summary about the corresponding estimation (Fig. 2).

Smartwatch. These devices follow the states defined in Fig. 2a. Then, the three explained contexts may occur. However, in the case of the smartwatches, contexts 2) and 3) can happen at the same time. Thus, the required energy is potentially the highest in the scenario. As a result, the current requirement becomes a relevant issue for these devices because of the battery limitations. Currently, the average battery capacity for smartwatches, B_{sw}, is about $B_{\mathrm{sw}} = 400$ mAh [14]. **Smartphone.** The smartphones follows the states defined in Fig. 2b in the architecture. This way, the communication operations it performs are mainly scanning and transmitting the stored User ID. This way, the energy required is limited. Also, the average battery capacity for a smartphone, B_{sp}, is $B_{\mathrm{sp}} = 5000$ mAh [14]. **Bluetooth Beacon.** This element performs the reception of information from smartwatches (Fig. 2c). Bluetooth Beacons are fed with energy by a solar panel. Thus, a battery of $B_b = 2300$ mAh is considered to provide power to the device [17].

Considering this, it is possible to perform estimations about the energy requirements and the power consumption, following an equation which relates the varibles. As a result, the equations provides potential calculation of the energy model. In the next subsection, an energetic cost estimation is done, comparing the potential outcomes under three different scenarios.

4.2 Energy Consumption Estimation

The architecture proposed in this work draws on the collaboration of a set of heterogeneous devices. However, this distributed approach requires the autonomous operation of the elements. Therefore, the battery and energy consumed for the different tasks become critical to the working of the solution. Thus, based on the energy consumption model detailed in the previous subsection, a set of potential scenarios are applied to the formulated equations.

The consumption model provides a relation between the tasks, the energy required and the communications that the devices perform. This way, the consumed power varies, depending on the interactions. Therefore, the number of considered devices are defined following a realistic proportion of inhabitants in a rural village: the number of smartwatches is 50, the smartphones are 30 and only one Bluetooth Beacon is defined. Considering the potential interactions that the devices can perform, three main scenarios can be identified: 1) a context where a large number of interactions takes place, C_1; 2) a context where the number of

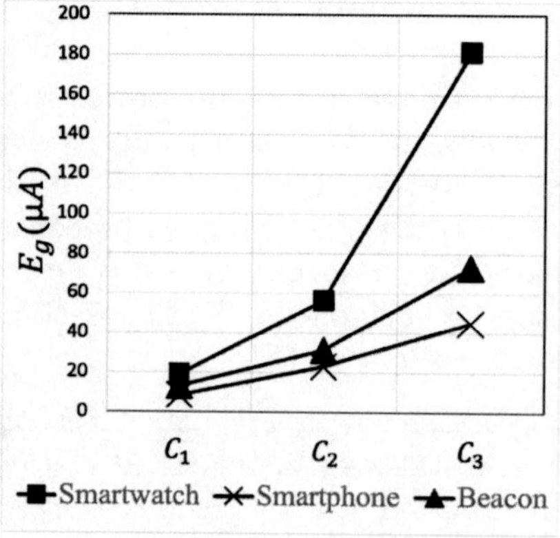

(a) Global energy consumption, E_g, as function of the three scenarios, C_1, C_2, C_3

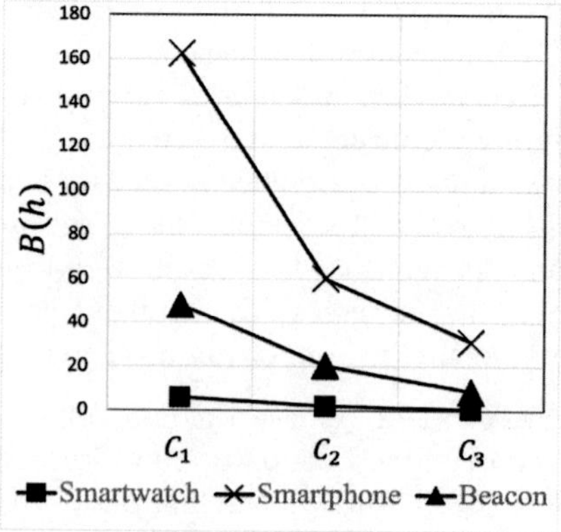

(b) Battery life in hours, B, as function of the three scenarios, C_1, C_2, C_3

Fig. 3. Estimated results for the energy consumption model

interactions is moderated, C_2; and 3) a context with few transmissions are performed, C_3. These distributions allows the identification of the impact between the battery consumption requirements and the estimated interactions. Therefore, it is possible to identify the viability of the proposed architecture. Also, the numbers for each scenario are estimated considering the potential encounters in the given population during an ordinary day.

The first scenario, C_1, defines a context where the interactions in a day are low. For this, the considered number of scanning, transmitting and receiving operations for each device are minimum. Therefore, the smartwatches receive an average of 13 encounters while transmit an average of 3 messages. This setup supposes that every smartwatch performs at least three data transfers and experiences 13 information receptions from other smartwatches or smartphones. In the case of the smartphones, only 10 messages are sent as average whereas the Bluetooth beacon receives an average of 25 messages. This reflects that at least the 20% of the smartwatches communicate with destination. In the second scenario, C_2, the average of encounters for the smartwatches is 30, defining a delivery rate of messages of 10. For the smartphones, the average number of transfers is 30 and, in the case of the beacon, it receives an average of 25 messages. Thus, this scenario reflects a context where a half of smartwatches have been able to communicate with destination. Finally, in the third scenario, C_3, the consumption values are the highest. For the smartwatches, an average of 120 encounters are defined, with 50 data transfers. In smartphones, a total of 60 data sends are set and, for the beacon, 60 messages received.

These explained estimations allow the assessment of the potential energy requirements associated to each device. In order to resume the variables, Table 2 includes the details of these scenarios, whereas Fig. 3 provide the obtained results.

Table 2. Variables considered for estimations

Variable	Value
Length of estimations (h)	24
# Smartwatches	50
# Smartphones	30
# Bluetooth Beacon	1
B_{sw} (mAh)	415
B_{sp} (mAh)	5000
B_b (mAh)	2500
I (ms)	1000

Figure 3a shows the energy requirements of the devices as function of the three considered scenarios. As can be seen, the intensification of the interactions in the third scenario reflects how the consumption increases. The smartwatches experiences the highest impact in the requirements, since they perform sending and receiving operations while the other entities do not implement both. Thus, it is important to consider this consumption in smartwatches as a key factor in the potential viability of the architecture. Besides, these results can be crossed with the life estimation of the batteries for each device given in Fig. 3b.

Figure 3b reflects the average battery life in hours as function of the three considered scenarios. As can be seen, the expected length for the battery in the smartwatches is very low respecting the smartphones and the beacon. This is mainly due to the high requirements in energy and the limited battery capacity. Thus, the average duration finds special limitations to provide services during a complete day. In the case of smartphones and the beacon, the technical viability is solid since the estimated length for the batteries is reasonable for the considered scenarios. Nevertheless, the Bluetooth beacon faces limitations to satisfy the energy requirements of scenario three. However, considering the device is fed by a solar panel, it may provide energy to the battery during continuous periods.

Considering the estimations calculated from the proposed energy consumption model, the architecture finds relevant limitations at the power consumption, concretely in the smartwatches. The average consumption for these devices in an intense scenario disgorges into a very limited battery life which may endanger the architecture performance and operability. This event is mainly caused by the short capacity of the current batteries for the smartwatches. However, considering a future potential improvement in the life for these devices will enhance the duration and will enable the deployment of the proposed architecture. As a response for this, we have estimated the consumption in a smartwatch if the battery capacity would increase up to $B_{sw} = 1500$ mAh. Thus, Fig. 4 shows this hypothetical calculus for the previous described scenarios.

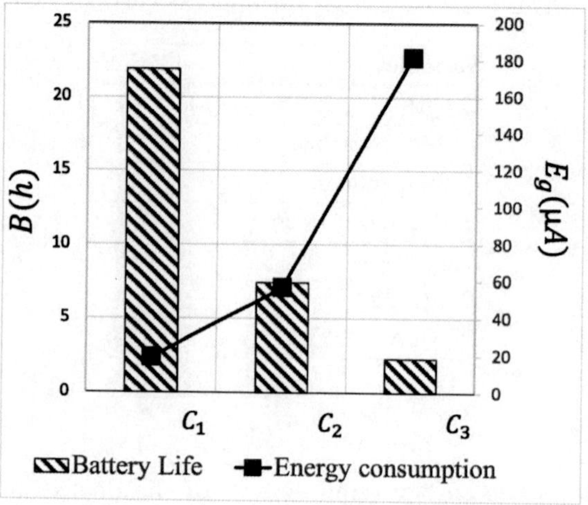

Fig. 4. Battery life for a smartwatch with the battery capacity increased

As Fig. 4 describes, smartwatches would provide a sustainable operability if they are equipped with a larger battery length. Thus, contexts as C_1 and C_2, where the number of interactions are limited, the devices would perform succesfully. In conclusion, the architecture achieves a technical viability which allows the distributed interaction of the different IoT devices involved in the solution. Then, the proposal satisfies the raised requirements and provides a potential tool to detect loneliness among ageing people in a rural area. For this, Internet is not required, finding on BLE an useful resource to perform data transmissions while detecting encounters. In the next section, these conclusions are extended with the future works opened in the research line.

5 Conclusions and Future Works

Loneliness among ageing people has become a significant issue for society, specially on isolated rural areas that lack of Internet connection. In this work, we propose a distributed sustainable IoT architecture to detect potential candidates of suffering loneliness among elderly population of a rural area. The proposal is based on the identification and registration of encounters of elderly people, tracing a graph of the contacts they have. For this, ageing people are equipped with a smartwatch which is able to recognise devices such as other smartwatches and smartphones. Thus, it is possible to store in the individual smartwatches the historical encounters that the elderly has experienced. Finally, a Bluetooth beacon is in charge of receiving the contacts to build a social graph of encounters.

As the collaboration between autonomous devices become essential, it is important to study the technical viability of the proposal. For this, a section with an estimated energy consumption model is provided, analysing the impact of the architecture operation in the battery of the involved devices. As a result, the study manifests how, under certain conditions, the solution is currently viable and deployable in a real context. Then, the work achieves successful results at power sustainability but finding some limitations at the battery life of smartwatches. Then, considering a future increase in these parameters, the architecture may find plenary operability. The presented paper opens an interesting research line which enables a significant enhance in the study of loneliness. For this, next works will be focused on developing a realistic implementation of the architecture, aiming to analyse the real requirements of the solution before a real-life deployment.

Acknowledgment. This work was supported by the 4IE+ Project (0499-4IE-PLUS-4-E) funded by the Interreg V-A España-Portugal (POCTEP) 2014–2020 program, the project RTI2018-094591-B-I00 (MCI/AEI/FEDER, UE), by the Department of Economy, Science and Digital Agenda of the Government of Extremadura (GR18112, IB18030), and by the European Regional Development Fund.

References

1. Steptoe, A., Owen, N., Kunz-Ebrecht, S.R., Brydon, L.: Loneliness and neuroendocrine, cardiovascular, and inflammatory stress responses in middle-aged men and women. Psychoneuroendocrinology **29**(5), 593–611 (2004)
2. Ventura-León, J., Sánchez-Villena, A.R., Caycho-Rodríguez, T., Barboza-Palomino, M., Rubio, A.: Fear of loneliness: development and validation of a brief scale. Front. Psychol. **11**, 2768 (2020)
3. Nzabona, A., Ntozi, J., Rutaremwa, G.: Loneliness among older persons in uganda: examining social, economic and demographic risk factors. Ageing Soc. **36**(4), 860 (2016)
4. Galán-Jiménez, J., Moguel, E., García-Alonso, J., Berrocal, J.: Energy-efficient and solar powered mission planning of UAV swarms to reduce the coverage gap in rural areas: the 3D case. Ad Hoc Netw. **118**, 102517 (2021)
5. Phillips, C., Gazo-Cervero, A., Galán-Jiménez, J., Chen, X.: Pro-active energy management for wide area networks. In: IET International Conference on Communication Technology and Application (ICCTA 2011), pp. 317–322 (2011)
6. Galán-Jiménez, J.: Minimization of energy consumption in IP/SDN hybrid networks using genetic algorithms. In: 2017 Sustainable Internet and ICT for Sustainability (SustainIT), pp. 1–5 (2017)
7. Domènech-Abella, J., et al.: Loneliness and depression in the elderly: the role of social network. Soc. Psychiatry Psychiatr. Epidemiol. **52**(4), 381–390 (2017). https://doi.org/10.1007/s00127-017-1339-3
8. Ige, J., Gibbons, L., Bray, I., Gray, S.: Methods of identifying and recruiting older people at risk of social isolation and loneliness: a mixed methods review. BMC Med. Res. Methodol. **19**(1), 1–11 (2019)
9. Hagan, R., Manktelow, R., Taylor, B.J., Mallett, J.: Reducing loneliness amongst older people: a systematic search and narrative review. Aging Ment. Health **18**(6), 683–693 (2014)
10. Chen, Y.-R.R., Schulz, P.J.: The effect of information communication technology interventions on reducing social isolation in the elderly: a systematic review. J. Med. Internet Res. **18**(1), e18 (2016)

11. Wilson, C.: Is it love or loneliness? Exploring the impact of everyday digital technology use on the wellbeing of older adults. Ageing Soc. **38**(7), 1307–1331 (2018)
12. Rivero Jiménez, B., Conde-Caballero, D., Juárez, L.M.: Loneliness among the elderly in rural contexts: a mixed-method study protocol. Int. J. Qual. Methods **20**, 1609406921996861 (2021)
13. Galán-Jiménez, J., Berrocal, J., Garcia-Alonso, J., Azabal, M.J.: A novel routing scheme for creating opportunistic context-virtual networks in IoT scenarios. Sensors **19**(8), 1875 (2019)
14. Min, C., et al.: Exploring current practices for battery use and management of smartwatches. In: Proceedings of the 2015 ACM International Symposium on Wearable Computers, pp. 11–18 (2015)
15. Punjabi, G., Shrivastava, V., Govindarajan, M.J.: Best practices for developing rest API (2020)
16. Kamath, S., Lindh, J.: Measuring bluetooth low energy power consumption. Texas instruments application note AN092, Dallas (2010)
17. AGM battery 2.3ah 12v table comparison. https://merkasol.com/epages/62387086.sf/es_ES/?ObjectID=164402087. Accessed 14 Dec 2021

Software Product Lines for Industrial Robots: A Pilot Case with Arduino

Andrés Felipe Solis Pino[1,3(✉)], Jose García Alonso[2], Enrique Moguel[2], Cristina Vicente-Chicote[2], Julio Ariel Hurtado Alegria[3], and Pablo H. Ruiz[1]

[1] Corporación Universitaria Comfacauca, Cl 4 N 8-30, Popayán, Colombia
{asolis,pruiz}@unicomfacauca.edu.co

[2] Universidad de Extremadura, Av. de Elvas, s/n, 06006 Badajoz, Spain
{jgaralo,enrique,cristinav}@unex.es

[3] Universidad del Cauca, Cl 5 #4-70, Popayán, Colombia
ahurtado@unicauca.edu.co

Abstract. Software reuse approaches in industrial robots are little exploited by industry, which often leads programmers to continue coding the same solutions, wasting time, effort, and cost. This paper describes the construction of a Software Product Line (SPL) to determine the feasibility of this approach as a reuse strategy for industrial robots. For the definition of the SPL, we followed the fundamental activities of domain engineering and application engineering. In addition, we identified its limitations and possible future work. As a result, it was got that the SPL approach is viable because a derivation of a product was made from the SPL applying some software reuse metrics, where it was found that 33% of the code needed for the operation of the robot was generated by the proposal, which represents a potential improvement in the time that developers take to program industrial robotics solutions with Arduino. In addition, it identified the potential of this approach in solutions to support the elderly in their homes and care centers, as well as some limitations related to the SPL and the domains involved.

Keywords: Software product lines · Arduino · Gerontechnology

1 Introduction

Aging is a natural and irreversible process in human beings. In recent years, the population aging figures have increased in most regions of the world. It is expected that one in five inhabitants of the planet in 2050 will be over 65 years old [1]. In this context, ensuring that older adults enjoy the best possible living conditions becomes a challenge for society [2]. Technologies are expected to play a fundamental role in the efforts to ensure a better quality of life for older adults [3]. Industrial Robotic Systems (IRS) in the domain of gerontechnology have been employed as service robots that support basic tasks such as manipulation and transportation of objects at the request of older adults [4]. These types of

J. García-Alonso and C. Fonseca (Eds.): IWoG 2021, LNBE, pp. 55–66, 2022.
https://doi.org/10.1007/978-3-030-97524-1_6

electromechanical devices are multipurpose, automatically controlled, and reprogrammable devices that can perform various tasks in different domains [5]. For this reason, these types of robots are becoming more and more complex as they play an increasingly important role in society [6].

It is now widely accepted that traditional methodologies for building software in industrial robots are reaching their limits [7] and have not been adopted as expected in the industry [8]; therefore, neither hardware nor software needs are being met, recognizing that novel approaches and strategies must ensure that these types of robots meet current and future societal expectations [9]. Software Engineering (SE) and specifically software reuse approaches have emerged as tactics to improve the development of this type of system at the application level, having punctual approaches but without extending the use of these techniques [10]. Therefore, specific proposals that try to solve specific problems of a punctual domain could generalize the use of reuse in IRS [11,12]. One of the reuse alternatives that could help to remedy the above is the SPL's because this strategy systematically defines a set of software products that share common and variable assets, which are configured and reused in a planned way to meet the needs of a specific domain [13]. Finally, the correct implementation of these methodologies would allow building better software applications for different domains, as is the case of gerontechnology, allowing developers to address other problems specific to these devices, and facilitating the fulfillment of the expectations that are held about this type of robot.

To the best of the authors' knowledge, SE has not been widely adopted to improve the construction of gerontechnology applications, so specific proposals to support or optimize software development in industrial robots would affect the domain and thus robotic assisting technologies to improve the quality of life of older adults. Considering the above, it becomes clear the need to reward and apply reuse approaches that allow improving the software development process for industrial robots, so that developers can benefit from its advantages. Therefore, this paper aims to expose, through a proof of concept, the feasibility of a software reuse proposal based on software product line engineering on IRS with Arduino, called IRArduino-SPL.

2 Related Work

To the authors' knowledge, there have been limited approaches between IRS and gerontechnology using SE as a means of improvement in the construction of applications or technologies for this type of device. A work that relates these fields is that of Alves-Oliveira *et al.* [14], in which they propose an activity management framework that specifies when older adults require a robot to achieve independent living, allowing setting goals and challenges for future research. It shows that one-off situations such as medication management and nutritionally adequate may be scenarios where industrial robots can play a key role.

Another relevant research is by Takeda *et al.* [15], where they show that most robots proposed to assist elderly people are unreliable and programmed for very specific situations, so they propose a design architecture for learning-based robotic support systems. They implement the proposal using an autonomous robot, getting positive results and exposing that the architecture is functional.

Chen *et al.* [16] focus on Alzheimer's disease, showing that Chinese chess is a good measure to strengthen neural links and preserve cognitive functions in the elderly. Therefore, they propose a robotic chess system that uses elements of computer vision and neural networks to work collaboratively with this population group. This system helps people to train their thinking and to have a distraction, elements accepted as conducive to prevent the onset of this disease.

In [17] they report a framework for the evaluation and design of assistive robots to improve the quality of life of people in disadvantaged situations. For this, they implement the framework in industrial robots that work as assistants to reach objects.

A wider range of results is found, as with Anzari *et al.* in [18] where a help manipulator robot is proposed to automate the personal bathing tasks of senior citizens. Another important research is that of Jardon *et al.* in [19], where they propose an autonomous robot with an arm, which allows performing the main tasks of daily life in patients admitted to hospitals.

Finally, previous works show different perspectives and implementations of software reuse to improve the development of gerontechnology applications in IRS, but none of them report SPLs to materialize reuse, so there is a knowledge gap that this article aims to fill.

3 Materials and Methods

To determine the potential of the proposed SPL approach, it applies to a proof of concept in the context of IRS construction with Arduino. We follow the activities proposed in the process Small-SPL [20] and we use some guidelines suggested by the SPL framework of the Software Engineering Institute to perform domain engineering and application engineering [21]. The percentage of reuse was used as a metric for measuring the reuse level achieved (Eq. 1) as is proposed by Frakes and Terry [22], was used; where *LR* is the number of reused Source Lines of Code (SLOC), *TL* is the total lines of code in the system, and *R* is the software reusability of the proposal in terms of a percentage of the total lines of code.

$$R = (LR/TL) * 100 \quad (1)$$

The main materials used in the strategy's construction were IRS source codes with Arduino, software similarity analysis tools such as Code Compare, SemanticMerge, and a Python script. We used the S.P.L.O.T tool [23] for variability modeling and analysis, and Arduino as the underlying technology.

3.1 Domain Engineering

Domain Modeling. For SPL building, it is essential to analyze its application domain to determine the scoping, the relevant abstractions, and variability. From the programming viewpoint of IRS with Arduino, we determine the main programming idioms. We used Code Compare, SemanticMerge, and a customized Python script configured with reserved words of the Arduino environment proposed by the Arduino language [24]. With these tools, a lexicographic analysis of 10 IRS source codes was carried out. We identified that the syntax for Arduino is organized in structures, values (variables and constants), and functions. Moreover, we found the most used statements, allowing us to establish which are the recurring programming idioms in Arduino for IRS.

The analysis performed allowed us to verify that a template-based software reuse strategy in Arduino is called *BareMinimum*, which is the minimum Source Code (SC) to compile a program on the platform. This template uses abstractions, function calls, and a hardware abstraction layer that provides a foundation for developers to work with. This template is insufficient, as it omits important elements that structure programming for IRS and is not adaptable to the domain. Templates focused on these devices could facilitate reuse in the domain.

In the semantic analysis carried out with Code Compare and SemanticMerge, we found that there are three blocks of frequent statements in the analyzed codes. The first block contains the variable declarations, libraries, and headers; these statements are found before *void setup()*. In the second block, we found all those related to the initialization of variables and ports, the declaration of library objects. This block of code is usually inside *void setup()*. The third block is related to the logic adjacent to the operation of the IRS in Arduino; the code in this section determines the trajectories, motion planning, and operation of the sensors and actuators; its position in the SC is inside *void loop()*. We also determined that the codes of the IRS refer to two important blocks of programming statements, the first related to the algorithms that govern the robot (called, algorithm block), and the other referring to the control hardware devices (called, hardware block).

The algorithm block contains statements related to the logic adjacent to the operation of the device, expressed through an action and reaction pattern. For each stimulus perceived by the sensors, there is an action by the actuators. This block of statements lacks important software elements as kinematics or user interface. The second block of statements belongs to the hardware drivers, which is the code implemented for the correct functioning of the physical devices; Here, the developers strive to make the sensors and actuators work in accordance and sync with the algorithm block. In the semantic analysis, it was found that the most used electronic elements in IRS with Arduino are sensors and actuators. These allow the robot to perceive the environment (sensors) and acting (actuators). They dictate its operation based on software premises. Therefore, a specific abstraction process was carried out on these devices to limit the variability in the programming of these elements. For this, we carried a lexicographic analysis of the SC of 10 types of sensors and 5 types of actuators, constituting the study of almost 40 codes to determine which common software elements can be modeled on these elements. According to the analysis, it was established that most sensors have four main and common code blocks in their programming. The first block of statements (called *header*) is related to the declaration of variables, constants, and libraries. The second block (named *body*) contains all the actions related to the initialization of the internal and external Arduino modules, the initialization of variables, the determination of the input pins, and exit. The third block (called *footer*) identified, has the statements that send the sensing signals to determine the current state of the robot functions. Finally, the fourth block (named *logic*) contains all those decisions and actions that the sensor performs after receiving information from the environment. The robot developer will implement these logics, such as actuator operations or orders to internal modules to continue the normal operation of the system.

As for the actuators, they use different statements but the same methods as the sensors in *header*, *body*, and *logic* since they base their operating instructions on the same programming structures. The main difference lies in *footer* because the sensors in this abstraction have the logic related to signaling the environment, while the actuators do not perform this function, but execute actions that are usually preceded by a change in the environment. For sensors and actuators, we based the determination of the attributes in the class diagram on what was proposed by Adafruit Industries, which structures the software development in its sensors in Vaut *et al.* [25]. Finally, Fig. 1 shows a class diagram in the Unified Modeling Language, as a result of the domain model abstracted.

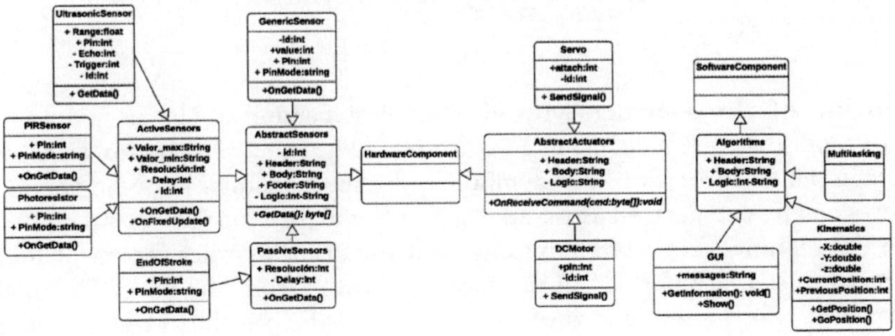

Fig. 1. A conceptual model of IRS with Arduino through a class diagram.

Identification of the Common and Variable Characteristics. The characterization of the SPL was carried out by identifying the variability, where the variable elements and the common characteristics. A common characteristic is an element that all SPL-derived products must consider. In this case, the operating platform of all the derivatives of the SPL is Arduino, so the elements that compose the proposal have a similar operating logic. All industrial robots have in common that they use sensors, actuators, and end effectors. The programming idioms collected in the IRS with Arduino have in common that they are structured under three main blocks of SC. Now, the products that will be generated from the SPL have different characteristics and configurable elements (sensors, actuators, or functionalities), but within these several common characteristics were found in the software that can be abstracted and facilitate code creation. In the sensors, there are four sections of code, while in the actuators, three code blocks were determined. The establishment of abstractions for sensors and actuators facilitates the construction of the software in the SPL because it structures and simplifies the transformation from abstraction to text.

The elements that can vary in the domain are numerous because IRS are complex and comprise multiple components and configurations. These comprise different types of actuators, sensors, and end effectors, so it is necessary to limit the variability. Another variant element in the domain is the algorithms that govern the robot because the use or not of direct and inverse kinematics are decisions that affect the development and operation of these systems. It was found that in the domain the developers of IRS with Arduino do not make use of this type of equations or algorithms, which controlling the motion planning of the robot. Finally, other elements that vary in the domain are the functions that these types of systems have, because the jobs to which they can be adapted are diverse, being difficult to abstract and cover the robot tasks for the proposed software reuse proposal. This is also reflected at the programming level of the electronic devices, by the case of, once they fulfill their function, it is complicated to determine what is the next step to follow with the information collected with sensors, or what is the subsequent action of an end effector once it's the task has been fulfilled.

Definition of the Feature Model. The first version of the IRArduino-SPL feature model was defined using FeatureIDE [26]. In Fig. 2, rectangular nodes represent the features and lines symbolize the relationships between them. The Features can be categorized as mandatory, optional, or alternative. An empty circle on the rectangle represents optional features. Black circles represent mandatory features and are part of all products generated from the SPL. The alternative features are the leaf nodes of the model that denote that at least one must be selected as part of a product.

The scoping of IRArduino-SPL was supported in S.P.L.O.T. [23]. For the feature model defined above, we found that there are 36 features in the diagram, of which 8 are mandatory, 3 are optional and 6 are alternatives, while 24 are grouped. S.P.L.O.T. validates that the proposed feature model is consistent. Furthermore, 9 core assets make up the most important reusable elements of the proposal. Also, the tool allowed us to determine 58,590 valid product configurations derivable from the feature model. Also, it was found that it must make a minimum of 36 decisions to have a functional product. Finally, 6 constraints were defined for the proposed model.

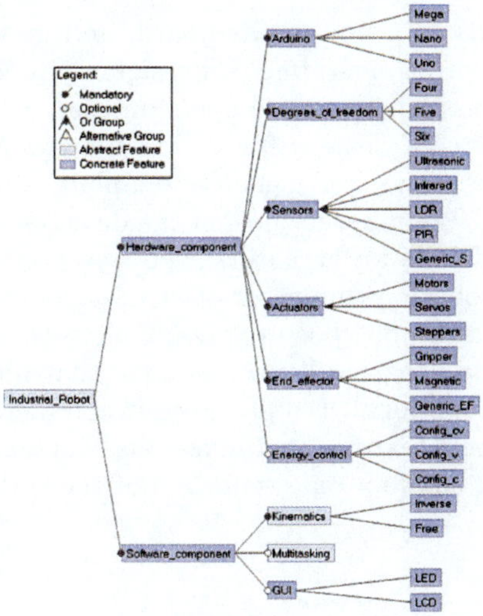

Fig. 2. The feature model proposed for the SPL developed for IRS with Arduino.

3.2 Application Engineering

Code Generation in IRArduino-SPL. Once the domain model was materialized, we identified, built, cataloged, and applied the software components developed in the SPL domain. IRArduino-SPL is based on the abstractions and the domain model conceived, therefore, as a tool for creation and reuse a code generator was defined. The generator supports the core asset development and product development. This generator implements the class model in Fig. 1 using the programming language Python, because of its versatility and successful track record for the development of this type of tool.

The internal code generation process comprises two principal activities. In the first one, the user's needs are established according to a workflow, presenting some decisions for resolving the variability. The second activity is the transformation of user requirements into code for the Arduino platform, through the Object-Oriented Programming (OOP) paradigm. The classes are a description of the domain model, where the attributes that capture the behavior of its instances are implemented. There are also derived classes that allow for extending the possibilities of the objects instantiated with new attributes and methods, as well as inheriting other pre-existing ones. The objects created can manipulate the input data in the function of obtaining specific output data. This is important because once the objects are instantiated, it must transform them into a programming format that can be readable by Arduino. For this, we use templates based on the programming idioms found in the domain analysis process. Finally, it should be noted that the code generator can assign pins to avoid conflicts between sensors and actuators, for this a representation of the development boards (Arduino Uno, Nano, and Mega) was conceived as dictionaries in Python, where each dictionary key corresponds to a pin on the board, and its equivalent value is the state of this so that the tool each time you assign a pin changes the state of the value so that it is not assigned in more opportunities.

The code generator can create software for ultrasonic sensors, infrared sensors, and photoresistors, as well as a generic template or exoskeleton for generic sensors, regardless of the number of pins on the development board. It also supports the generation of code for actuators such as servos and motors, as well as end effectors such as robotic grippers or electromagnets. The attribute *logic* in both sensors and actuators has been expressed in such a way that, if the user chooses this option, the program generates code that allows checking whether the selected device is functional. Finally, once it completes the code generation process, the tool creates a text file containing the source code with all the user's specifications. Figure 3 shows a representation of the code generation process.

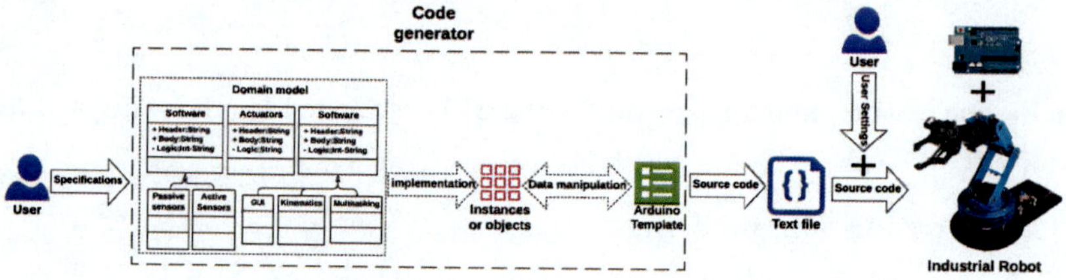

Fig. 3. Reference architecture for source code generation process in IRArduino-SPL.

For the user to generate the code, a command-line menu is used where you can choose the Arduino board to be used. For now, the tool supports the Arduino Uno, Nano, and Mega 2560. We made this choice because each of the boards has different PINs, so the tool needs to assign them correctly. Afterward, the user is asked if he/she wants the created elements to have code to determine if the operation of the element is correct, as part of the mentioned *logic* attribute. Then, choose among the supported actuators, sensors, and end effectors, remembering that there is no limit number for the creation of the software for these devices. Finally, the program will generate the SC in a text file. It then transferred this to the Arduino IDE to be compiled on the platform.

Proof of Concept. We develop a proof of concept for illustrating and evaluating the implementation of an IRS with Arduino with 5 degrees of freedom, 2 types of sensors, and 1 robotic gripper, derived as a product through the defined reuse strategy. We performed the test in an experimental environment to verify the feasibility of IRArduino-SPL. First, we built the robot (Fig. 4a) then we generated code by the SPL (composed of the determination of robot requirements, the transformation of abstractions to code through templates, adaptations to the code to adjust the operating *logic*, and compilation on the development board). To calculate the percentage of reusability, we use the metrics proposed in [22].

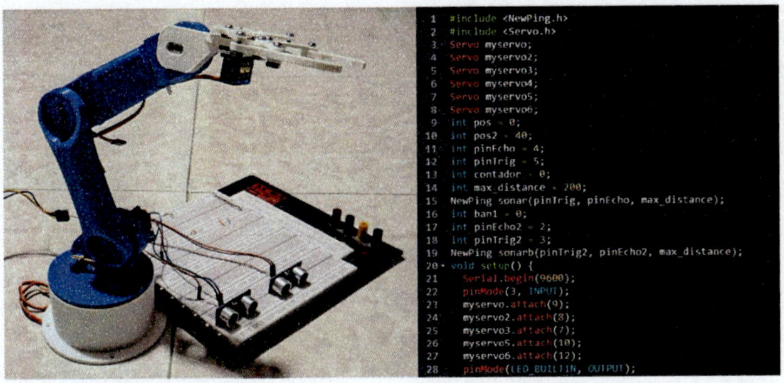

Fig. 4. (a) IRS with Arduino employed in the proof of concept. (b) A snippet of SC generated by IRArduino-SPL.

Based on Eq. 1, it was determined that IRArduino-SPL provides the developer with 33.3% reusable software code (in terms of SLOC) by using the domain model (Fig. 4b). The remaining 66.7% were developer construction concerning the robot operation, filling the code got for the IRS to perform a concrete action. Here, we programmed the transport of an object from one place to another, depending on an ultrasonic sensor and a limit switch. It can be highlighted that reused Source lines of code in *header*, *body*, and *footer* account for 86% of the total SLOC used in these attributes, the remaining 14% being programmed by the robot developer. Now, concerning the *logic* attribute, the reused SLOC accounts for 17% of the total lines in this section, while the programmer develops the remaining 83%. This is an obvious example that better abstractions should be made on this specific attribute, to increase the possibilities of reuse. It can access here a video of the proof of concept and the materials used in the research (https://cutt.ly/jlk8AmV).

4 Discussion

In the development of the proof of concept, we established that IRArduino-SPL assets are compatible and work coherently, generating a functional product by reusing them. Thus, we verified that conceptually the reuse proposal in the context of an IRS with Arduino has a lot of potentials and is viable. During the execution of the proof of concept, an IRS with Arduino was got, including the task programming for which it was built (transporting an object from one place to another). Furthermore, IRArduino-SPL achieved a correct synergy between hardware and software, facilitating to the developer implement specific activities such as robot task logic or kinematics. With the reuse materialized in the proof of concept, we found that the code provided by the tool allows the programmer to save development time.

As it is the first version of implementing a reuse proposal in a little-explored domain, some shortcomings can be corrected. There are limitations related to the generation of SC for programming robot functions, so the developer must take care of this task. In future versions, it can make abstractions in the behavior of IRS, so that it can integrate the main functionalities offered by these systems using some patterns such as template method, strategy, and method factory. For complex aspects such as the planning and control of the robot's movement, they require a detailed study to adapt them and incorporate them into the model, because each robot is different with different equations and algorithms.

IRArduino-SPL in the domain of gerontechnology is a contribution that facilitates the creation of software for different hardware elements (sensors and actuators) so that developers can focus on other topics related to industrial robots and elderly people. However, in future iterations of the proposal, proposing high-level abstractions that do not focus on hardware, but on the functionalities that industrial robots can perform would be an interesting contribution, as repositories of common functions (grasping items or bipedetation help) that occur when elderly people and industrial robots interact could be created, so that developers can save time in creating these functionalities and worry about other common issues in the domain of robots.

This proposal is in an initial state, there are some limitations. The first is the code generator and its scalability because the tool was developed with the OOP, which makes it difficult to create and develop software assets for specific elements (actuators or sensors), since this paradigm is not focused on this aim, unlike the Model-Driven Engineering which enabling automatic code generation, providing customization and interoperability capabilities using more reflexive models (metamodels). Finally, using tools such as Acceleo or Telosys in the proposal would facilitate the creation of software for specific elements, thus increasing the possibilities of the SPL.

5 Conclusions

This work presents IRArduino-SPL as a software reuse proposal based on the concept of software product lines. For the proposal definition, we followed domain and application engineering activities applied to the context of IRS. First, we defined fundamental assets, such as the domain model, the feature model, the scope, and a production strategy based on the generation of code. Furthermore, we developed an IRS with Arduino with 5 degrees of freedom, 2 types of sensors, and 1 robotic gripper for the Arduino platform. As a main result, IRArduino-SPL is a coherent, viable, and implementable and with great potential reuse strategy. The major contribution of this research is to generate empirical evidence of a specific reuse proposal, such as SPLs, in a domain little explored from the point of view of software reuse. IRArduino-SPL implementation contributes to the Arduino domain, bringing knowledge and experience where evidence is limited and unclear. Allowing the researcher to establish the foundations for future and more complete reuse strategies in the context of IRS with Arduino. Also, this work shows the software reuse for IRS in a field in which there are no solid foundations, so the first version of IRArduino-SPL must be refined to help the maturation of the area in this specific context.

IRArduino-SPL faces challenges in how to achieve the abstraction of common robot functions or includes new software elements, such as motion control or user interfaces. These challenges may have arisen from the abstraction done in the domain, which perhaps focused more on hardware and did not consider core software elements such as trajectories, cinematics, conceptual and particular elements own of its domain. The first domain abstraction helps to materialize reuse but does not incorporate important elements (functions, robot control, and variability limitation) that should be considered for future versions of IRArduino-SPL. Also, better management of variability over SPL needs to be done, as there are too many configurations, which could make it difficult to develop and support core assets in the future.

References

1. He, W., Goodkind, D., Kowal, P.R., et al: An aging world: 2015 (2016)
2. van Hoof, J., Kazak, J., Perek-Białas, J., Peek, S.: The challenges of urban ageing: making cities age-friendly in Europe. IJERPH **15**(11), 2473 (2018)
3. Li, J., Ma, Q., Chan, A.H., Man, S.: Health monitoring through wearable technologies for older adults: smart wearables acceptance model. Appl. Ergon. **75**, 162–169 (2019). https://doi.org/10.1016/j.apergo.2018.10.006
4. Thach, K.S., Lederman, R., Waycott, J.: How older adults respond to the use of virtual reality for enrichment: a systematic review. In: 32nd Australian Conference on Human-Computer Interaction, pp. 303–313. ACM, Sydney (2020)
5. Pagani, R., Nuzzi, C., Ghidelli, M., Borboni, A., Lancini, M., Legnani, G.: Cobot user frame calibration: evaluation and comparison between positioning repeatability performances achieved by traditional and vision-based methods. Robotics **10**(1), 45 (2021)
6. Moniz, A., Krings, B.J.: Robots working with humans or humans working with robots? searching for social dimensions in new human-robot interaction in industry. Societies **6**(3), 23 (2016). https://doi.org/10.3390/soc6030023
7. Heineck, T., Goncalves, E., Sousa, A., Oliveira, M., Castro, J.: Model-driven development in robotics domain: a systematic literature review. In: 2016 X Brazilian Symposium on Software Components. Architectures and Reuse (SBCARS), pp. 151–160. IEEE, Maringá, September 2016
8. Heikkila, T., Dobrowiecki, T., Dalgaard, L.: Dealing with configurability in robot systems. In: 2016 12th IEEE/ASME International Conference on Mechatronic and Embedded Systems and Applications (MESA), pp. 1–7. IEEE, Auckland, August 2016
9. Siepmann, F., Ziegler, L., Kortkamp, M., Wachsmuth, S.: Deploying a modeling framework for reusable robot behavior to enable informed strategies for domestic service robots. Robot. Auton. Syst. **62**(5), 619–631 (2014)
10. Brugali, D., Siciliano, B., Khatib, O., Groen, F. (eds.): Software Engineering for Experimental Robotics. Springer Tracts in Advanced Robotics, vol. 30. Springer, Heidelberg (2007). https://doi.org/10.1007/978-3-540-68951-5
11. Gherardi, L., Brugali, D.: Modeling and reusing robotic software architectures: the HyperFlex toolchain. In: 2014 IEEE International Conference on Robotics and Automation (ICRA), pp. 6414–6420. IEEE, Hong Kong, May 2014
12. Solis, A., Hurtado, J.: Reutilización de software en la robótica industrial: un mapeo sistemático. Rev. Iberoamericana Autom. Inform. Ind. **17**(4), 354–367 (2020)

13. Rodas-Silva, J., Galindo, J.A., Garcia-Gutierrez, J., Benavides, D.: Selection of software product line implementation components using recommender systems: an application to wordpress. IEEE Access **7**, 69226–69245 (2019)
14. Alves-Oliveira, P., Petisca, S., Correia, F., Maia, N., Paiva, A.: Social robots for older adults: framework of activities for aging in place with robots. In: ICSR 2015. LNCS (LNAI), vol. 9388, pp. 11–20. Springer, Cham (2015). https://doi.org/10.1007/978-3-319-25554-5_2
15. Takeda, M., Hirata, Y., Weng, Y.H., Katayama, T., Mizuta, Y., Koujina, A.: Accountable system design architecture for embodied AI: a focus on physical human support robots. Adv. Robot. **33**(23), 1248–1263 (2019)
16. Chen, P.J., Yang, S.Y., Wang, C.S., Muslikhin, M., Wang, M.S.: Development of a Chinese chess robotic system for the elderly using convolutional neural networks. Sustainability **12**(10), 3980 (2020)
17. Tanaka, H., Yoshikawa, M., Oyama, E., Wakita, Y., Matsumoto, Y.: Development of assistive robots using international classification of functioning, disability, and health: concept, applications, and issues. J. Robot. **2013**, 1–12 (2013)
18. Ansari, Y., Manti, M., Falotico, E., Cianchetti, M., Laschi, C.: Multiobjective optimization for stiffness and position control in a soft robot arm module. IEEE Robot. Autom. Lett. **3**(1), 108–115 (2018)
19. Jardón, A., Giménez, A., Correal, R., Martinez, S., Balaguers, C.: Asibot: robot portátil de asistencia a discapacitados. Concepto, arquitectura de control y evaluación clínica. Rev. Iberoamericana Autom. Inform. Ind. RIAI **5**(2), 48–59 (2008)
20. Camacho, M.C., Hurtado-Alegria, J.A., Ruiz-Melenje, P.H.: Un Método Incremental para el Análisis visual de modelos de Proceso software. Rev. Gerencia Tecnol. Inform. **15**(43), 79–91 (2016)
21. Northrop, L., Clements, P.: A framework for software product line practice, version 5.0. Technical report, Software Engineering Institute, Carnegie Mellon University, Pittsburgh, Pensilvania (2012)
22. El-Sharkawy, S., Yamagishi-Eichler, N., Schmid, K.: Metrics for analyzing variability and its implementation in software product lines: a systematic literature review. Inf. Softw. Technol. **106**, 1–30 (2019)
23. Bashroush, R., Garba, M., Rabiser, R., Groher, I., Botterweck, G.: CASE tool support for variability management in software product lines. ACM Comput. Surv. **50**(1), 1–45 (2017)
24. Dunbar, N.: Arduino Software Internals: A Complete Guide to How Your Arduino Language and Hardware Work Together. Arduino Software Internals (2020)
25. Vaut, L., Scarano, E., Tosello, G., Boisen, A.: Fully replicable and automated retention measurement setup for characterization of bio-adhesion. HardwareX **6**, e00071 (2019)
26. Berger, T., Steghöfer, J.-P., Ziadi, T., Robin, J., Martinez, J.: The state of adoption and the challenges of systematic variability management in industry. Empir. Softw. Eng. **25**(3), 1755–1797 (2020). https://doi.org/10.1007/s10664-019-09787-6

Technologies to Increase the Quality of Life of the Elderly Population

Accessible and Personalised Environments for the Care of Older People in the Home Environment

María Pilar Aguera-Boves[1], Estibaliz Jiménez-Arberas[2], and Carmen Cipriano-Crespo[3](✉)

[1] Accessibility Expert, Goberment of Principality from Asturias, Asturias, Spain
[2] Faculty Padre Osso (centre attached to the University of Oviedo), Oviedo, Spain
estibaliz@facultadpadreosso.es
[3] Faculty of Health Sciences, Universidad de Castilla-La Mancha, Talavera de la Reina, Toledo, Spain
Mariacarmen.cipriano@uclm.es

Abstract. The relationship between the characteristics of physical environments with the characteristics of older people facilitates or limits social participation and optimal occupational performance.

The ageing process produces a series of anatomical, physiological and functional modifications that lead to changes in the daily occupational performance of older people. This makes it more necessary to assess and adapt environments to support the adaptation process of older people and to facilitate their independence and safety in their usual environment.

Keywords: Adaptation of the environment · Accessibility · Ageing · Occupational performance · Older people

1 Introduction

Ageing is a universal biological process that accompanies us throughout life, resulting from the accumulation of a variety of molecular and cellular changes over time, leading to a gradual decline in physical and cognitive abilities, an increased risk of disease, and ultimately death [18, 19, 28]. Common conditions of old age include hearing loss, decreased visual acuity, back and neck pain and osteoarthritis, diabetes, depression and dementia [19]. As people age, the likelihood of experiencing several conditions at the same time increases.

Old age is also characterised by the emergence of several complex health conditions that usually occur only in the later stages of life and do not fall into specific morbidity categories. These health conditions are commonly referred to as geriatric syndromes [21]. They are usually the result of multiple underlying factors including, but not limited to: frailty, urinary incontinence, falls, delirium, and pressure ulcers [2].

But it should not be forgotten that this ageing process is also clearly influenced by how the person is; their physical condition, their psychological characteristics, the

J. García-Alonso and C. Fonseca (Eds.): IWoG 2021, LNBE, pp. 69–77, 2022.
https://doi.org/10.1007/978-3-030-97524-1_7

level of social participation, the support that the person has [15, 19]. Older people's occupational performance is affected as the person ages, occupations, roles and activities to be performed on a daily basis change [26, 27]. While some of the variations in older people's health are genetic, the physical, social and economic environments in which they live can also influence how they participate in society. These environments are of great importance, in particular housing, neighbourhoods and communities. Each person with his or her specific abilities and each dwelling, building or neighbourhood makes different occupational performance and functional demands according to its design and existing access barriers [17].

From the characteristics of the ageing process and from the point of view of the musculoskeletal system and specifically during walking, in which there is an increase in kyphosis, a decrease in the base of support and stride length, an increase in instability in balance and postural alignment, a decrease in braking, etc., there are alterations in walking that lead to instability and the possibility of producing falls and accidents [11, 12]. In addition to other characteristics that originate in the decline of the cardiovascular, respiratory, digestive, nervous and sensory systems, among others, which make it difficult for older people with greater fragility to adapt to the characteristics of the environment. Therefore, it is necessary that the environment facilitates their functionality, adjusted to these characteristics, and it is essential for the reduction of risks to achieve simplicity in the use and handling of the environment; simplifying the demand for tasks, favouring safety, thus promoting interaction and relationship with the environment and increasing their performance in daily activities [17]. The adaptation of the person to the environment and the use of the environment in a safe way is a fundamental feature that an accessible environment must offer to older people [9]. From the Occupational Therapy point of view, it is important to accompany the person in this process in order to detect the person's needs and how to find solutions to them [14, 19, 24].

2 Definition of Occupational Therapy

Occupational Therapy is defined by the European Committee of Occupational Therapists as follows [33] as the health profession that is based on knowledge and research into the relationship between health, occupation and environment in the well-being of the person in the presence of physical, cognitive, social, affective and/or environmental limitations that alter their development potential and their occupational performance; that uses meaningful activities for the person with the ultimate aim of restoring, maintaining and/or developing the skills necessary to integrate and participate in their biopsychosocial sphere".

Theoretical and practice models of Occupational Therapy, as a model of human occupation, [13] Biopsychosocial model. A. Mosey [23], Personal adaptation through occupation, [29] among others, include as a fundamental part of the Occupational Therapist's intervention the physical environment, which is an essential part of the person, and in accordance with the Framework for the Practice of Occupational Therapy: Domain and Process 4th edition of the American Occupational Therapy Association [5] assuming the context and environment aspects of the Occupational Therapy Domain interact with the; areas of occupation, person factors, skills and performance patterns, and activity demands that make up the person dimension for the Occupational Therapist.

3 Universal Accessibility

Universal accessibility is the condition that environments, processes, goods, products and services, as well as objects or instruments, tools and devices, must meet in order to be understandable, usable and practicable by all people in conditions of safety and comfort and in the most autonomous and natural way possible. It presupposes the "design for all" strategy and is without prejudice to reasonable accommodation" [22].

When an environment is accessible it provides a number of benefits to the people who use it, comfort and safety in use will help people by improving the conditions of use and habitability of buildings [17].

4 Environmental Assessment as a Tool for Performance Improvement

The Occupational Therapy discipline aims to understand the needs for adaptation of environments and simplification of tasks. It is essential to carry out an analysis of the activities, characteristics and functional needs of the person [31]. As well as assessing the different environments in which the elderly person develops in order to be able to conclude with both in a process of intervention that may be aimed at:

- Improving occupational performance: the way and manner in which older people carry out tasks that cause interaction with the environment [3].
- Adaptation of the environment: Physical, cognitive and sensory, as well as use of assistive technologies and products.
- Simplification and adaptation of activity requirements.

These actions will compensate for the small and/or large limitations that the elderly person may have when carrying out their daily activities. Increasing, therefore, the skills and abilities that the person retains, and carrying out an intervention in the environment that facilitates the execution of activities in an independent and safe manner [20].

The Occupational Therapist is the professional trained and qualified to carry out these functions, having extensive training in the physiology and biomechanics of the human being, and of the ageing process in particular. They also have knowledge of the aspects of occupational performance, in order to evaluate the interaction of the person with the environment [25, 30].

Through the knowledge and analysis of the activity, the Occupational Therapist carries out the occupational assessment by means of which he/she will determine the factors that influence the functioning of the person and sets intervention objectives to promote his/her independence in daily activities and occupations.

Focusing on the assessment aspect of the environment, it is necessary for the therapist to be able to analyse the different steps that are necessary in each of the activities of daily living, while analysing the influence of the environment: furniture and products, analysing the functionality and correspondence of these in the independence of the person [16]. Starting with the environment close to the home, analysing the layout of pavements, studying the possibilities of access to establishments, and reviewing the means of signposting and orientation in the area, auditory, visual, etc. Proposing actions that allow the independence of the person, with the aim of promoting their autonomy and independence in their community environment and facilitating participation with the people and activities that take place in their immediate environment [10].

The access portal to the building must be free of architectural barriers, allowing for easy access and movement, but it is also necessary to take into account the integral characteristics of the environment, bearing in mind universal accessibility. To this end, we can use the DALCO requirements to facilitate accessibility to the environment, these requirements are: Ambulation, Apprehension, Localisation, Communication, and they are included in the UNE standard 170001-1:2007 of Universal Accessibility [1]. Each of the requirements is made up of different elements which are briefly described below:

- Wandering: The action of moving from one place to another, including the analysis of: maneuvering spaces, pavements, circulation area, changes of plane.
- Grasping: The action of picking up or grasping an object. It includes the analysis of: reach, actuating elements, grasping and transport of the object.
- Localizations: The action of identifying a place to be reached. It includes signaling, lighting and location.
- Communication: The action of exchanging information, consisting of: verbal, written, audio, visual and other means of communication through graphics, symbols and signs.

By means of a descriptive study where the observation and analysis of each of these actions and the way in which they interact with the elderly stands out, it can be affirmed that the elderly usually present the following difficulties in the accessibility of the portal:

- Difficulties in manipulation with the door lock, in the action of inserting the key, due to limitations in fine coordination, in the execution of the gripper, in the precision of the action due to some symptomatology associated with tremor, vision difficulties, etc.
- Restrictions due to the provision of steps in the doorway, and/or stairs, which limit access to people with hip fractures, who are afraid of previous falls, people who lack sufficient strength to lift the lower limb, gait disorders, etc.
- Limited access to the letterbox area, as it is located in poorly lit and/or inaccessible spaces, or with designs that are difficult to handle.
- Difficulty in circulation, due to the arrangement of furniture in inadequate spaces, or mats that are not flush, which can cause falls, trips and blows in people with insecure walking, vision problems, etc.

Some of the possible solutions to these difficulties consist of adapting the environment to the performance characteristics of people, trying to implement universal accessibility measures that allow the greatest number of needs and characteristics to be considered. These include facilitating access to the doorway without unevenness; card-operated opening systems; automatic and/or easy-to-open doors; aligned placement of furniture to allow free movement; indicative signs and posters, with legible, contracted lettering and pictograms that allow location and orientation inside the doorway; access to a barrier-free lift. These actions cannot always be carried out, so in these cases the objective will be to provide the person with support products that allow them to be as independent as possible. An assistive product is any product (including devices, equipment, instruments, technologies and software) specially manufactured or available on the market to prevent, compensate for, control, mitigate or neutralize impairments, activity limitations and participation restrictions [8].

Since training in the use of these products is necessary in order to make the adaptation as functional as possible, some of the support products that can be of great use in accessing the doorway are: Key aid, a support product that facilitates gripping and clamping of the key; Stair climber; Platform lift; Portable ramp.

The person's home must be carefully analysed, as it is the space where they carry out their daily life activities and those that provide them with a greater sense of autonomy and value [7]. Therefore, it is essential to carry out a diagnosis of the different rooms and the activities that the person carries out in them, analysing occupational performance [4].

We will now define some of the main rooms: bathroom and kitchen, which are where the greatest number of accidents occur and where we must focus a large part of our intervention in order to prevent possible risks.

Bathroom: the space where the greatest number of accidents occur, which can sometimes be fatal, and in the smallest of cases disabling, so we must evaluate the room and especially:

- Flooring, avoiding slippery floors that can cause precipitation.
- Bathtub/shower, in many cases the elderly still has a bathtub, so in addition to trying to guide them towards changing to a flush shower, it will be necessary to place bars and handles at different points to facilitate support and safety. Shower seats are also a very stable alternative for anyone who may be unstable. In the event that this modification is not possible, there are different support products that facilitate safe access to the bathtub, such as: transfer benches, transfer chairs, swivel chairs. In addition to these adaptations, it is necessary to train with the person the different steps to be taken, in order to facilitate the basic techniques of safe transfers.
- Toilet, the height of the toilet must be appropriate to the person's abilities, so a toilet seat can be included to facilitate the act of sitting down and getting up. Likewise, and to ensure safety and facilitate incorporation, handholds and support bars can be installed at the appropriate height for the person's grip.
- Washbasin. Depending on the needs and characteristics of the elderly person, a space below the washbasin will be provided to enable them to access and position themselves appropriately to carry out the activities. On some occasions, a chair, handholds, a single-lever mixer tap, etc. will be provided.
- Arrangement of furniture and utensils. A space for passage and maneuverability of the person free of obstacles shall be provided, as well as the placement of utensils in spaces within reach, allowing access to them without the need to make unsafe gestures.
- Other issues to be analysed are the thermal capacity of the person and the possibility of installing automatic water temperature regulators, which prevent burns.

Depending on the specific needs of each person, which must be analysed, some of the existing products that facilitate the performance of the different activities can be proposed in order to achieve maximum independence for the person and prevent possible risks during the activity: soaping brushes, long reach brushes, suction brushes, soap dispensers, etc.

Kitchen: Like the bathroom, this is one of the spaces in the house where the greatest number of accidents and injuries occur, so it is important to evaluate this space and the activities that take place in it, making a diagnosis of the difficulties encountered and proposing improvements in functionality. Some of the issues to be analysed in the environment are as follows:

- Non-slip and even flooring.
- Arrangement of objects and design features to facilitate their reach, use and handling. Trying to place them in easily accessible spaces and prioritising the placement of the heaviest items in the closest spaces.
- Use of gas-induction cooker, among the many benefits provided by the induction cooker, is the advantage of not having carbon monoxide leakage in case of forgetting to turn off the tap, therefore, we will always try to modify it.
- Possibility of introducing contrast in handles and knobs, as it facilitates the location of the different mechanisms.
- During the different kitchen activities, there are a series of recommendations that we can use depending on the needs of each person, such as:
- In people with cognitive impairment, it may be advantageous to use reminder systems, alerts, lists, etc., with a description of the different steps for carrying out the activities. Likewise, the use of signs with the name and/or images, pictograms of the utensils found inside the cupboards.
- -For people with impaired vision, audio systems can be introduced, voice announcers, kitchen robots, which allow them to interact with the different utensils and electrical appliances. As well as the maintenance of the order and placement of the products that allows them to remember their location at all times.
- For people with motor and/or mobility limitations, the use of support products that make it easier for them to carry out the activities, such as automatic peelers, different plastozote grips, can openers, non-slip tablecloths, etc. As well as passageways and obstacle-free spaces that allow them the necessary mobility and manoeuvrability, such as: free space under the worktop to allow them to approach, etc.
- For people with hearing difficulties, the sound systems should be replaced by pilot lights and light indicators.

Once the areas of the environment and the person's performance have been analysed, an intervention will be carried out, comprising a series of proposals personalised to the abilities and needs assessed, on an individual basis, including some of those listed above and training them for safe, satisfactory and secure performance, always with the aim of maintaining the person's autonomy and independence and preventing accidents in the home.

5 Instruments

Occupational therapists use their theoretical/practical knowledge of their profession, scientific evidence, experience, as well as the tools inherent to their professional profile, which are the analysis and understanding of the activity, the evaluation of occupational performance and knowledge of the principles of the relationship between the person and the environment. The occupational therapist has extensive knowledge of the adaptation of tasks and environment, of universal accessibility, and has the necessary skills to prescribe and train in the use of assistive products and technologies that facilitate the execution of the activity.

In order to carry out the assessment of the home environment, different measuring instruments are necessary, as well as a photographic camera, which facilitates the collection of data for subsequent analysis. By means of observation, measurement and interview, data will be collected to enable the development of an intervention proposal, and the therapist can use different standardised assessment scales such as Romero's Occupational Therapy Home Assessment [32] or Safety Assessment of Function and the Environment for Rehabilitation [6] among others.

For the assessment of the person's capabilities, the occupational therapist relies on standardised scales to evaluate the person's dimensions in a holistic manner. To evaluate the performance of activities of daily living, he/she can use: Barthel Index, Katz, FIM, etc., as well as those evaluation scales necessary to evaluate other areas such as: cognitive, social and affective, such as Mini Mental, Pfeiffer SPMSQ, Goldberg Anxiety and Depression Scale, OARS, etc.

6 Conclusions

The accessibility of the elderly person's home environment allows and facilitates the continuity of the development of their life project in their usual environment, this being one of the main concerns of the elderly. Therefore, the evaluation of the spaces, activities and performance of the person in their environment is one of the main objectives of the Occupational Therapist, as the basis of the principles that underpin the principles of their profession; attending to the quality of life and promoting autonomy and personal independence.

References

1. Aenor (2021): Certificación Accesibilidad Universal UNE 170001–AENOR. https://www.aenor.com/certificacion/responsabilidad-social/gestion-accesibilidad-universal. Accessed 10 Oct 2021
2. Alarcón, T.A., Montalvo, J.I.G.: Grandes síndromes geriátricos Concepto y prevención de los más importantes. Medicine Programa de Formación Médica Continuada Acreditado **8**(108), 5778–5785 (2003)
3. Algado, S.S., Urbanowski, R.: El modelo canadiense del proceso del desempeño ocupacional. Revista electrónica de terapia ocupacional Galicia TOG **3**, 6 (2006)

4. Alonso, F., et al.: Adaptación de la vivienda en la población dependiente: necesidades, programas y casos. Equipo ACCEPLAN Institut Universitari d'Estudis Europeus, Barcelona (2007)
5. AOTA: Occupational therapy practice framework: domain and process–fourth edition. Am. J. Occup. Ther. **74**(Supplement_2), 7412410010p1–7412410010p87 (2020). https://doi.org/10.5014/ajot.2020.74S2001
6. Backman, C.: SAFER tool: safety assessment of function and the environment for rehabilitation. Can. J. Occup. Ther. **69**(5), 303 (2002). Page count = 1
7. Bocanegra, N.M., Pérez, M.G., Torres, M.P.D.H.: Atención en el hogar de personas mayores: manual de terapia ocupacional (2004). https://dialnet.unirioja.es/servlet/libro?codigo=249447. Accessed 15 Oct 2021
8. Castelao, G.S., Faes, R.F.: Productos de apoyo para personas con discapacidad.Clasificación y terminología. Revista asturiana de Terapia Ocupacional **6**, 11–13 (2008)
9. Cuenot, M.: Clasificación internacional del funcionamiento, de la discapacidad y de la Salud. EMC Kinesiterapia Medicina Física **39**(1), 1–6 (2018). https://doi.org/10.1016/S1293-2965(18)88602-9
10. De-Rosende, I., Santos-del-Riego, S.: Influencia de la terapia ocupacional en la realización de adaptaciones en el hogar de las personas en situación de dependencia. Revista Terapia Ocupacional Galicia **2013**(18) (2013). https://ruc.udc.es/dspace/handle/2183/16622. Accessed 12 Oct 2021
11. Fernández Pérez, T.P., Ruiz Sarmiento, J.E.: Efectos de la actividad física en la estabilidad del equilibrio de los adultos mayores del Centro Geriátrico Diurno (2017). http://dspace.ups.edu.ec/handle/123456789/14439. Accessed 6 Oct 2021
12. Herrero Larrea, A.: Estudio de los parámetros espaciales de la marcha en la población anciana española y su asociación con resultados adversos de salud., TDX (Tesis Doctorals en Xarxa). Ph.D. Thesis. Universitat Internacional de Catalunya (2017). http://www.tdx.cat/handle/10803/461171. Accessed 6 Oct 2021
13. Kielhofner, G.: Terapia ocupacional. Modelo de Ocupación Humana. Teoría y aplicación. Ed. Médica Panamericana (2004)
14. Krzemien, D., Miranda, C.M., Martin, N.G.: La ocupación en la Gerontología: una perspectiva crítica del Modelo de Ocupación Humana (2020). https://doi.org/10.25214/25907816.268
15. Leiton Espinoza, Z.E., Leiton Espinoza, Z.E.: El envejecimiento saludable y el bienestar: un desafío y una oportunidad para enfermería. Enfermería universitaria **13**(3), 139–141 (2016). https://doi.org/10.1016/j.reu.2016.06.002
16. López, B.P., Molina, P.D., Arnaiz, B.N.: Conceptos Fundamentales de Terapia Ocupacional. Ed. Médica Panamericana (2001)
17. López, F.A.: La accesibilidad en evolución: la adaptación persona-entorno y su aplicación al medio residencial en España y Europa (2016). http://purl.org/dc/dcmitype/Text. Universitat Autònoma de Barcelona. https://dialnet.unirioja.es/servlet/tesis?codigo=84882. Accessed 6 Oct 2021
18. Luna, M., et al.: Síndromes geriátricos, los grandes ausentes en los índices de comorbilidad usados para determinar el riesgo de desarrollar demencia. Acta Médica Peruana **35**(3), 189–190 (2018)
19. Martínez Pérez, T., et al.: El envejecimiento, la vejez y la calidad de vida: ¿éxito o dificultad? Revista Finlay **8**(1), 59–65 (2018)
20. Méndez, S.F., García, A.G.: Adaptaciones del entorno y de las actividades de la vida diaria en enfermos con Alzheimer desde terapia ocupacional. Revista Terapia Ocupacional Galicia **16**(30), 265–271 (2019)
21. Menéndez Colino, R., et al.: Aspectos terapéuticos de los grandes síndromes geriátricos. Tratamientos farmacológicos y no farmacológicos. Indicaciones. Medicine **12**(46), 2743–2754 (2017). https://doi.org/10.1016/j.med.2017.12.002

22. Ministerio de Presidencia (2013): BOE-A-2013–12632. https://www.boe.es/buscar/act.php?id=BOE-A-2013-12632&p=20171109&tn=3. Accessed 15 Oct 2021
23. Mosey, A.C.: An alternative: the biopsychosocial model. Am. J. Occup. Ther. **28**(3), 137–140 (1974)
24. Muñoz, C.G.M.: La terapia ocupacional y la promoción de la salud emancipadora para personas mayores. Revista Chilena de Terapia Ocupacional **17**(2), 111–117 (2017). https://doi.org/10.5354/0719-5346.2017.48091
25. De Terapia Ocupacional, C.C.: VI Congreso Latinomericano, XIV Congreso Colombiano: Terapia Ocupacional crea en torno al entorno. Revista Ocupación Humana **12**(1 y 2), 1–8 (2007). https://doi.org/10.25214/25907816.91
26. Paredes Maseda, U.: Perspectiva ocupacional de personas cuidadoras vinculadas a un centro de día de mayores: estudio mixto (2020). https://ruc.udc.es/dspace/handle/2183/26570. Accessed 6 Oct 2021
27. Ponte Loureiro, A.: Terapia ocupacional en personas mayores: cambio de roles (2018). https://ruc.udc.es/dspace/handle/2183/20271. Accessed 6 Oct 2021
28. Rebollido, J.M.R., del Rey, M.M.L.R., Viera, M.G.: La actividad física y envejecimiento exitoso: consideraciones de una relación necesaria. Revista Conrado **16**(74), 231–239 (2020)
29. Reed, K.L., Sanderson, S.N.: Concepts of Occupational Therapy. Lippincott Williams & Wilkins (1999)
30. Revuelta, F.F.: Vida asisitida por el entorno Terapia ocupacional. Revista informativa de la Asociación Profesional Española de Terapeutas Ocupacionales **47**, 12–17 (2008)
31. Rodríguez, R.G.: El análisis de la actividad en el proceso de valoración de la situación de dependencia. Revista Electrónica de Terapia Ocupacional Galicia TOG **2**(7 (Monográfico Octubre)), 5 (2015)
32. Romero, D., Moruno, P.: Terapia ocupacional: teoría y técnicas. Masson (2003). https://dialnet.unirioja.es/servlet/libro?codigo=79695. Accessed 15 Oct 2021
33. Toribio, C.L.: Comité Europeo de terapeutas ocupacionales: resumen de la reunión 32: 14–15 abril 2000. Terapia ocupacional: Revista informativa de la Asociación Profesional Española de Terapeutas Ocupacionales **23**, 36–38 (2000)

Acceptance of Digital Tools for Healthy Aging. New Challenges for Nursing

Jerónimo Luengo Polo, Adriana V. Muñoz Ortega, Borja Rivero Jiménez(✉), David Conde Caballero, and Lorenzo Mariano Juárez

University of Extremadura, Cáceres, Spain
brivero@unex.es

Abstract. The fast evolution in the implementation of new technologies in the healthcare environment has created a wide range of new tools for applying patient care and their pathologies' control. In the hospital background, this implementation has been continuous and adapted to each category, easing the learning and acceptance. It has not happened likewise in the Primary Care environment because the degree of acceptance of the new digital tools and their use being ignored. By this narrative review of the literature, the aim is to objectify the need to carry out research studies for assessing the attitudes and skills of Nursing professionals in the primary care setting in the acceptance of new technologies by means of validated tools, for, with their correct implantation, apply nursing care that facilitates healthy aging for patients through new digital tools. The limited literature on research previous to the implementation of new digital tools focused on health for professionals makes it necessary to evaluate the health population to identify facilitators and barriers in the implementation of new tools. This seems to be a previous step for a correct implementation in favor of quality nursing care for the population attended through the new information and communication technologies.

Keywords: Nurse acceptance · IT acceptance · UTAUT · Information technology

1 Introduction

The implementation of new digital technologies has been regular in the last 10 years, where they have come to be implemented in different areas such as work, communications, administration and management, and also health and care space [1]. The process is online with the recommendations of the United Nations through its agency for information and communication technologies [1, 2]. It is a transformation that is part of a global digitalization framework that has reached most professional sectors, including healthcare.

The WHO has shown that is necessary a health digital transformation to improve their outcomes [5]. Likewise, the European Commission has opted for training people, the transformation of companies and the digitization of public services, including health services [6]. Because of that, the health systems reality in general and care practices in

J. García-Alonso and C. Fonseca (Eds.): IWoG 2021, LNBE, pp. 78–83, 2022.
https://doi.org/10.1007/978-3-030-97524-1_8

particular are increasingly directed towards the use of technology. Medicine is closer and closer to diagnoses based on technological evidence. Nurses have at their disposal a wide and growing range of tools to provide care: applications to control therapeutic adherence [7], mental health applications [8], barcode medication administration [11], sensor-based medication systems [12], use of automated storage and distribution systems for medication by units [13]. Also the efforts that being made for professionals to acquire digital skills are remarkable [14], for example in the use of digital medical records, telehealth, videoconferences or the application of virtual assistants. The training plans for nurses also seem deficient in this regard, requiring an assessment and adaptation to the current situation [15–17]. The university degree programs in Spain hardly pay attention to digital care, which requires specialized training through courses or masters.

However, the way is not proving easy. A lot of barriers are making the process more difficult. There are, for example, educational barriers of the population as to acceptance of the need to use new technologies, despite the evidence that their incorporation would imply higher levels of efficiency and effectiveness [18–20]. In his model of technological acceptance, Davis carries out an exhaustive study of the causes that help or hinder the technological acceptance by society [21], concluding that the cultural variable also influences the greater or lesser implementation of certain tools [22]. Cultural resistance must be evaluated and diagnosed in order to apply policies and educational lines that help to implement it. Structural barriers must also be consider. It is well known that these new technologies appear mainly in hospital environments where training recycling is continuous. However, in primary care, where professionals have a high age average, with job characteristics that make them peculiar, the use of technological devices is lesser.

Traditionally, much of the research on acceptability has focused on the population that receives care and technology [23, 24], trying to join the technology's use and function to environment's culture that receives care through these new tools, but the barriers and difficulties of the professional population have rarely been addressed [25]. This research approaches this part of the population spectrum until now little studied, especially in the case of the situation of Nursing in primary care, through lines of research based on the technological acceptance model of Davis et al. which is based on the theory of reasoned action proposed by Azjen and Fishbein [26].

2 Objectives

By the aim of knowing the possible resistance of Nursing professionals to the incorporation of this type of new tools, we are wondering a series of questions: What are the nurses impressions about the use of technology or technological applications in their daily praxis? Are they open or do they lay to rejection? How does it vary depending on the type of technology, issues such as gender, age or education received?

3 Methodology

A review of the published literature is carried out. A bibliographic search is applied through databases Pubmed, Scopus, Web of Science, SciELO. Searches were carried out, according to each database, using keywords:

Boolean descriptors and operators for searching

(Nurse OR Nursing) AND (Technology) AND (IT Acceptance OR UTAUT)

TOTAL ITEMS SEARCH: 372 (12 + 133 + 235 + 2)

Based on a narrative review of the literature found, we evaluate the published studies on the acceptability by nursing of the new digital tools, excluding articles' repetitions and those that were not focused on the assessment of the acceptance of the new tools by health professionals, identifying types of studies, assessment of the results obtained and validated tools for their obtaining and standardized application on the personnel for the implantation in the environments of the workers. We approach some of the issues that facilitate or hinder the acceptance of technology by nurses in various fields of clinical practice.

Our final objective is to make a revision of the articles previously posted for later do a methodological proposal that aims to identificate the issues that mediate these processes of acceptance and rejection of technology in a population of primary care nurses, looking for cultural barriers that difficulties new tools' implementation, by that the care application and facilitate concepts pin up a positive demeanor used for these new tools.

The population we want to evaluate are primary care nurses from rural environment. We will review research work that focused in the identificacion of the barriers that limits the acceptance of the new digital tools and the facilitators of their implementation through through making validated identified questionnaires.

4 Results

The research carried out focuses on satisfaction polls of use by health professionals after the implementation of digital tools [27], obviating that for the implementation and acceptance of new tools, it will be necessary to evaluate the availability of professionals through diagnostic and efficacy evaluation tools that indicate the using and intentionality of the evaluated technology for a correct implementation and employ [28].

Other studies have focused on the sights of nursing community on technology uses in health systems [29], where a part of the participants were convinced of the importance on information technologies in the provision of health and medical services; nevertheless, there was a significant group that set forth their skepticism about the need to develop e-health services in the specific context of nursing in Poland.

The first works focused on use's problems or nurses' barriers are interested on the use and management of the internet and computers. The work of Eley et al. [30] through questionnaires distributed in the Australian Federation of Nursing described about 20 possible barriers that would hinder information use of technologies in the workplace, these are the firsts works that concrete the identification of cultural barriers and facilitators behaviors of professionals that are going to apply cares though digital tools.

That is why new digital tools evaluation processes must be standardized before their implementation, in search of the disposal of the professionals who will work with them to evaluate their use and the intention, following the results obtained in other fields when they apply the Unified Theory of Acceptance and Use of Technology (UTAUT), formulated by Venkatesh, Morris and Davis [31, 32] and applied in health studies to evaluate Digital Medical Records [33], to put on optimal health care to the population that result in a real and evaluated benefit of the new tools given in view of the great applications diversity that coexist in the mart.

Therefore, it is necessary to prepare validated questionnaires for each population with its cultural bias that indicate the barriers that limit the acceptance of the new tools in the nursing care environment for patients in the home background, as well as identify facilitating devices for implement correctly new technologies, as well as acceptance and use of the same at less cost for the health system, at once that we improve the population care.

5 Conclusions

New technologies' uses applied to healthcare deal several difficulties and barriers. Although most of the efforts are focused on identify and facilitate adaptability and the use of the population care – patients, their families and formal and informal caregivers -, the health professional culture itself is a central issue to consider. In the case of nurses, the available experience has revealed cultural attitudes of rejection and difficulties in moving from analog to virtual healthcare settings, in addition to the need to evaluate skills that professionals have to enforce and knowledge that will support implementation of new work environments, through specialized postgraduate training and reinforcement in university degree studies, in the specific technology. Issues such as age, gender or training received are crucial to do a correct previous appreciation and then programate a specialized training.

There are no specific studies that address the contemporary training scene in Spain as an object of study. Anyway, it seems clear that we must focus more and more on this professional group if we want to carry out an e-health revolution and get a good level of specialized training in line with the rest of countries who follows us.

We must also offer technological solutions adapted to professionals after a standardized assessment of their culture, which must be part of the usability analysis for previously implementing to any technology acquirement to improve care. Issues such as gender, age, perception of technology, training plans of health institutions or universities are elements of an equation that must be solved in a concrete way, to obtain care with the maximum efficacy, efficiency and effectiveness guarantees for population and health systems.

Acknowledgments. This work was supported by 4IE + project (0499_4IE_PLUS_4_E) funded by the Interreg VA Spain-Portugal (POCTEP) 2014–2020 program.

Conflict of Interest. The authors declare that they have no conflict of interest.

References

1. Risling, T.: Educating the nurses of 2025: technology trends of the next decade. Nurse Educ. Pract. **22**, 89–92 (2017). https://doi.org/10.1016/j.nepr.2016.12.007

2. ITU (2021): Report on the Implementation of the Strategic Plan and the Activities of the Union, April 2019 – April 2021. April
3. UNCTAD (2021): Informe sobre tecnología e información 2021. Conferencia De Las Naciones Unidas Sobre Comercio Y Desarrollo, 29
4. Olarte, S.: Brecha digital, pobreza y exclusión social. Temas Laborales **138**, 285–313 (2017). https://dialnet.unirioja.es/servlet/articulo?codigo=6552396
5. Organization, W.H.: Estrategia Mundial Sobre Salud Digital, p. 42 (2020). https://www.paho.org/hq/index.php?option=com_docman&view=download&category_slug=56-directing-council-spanish
6. Comision Europea (2021): Brújula Digital 2030: el enfoque de Europa para el Decenio Digital. https://eur-lex.europa.eu/legal-content/es/TXT/?uri=CELEX:52021DC0118
7. Luengo-Polo, J., Conde-Caballero, D., Rivero-Jiménez, B., Ballesteros-Yáñez, I., Castillo-Sarmiento, C.A., Mariano-Juárez, L.: Rationale and methods of evaluation for acho, a new virtual assistant to improve therapeutic adherence in rural elderly populations: a user-driven living lab. Int. J. Environ. Res. Public Health **18**, 7904 (2021). https://doi.org/10.3390/ijerph18157904
8. Sprenger, M., Mettler, T., Osma, J.: Health professionals' perspective on the promotion of e-mental health apps in the context of maternal depression. PLoS ONE **12**(7), e0180867 (2017). https://doi.org/10.1371/journal.pone.0180867. PMID:28704442;PMCID:PMC5507525
9. Hsiao, S.J., Li, Y.C., Chen, Y.L., Ko, H.C.: Critical factors for the adoption of mobile nursing information systems in Taiwan: the nursing department administrators' perspective. J. Med. Syst. **33**(5), 369–377 (2009). https://doi.org/10.1007/s10916-008-9199-8. PMID: 19827263
10. Lee, T.T.: Nursing administrators' experiences in managing PDA use for inpatient units. Comput. Inform. Nurs. **24**(5), 280–7 (2006). https://doi.org/10.1097/00024665-200609000-00010. PMID: 16980781
11. Marini, S.D., Hasman, A., Huijer, H.A., Dimassi, H.: Nurses' attitudes toward the use of the bar-coding medication administration system. Comput. Inform. Nurs. **28**(2), 112–23 (2010). https://doi.org/10.1097/NCN.0b013e3181cd80f6. PMID: 20182162
12. Kummer, T.F., Schäfer, K., Todorova, N.: Acceptance of hospital nurses toward sensor-based medication systems: a questionnaire survey. Int. J. Nurs. Stud. **50**(4), 508–517 (2013). https://doi.org/10.1016/j.ijnurstu.2012.11.010. Epub 2013 Jan 24 PMID: 23352607
13. Escobar-Rodríguez, T., Romero-Alonso, M.M.: Modeling nurses' attitude toward using automated unit-based medication storage and distribution systems: an extension of the technology acceptance model. Comput. Inform. Nurs. **31**(5), 235–243 (2013). https://doi.org/10.1097/NXN.0b013e31828a0d81. PMID: 23478728
14. Kinnunen, U.-M., Heponiemi, T., Rajalahti, E., Ahonen, O., Korhonen, T., Hyppönen, H.: Factors related to health informatics competencies for nurses—results of a national electronic health record survey. CIN Comput. Inform. Nurs. **37**(8), 420–429 (2019). https://doi.org/10.1097/CIN.0000000000000511
15. Kaihlanen, A.M., Gluschkoff, K., Kinnunen, U.M., Saranto, K., Ahonen, O., Heponiemi, T.: Nursing informatics competences of Finnish registered nurses after national educational initiatives: a cross-sectional study. Nurse Educ. Today **106**(July), 105060 (2021). https://doi.org/10.1016/j.nedt.2021.105060
16. Kassam, I., Nagle, L., Strudwick, G.: Informatics competencies for nurse leaders: protocol for a scoping review. BMJ Open **7**(12), 1–4 (2017). https://doi.org/10.1136/bmjopen-2017-018855
17. Collins, S., Yen, P.Y., Phillips, A., Kennedy, M.K.: Nursing informatics competency as. J. Nurs. Adm. **47**(4), 212–218 (2017). https://doi.org/10.1097/NNA.0000000000000467
18. Monraz-Pérez, S., Pacheco-López, A., Castorena-Maldonado, A., et al.: Telemedicina durante la pandemia por COVID-19. Neumol. Cir. Torax **80**(2), 132–140 (2021). https://doi.org/10.35366/100996

19. Bermúdez, S.: Satisfacción del paciente de telemedicina durante la pandemia COVID-19, p. 1047492126. Disponible en: http://hdl.handle.net/10726/4093
20. Lorenzo Aparici, M.O.D.: La Telemedicina en España en la época de la postpandemia Covid-19. Revista: Toko-Ginecologia Practica **771**, 221–235 (2020). Periodo: 2
21. Davis, F.D., Bagozzi, R.P., Warshaw, P.R.: Extrinsic and intrinsic motivation to use computers in the workplace. J. Appl. Soc. Psychol. **22**(14), 1111–1132 (1992). https://doi.org/10.1111/j.1559-1816.1992.tb00945.x
22. Yong, L.A.: Modelo de aceptación tecnológica. Revista Internacional de Ciencias Sociales y Humanidades **1**(1), 42 (2004). http://www.redalyc.org/pdf/654/65414107.pdf
23. Wan Ismail, W.K., Chan, P.H.K., Buhari, N., Muzaini, A.: Acceptance of smartphone in enhancing patient-caregivers relationship. J. Technol. Manag. Innov. **7**(3), 71–79 (2012). https://doi.org/10.4067/S0718-27242012000300007
24. Kohnke, A., Cole, M.L., Bush, R.G.: Incorporating UTAUT predictors for understanding home care patients' and clinician's acceptance of healthcare telemedicine equipment. J. Technol. Manag. Innov. **9**(2), 29–41 (2014). https://doi.org/10.4067/S0718-27242014000200003
25. Yen, P.Y., Phillips, A., Kennedy, M.K., Collins, S.: Nursing informatics competency assessment for the nurse leader instrument refinement, validation, and psychometric analysis. J. Nurs. Adm. **47**(5), 271–277 (2017)
26. Ajzen, I.: The theory of planned behavior. Organ. Behav. Hum. Decis. Process. **50**(2), 179–211 (1991). https://doi.org/10.1016/0749-5978(91)90020-t
27. Ribeiro, O.M., Martins, M.M., Vandresen, L., Silva, J.M., Cardoso, M.F.: Utilidade das tecnologias de informação e comunicação: olhar dos enfermeiros portugueses. Texto Contexto Enferm [Internet] **30**, e20190139 (2021). [acesso MÊS ANO DIA]; Disponível em: https://doi.org/10.1590/1980-265X-TCE-2019-0139
28. Bennani, A.E., Oumlil, R.: IT acceptance by nurses in morocco: application of a modified unified theory of acceptance and use of technology. IBIMA Bus. Rev. **2014** (2014). Article ID 849383, https://doi.org/10.5171/2014.849383
29. Duplaga, M., Andrychiewicz, A., Dańda, J.: The opinions about e-health among nurses employed in hospitals located in an urban area in Poland. Comput. Inform. Nurs. CIN **31**(6), 281–289 (2013). https://doi.org/10.1097/NXN.0b013e31828a0d98
30. Eley, R., Fallon, T., Soar, J., Buikstra, E., Hegney, D.: Barriers to use of information and computer technology by Australia's nurses: a national survey. J. Clin. Nurs. **18**(8), 1151–1158 (2009). https://doi.org/10.1111/j.1365-2702.2008.02336.x. PMID: 19320784
31. Venkatesh, V., Morris, M.G., Davis, G.B., Davis, F.D.: User acceptance of information technology: toward a unified view. MIS Q. **27**(3), 425–478 (2003). https://web.archive.org/web/20060514100134/http://csdl.ics.hawaii.edu/techreports/05-06/doc/Venkatesh2003.pdf
32. Venkatesh, V., Bala, H.: Technology acceptance model 3 and a research agenda on interventions. Decis. Sci. **39**(2), 273–315 (2008). https://doi.org/10.1111/j.1540-5915.2008.00192.x
33. Huser, V., Narus, S.P., Rocha, R.A.: Evaluation of a flowchart-based EHR query system: a case study of RetroGuide. J. Biomed. Inform. **43**(1), 41–50 (2010). https://doi.org/10.1016/j.jbi.2009.06.001

Satisfaction: A Concept Based on Functionality and Quality of Life to Be Integrated in a Nursing Care Performance System

Margarida Goes[1], Henrique Oliveira[1,2](✉), Manuel Lopes[3], César Fonseca[3], and Lara Pinho[4]

[1] Polytechnic Institute of Beja, Beja, Portugal
hjmo@lx.it.pt
[2] Telecommunications Institute, Lisbon, Portugal
[3] Escola Superior de Enfermagem São João de Deus, Évora, Portugal
[4] Comprehensive Health Research Centre, Évora, Portugal

Abstract. Objective: The main objective of this research was to operationalize a nursing sensitive outcome, designated as *Satisfaction*, using a set of indicators sensitive to various aspects of the nursing care: (i) Functional capacity assessment (*Functionality*), which is considered an important indicator for elderly people's health and should be used to provide a robust data infrastructure on functioning and disability, allowing for national and international comparisons; (ii) Quality of Life assessment, which is another important health indicator that is strongly recommended by World Health Organization, as it includes multiple domains of functioning and well-being that are extraordinarily important in the assessment of health outcomes. **Methods**: Cross-sectional, descriptive study, with a final sample totaled 351 elderlies. Data collected by health professionals in the participants' houses, using a core set composed of items belonging to the International Classification of Functioning, Disability and Health and by the WHOQOL-BREF instrument. Structural equation modeling was the statistical methodology adopted. **Results**: The developed model presents favorable factorial validity and reliability, which allows to infer about the existence of an empirical strong relationship between both the *Functionality* and QoL theoretical models with *Satisfaction*. **Conclusions**: Both *Functionality* and QoL are determinants of *Satisfaction*, even though *Satisfaction* manifests itself with greater importance in QoL, rather than in *Functionality*.

Keywords: Elderly · Nursing care · Functionality · Quality of life · Nursing outcomes · Satisfaction

1 Introduction

Due to the aging of the Portuguese population, there has been an increase in chronic diseases and, consequently, a greater demand for healthcare, particularly in the case of the elderlies, who are among those who have multiple and complex chronic conditions (multimorbidity), and who require long-term healthcare [1].

J. García-Alonso and C. Fonseca (Eds.): IWoG 2021, LNBE, pp. 84–93, 2022.
https://doi.org/10.1007/978-3-030-97524-1_9

The World Health Organization (WHO) recognizes the inadequacy of the current health systems to care for people with multimorbidity, thus requesting a shift to a new paradigm, based on the following grounds [2]:

- Empowering and involving people, that is, fostering a equal and reciprocal relationship between clinical and non-clinical professionals and people who use health services, their families and communities, enhancing their experience in self-care;
- Strengthening clinical governance and accountability, that is, promoting transparency in decision-making, in order to generate robust systems of collective responsibility involving policy makers, managers, suppliers and users;
- Reorienting the healthcare model, in order to guarantee effective health services that prioritize community and primary care services in the co-production of health, investing in a change from a hospital internship regime to the one based on home care;
- Implementing coordination services in order to improve healthcare delivery by aligning and harmonizing processes between different health services around people's needs and preferences;
- Creating a favorable environment that promotes the necessary changes in legislative structures, agreements, financial incentives and formulation of new public policies.

The current Portuguese health system, as in many other countries, is mostly oriented to respond to acute health conditions, thus not guaranteeing to its users the maintenance of their overall health status, because it is not tailored to the needs of patients with multimorbidity. If no change is made, it will become increasingly fragmented, ineffective and untenable soon. According to Lopes [3], a fundamental shift in the way how the Portuguese health system is financed, managed and how healthcare are delivered, fostered by the concept of *patient-centered care* (PCC) and ensuring the integration and continuity of care, is becoming mandatory. Moreover, "*evidence shows that health systems oriented around the needs of people and communities become more effective, cost less, improve health literacy and patient engagement, and are better prepared to respond to health crises*", as stated by the WHO [4].

One way to make PCC more effective, empowering people and communities and making them the center of health systems, among other strategies, is to listen their expectations about how healthcare relieved discomfort and improved quality of life, that is, to what extent patients are "satisfied" with the healthcare provided and what were the outcomes achieved regarding their health status. According to the research work conducted by Kuipers and colleagues among 216 Dutch patients with multi-morbidity in the primary care setting [5], PCC was correlated significantly with satisfaction with care ($\beta = 0.425,\ p \leq 0.001$). PCC was also associated positively with patients' physical and social well-being. The authors concluded that if healthcare delivery is tailored to the needs of patients with multimorbidity, by paying attention to PCC, it will result in better patient outcomes.

Patient satisfaction with care has been considered worldwide as an important indicator to assess the performance of healthcare delivery, involving the quality of care provided by health professionals, the quality of health services themselves, and the context in which healthcare are provided [6].

In another research work conducted by Dubois and colleagues, the authors developed a nursing care performance framework (NCPF), which included a matrix of indicators covering the main functions of a nursing system, developed in accordance with three subsystems [7] (a more detailed view of the NCPF can be seen in Fig. 3 of the reference):

- Acquiring, deploying and maintaining nursing resources;
- Transforming nursing resources into relevant nursing services;
- Producing positive changes in patients' conditions.

The third subsystem addresses five dimensions, capturing the nursing sensitive outcomes in terms of the positive changes in a patient's functional status, disease state or evolving condition, namely:

- Outcomes reflecting patient safety (*risk outcomes and safety*);
- Outcomes reflecting patient comfort and quality of life related to care (*patient comfort and quality of life*);
- Outcomes reflecting changes in patients' knowledge, skills, and behaviors (*patient empowerment*);
- Outcomes reflecting patients' functional status (*patient functional status*);
- Outcomes reflecting patient satisfaction with the care experience (*patient satisfaction*).

In respect to the fifth dimension (here designated in short as *patient satisfaction*), Dubois and colleagues state that patient satisfaction is a subjective outcome made by patients that "*reflects the interaction of their expectations of care and their perceptions of actual outcomes resulting from provider services.*" Although all the work regarding the development of the NCPF is theoretical, it is important to make some development toward the operationalization of this fifth dimension, as described by Dubois and colleagues [7].

2 Objective

The aim is this article is to demonstrate how *patient satisfaction*, as modelled by Dubois and colleagues can be operationalized, and the proposal is to realize it by using two important health concepts: *Functionality* and *Quality of Life* (QoL). More details on how the work was done, are provided in the next sections of this article.

3 Methods

3.1 Ethical Considerations

The Health Ethics Committee of the Local Health Unit of Baixo Alentejo (HECLHUBA), was the institutional committee that approved the study protocol, including the study design, how the interviews were conducted, as well as the informed consent that was presented to each respondent. All the suggestions included in the HECLHUBA operating regulations were followed, which was developed under the Helsinki Declaration, with the aim of protecting the dignity, the privacy and freedom of participants in this study [8].

3.2 Sample Size and Inclusion Criteria

This research work involved 351 individuals residing in their own homes or at family members' or friends' homes, who had more than or equal to 65 years old. All the participants were registered in the database of the Local Health Unit of Baixo Alentejo (LHUBA). The adopted inclusion criteria were as follows: (i) individuals who were interested in participating in the study; (ii) were able to make their own decisions if they were sick or were hospitalized due to acute, short-term health care needs; and (iii) who signed the informed consent form and answered both instruments fully and correctly (with no missing data).

3.3 Instruments

To operationalize the patient satisfaction indicator, as described by Dubois and colleagues and belonging to the subsystem labelled as "Producing positive changes in patients' conditions" of their NCPF, the following correspondences were established (a more detailed view of the five dimensions included in this NCPF subsystem can be seen in Fig. 3 of [7]):

- data addressing the risk outcomes and safety, patient empowerment, and patient functional status are acquired using a coreset extracted from the International Classification of Functioning, Disability and Health (here designated in short as Functionality), based on the previous research work developed by Goes and colleagues [9];
- data addressing the patient comfort and quality of life are acquired using the instrument developed by the World Health Organization Quality of Life groups (WHOQOL), namely the WHOQOL-BREF instrument, based on the previous research work published by Goes and colleagues [10–12].

3.4 Statistical Methods

Sample data about *Functionality* and QoL were acquired using the structured interview methodology, and were considered as parallel samples, since the two instruments (Elderly Nursing Core Set for the *Functionality* [9] and WHOQOL-BREF for QoL [10]) were presented to the respondents simultaneously.

The factorial validity and reliability of the statistical model was verified through the confirmatory factor analysis (CFA), using the SPSS AMOS software version 23.0.0 (IBM, Armonk, NY), in accordance with the recommendations provided by Marôco [13] for this purpose, namely: (i) **individual reliability** of the items, through the analysis of the respective standardized factor loadings of the observed variables belonging to the *Functionality* and QoL models (λ_{ij}, where *i* is the index of the observed variables, while *j* is the index of the latent variables (unobserved variables), usually $\lambda_{ij} \geq 0.5$); (ii) **construct reliability**, through the analysis of composite reliability – *CR* (usually $CR_j \geq 0.7$); (iii) **construct validity**, by firstly verifying whether the items (observed variables) are a reflection of the latent variables that are intended to measured (**factorial validity**), and secondly by examining the value of average variance extracted (*AVE*) for each latent (**convergent validity** – usually $AVE_j \geq 0.5$); (iv) to check if *AVE* values is greater than the square of inter-construct correlations $-\phi^2_{j1,j2}$ (**discriminating validity** – usually by confirming if the output of the expression $\left(AVE_{j1} \bigwedge AVE_{j2}\right) \geq \phi^2_{j1,j2}$ is TRUE). The overall goodness of the model fit was based on the following indices, as suggested by Marôco [13]: (i) χ^2 statistic with correction by degrees of freedom χ^2/(df); (ii) *Comparative Fit Index* (CFI); (iii) *Parsimony Comparative Fit Index* (PCFI) (iv) *Goodness of Fit Index* (GFI); (v) *Parsimony Goodness of Fit Index* (PGFI); (vi) *Standardized Root Mean Square Residual* (SRMR); (vii) *Root Mean Square Error of Approximation* (RMSEA); (viii) *p*-value for the null hypothesis of RMSEA ≤ 0.05 (PCLOSE); (ix) *Modified Expected Cross-Validation Index* (MECVI).

4 Results

Figure 1 shows the initial CFA model (not adjusted) that was developed to obtain the scoring of the latent variable designated as "SAT" (*Satisfaction*), as a function of "Func" (*Functionality*) and "QoL" (QoL) latent variables. The fit indices shown at the top of Fig. 1 reveal that the model fit is poor, although $\chi^2/(df) < 3.0$. By correlating the item errors whose respective modification index (MI) values are greater than 11, a new (adjusted) model is obtained, which is shown in Fig. 2. This adjusted model presents a better overall model fit than the initial one (MECVI such that 8.688 < 10.152) and $\chi^2/(df) < 2.5$. The model presents individual reliability of the items (observed variables), as the respective standardized factor loadings (λ_{ij}) are almost all above 0.5 (only 8.3% are below 0.5 and none is below 0.3, this last threshold considered acceptable in case of exploratory studies [13]).

The structural equation model shown in Fig. 2 presents composite reliability since almost all *CR* values are greater than 0.7, except for the construct (latent variable) "SR(a)", whose value is equal to 0.585, see Table 1 (*CR* values between 0.7 and 0.5 are acceptable in exploratory research, which is the case here [13]). Construct validity is positively evaluated since all the items reflect the latent variables that are intended to be measured (factorial validity), and almost all *AVE* values are greater than 0.5 (convergent validity), except for the "SR(b)" and "Env" latent variables, with SR(a) being identified as the worst case (*AVE* values between 0.5 and 0.3 are acceptable in exploratory research, which is the case here [13]).

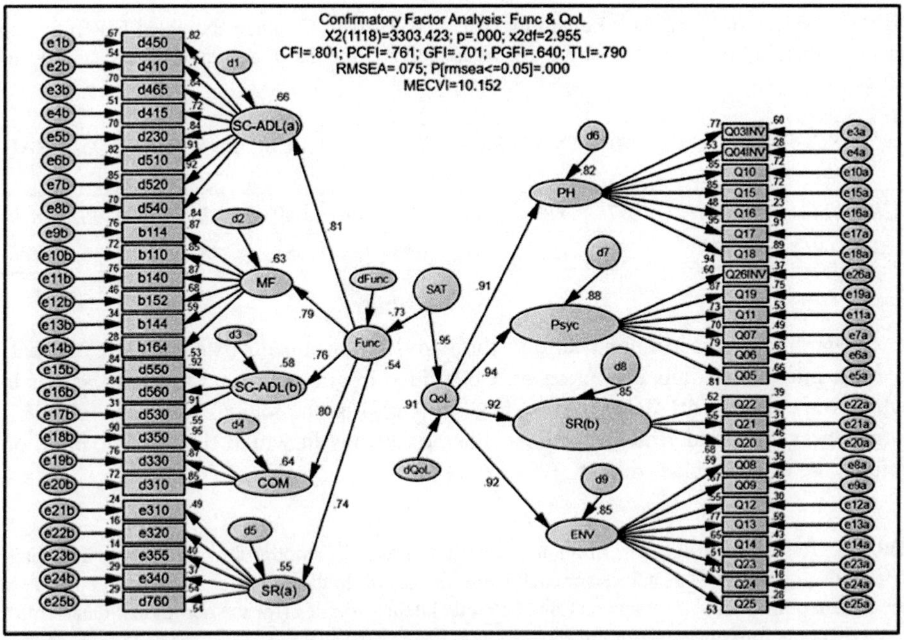

Fig. 1. Initial model (not adjusted) to capture whether *Satisfaction*, a sensitive dimension of nursing care, according to Dubois and colleagues [7] and designated as *patient satisfaction*, is a manifest variable either in *Functionality* and QoL.

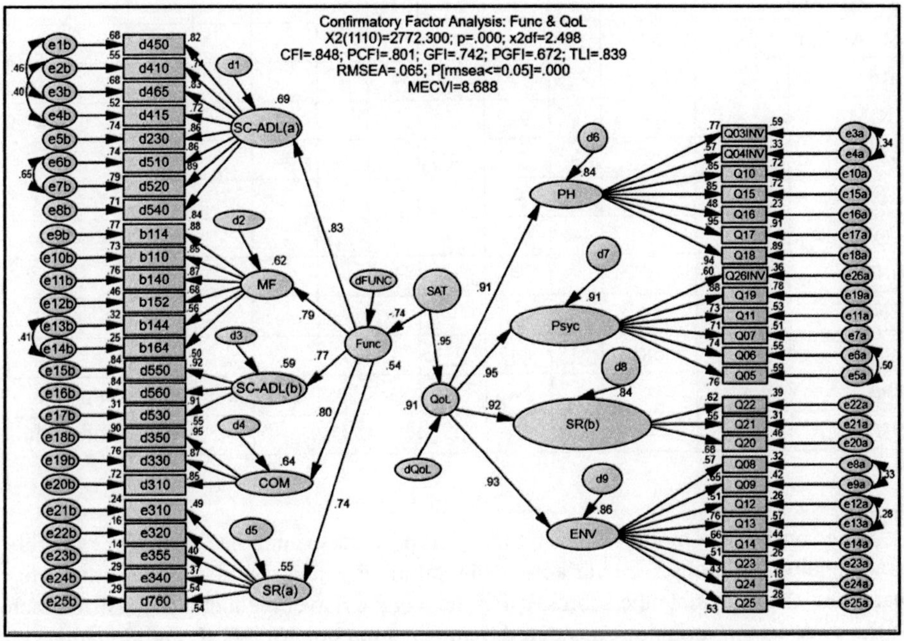

Fig. 2. Adjusted model to the one shown in Fig. 1.

Table 1. Values of Composite Reliability (*CR*) and Average Variance Extracted (*AVE*) for the model shown in Fig. 2 (for the acronyms, please refer to the list of acronyms at the end of this article).

	SC-ADL (a)	SC-ADL (b)	MF	COM	SR(a)	PH	Psyc	SR(b)	ENV	Func	QoL	SAT
CR	.943	.848	.875	.920	**.585**	.921	.899	.649	.802	.889	.962	.839
AVE	.676	.661	.548	.795	**.224**	.636	.600	**.382**	**.343**	.664	.863	.726

Regarding the discriminant validity, the analysis of the results listed in Table 2 reveals that the model only fails in four cases. Cells filled in gray represent those occasions in which the expression $(AVE_{j1} \bigwedge AVE_{j2}) \geq \phi^2_{j1,j2}$ returns the logical value of "FALSE", while the values underlined represent those occasions in which the same expression returns the logical value of "TRUE".

Table 2. Results regarding discriminant validation of the AFC model shown in Fig. 2. The diagonal cells present the *AVE* values for each latent factor, while the values at the last three lines are the square of inter-construct correlations between latent variables (for the acronyms, please refer to the list of acronyms at the end of this article).

	SC-ADL (a)	**SC-ADL (b)**	**MF**	**COM**	**SR(a)**	**PH**	**Psyc**	**SR(b)**	**ENV**	**Func**	**QoL**	**SAT**
SC-ADL(a)	.943	-	-	-	-	-	-	-	-	-	-	-
SC-ADL(b)	-	.848	-	-	-	-	-	-	-	-	-	-
MF	-	-	.875	-	-	-	-	-	-	-	-	-
COM	-	-	-	.920	-	-	-	-	-	-	-	-
SR(a)		-	-	-	.585	-	-	-	-	-	-	-
PH	-	-	-	-	-	.921	-	-	-	-	-	-
Psyc	-	-	-	-	-	-	.899	-	-	-	-	-
SR(b)	-	-	-	-	-	-	-	.649	-	-	-	-
ENV	-	-	-	-	-	-	-	-	.802	-	-	-
Func	.687	.585	.618	.637	.551	-	-	-	-	.889	-	-
QoL	-	-	-	-	-	.835	.908	.845	.865	-	.962	-
SAT	-	-	-	-	-	-	-	-	-	.543	.908	.839

Based on the CFA model shown in Fig. 2, it is possible to infer the *factor score* weights (*fsw* – one per each observed variable, in a total of 49 values), which represent weights that allow us to calculate the scores, using the weighted average methodology, for each of the three latent variables considered, namely: *Functionality*, QoL and *Satisfaction*. According to the *fsw* values inferred from the adjusted CFA model, it was possible to obtain the weighted average scores for the entire sample, for the three latent variables mentioned, whose result is shown in Fig. 3.

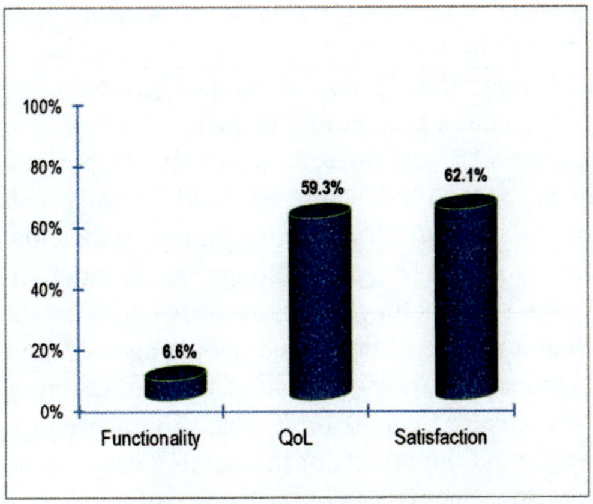

Fig. 3. Weighted average scores using the *fsw* values inferred from the CFA model shown in Fig. 2.

5 Discussion

The aim of this research work was to operationalize a measure of satisfaction with the nursing care delivery (here designated as *Satisfaction*), to individuals living in a rural area with low population density, residing in their own homes or at family members' or friends' homes, who had more than or equal to 65 years old. *Satisfaction* was considered here as a nursing sensitive outcome, on the production of positive changes in patients' conditions [7]. *Patient satisfaction* has been considered worldwide as an important indicator to assess the performance of healthcare delivery, involving the quality of care delivered by health professionals, the quality of health services themselves, and the context in which healthcare are delivered [6].

Individuals' health can be studied based on *Functionality*, which is a multidimensional concept that was developed by the WHO and includes the physical, social, psychological, and environmental dimensions of their lives [9], with these dimensions being used in this article as interconnected latent variables. On the other hand, QoL is another concept also developed by the WHO, which captures the individuals' own views of their well-being, based on the physical health, psychological, social relationships, and environment dimensions of their lives [10]. Therefore, there are some interconnections between the dimensions of *Functionality* and QoL, and for this reason, *Satisfaction* was measured in the scope of this research work based on the *Functionality* and QoL latent variables.

The results listed in Tables 1 and 2 shows that the CFA model of Fig. 2 presents favorable factorial validity and reliability, which allows to infer about the existence of an empirical strong relationship between both the *Functionality* and QoL theoretical models with *Satisfaction*. When determining the needs of nursing care according to the different levels of Functionality based on a self-care model [9], as well as when capturing the individuals' own views of their well-being [10], both *Functionality* and QoL latent variables are manifest variables of *Satisfaction*. It is important to note that such effect is statistically significant, although it does not imply a cause-effect relationship.

The model in Fig. 2 shows that *Functionality* and QoL are determinants of *Satisfaction*. However, *Satisfaction* has a greater impact on QoL, when compared to Functionality (explained variances of 91% and 54%, respectively). A possible explanation for the result found is that the proposed model captures what is similar between the three latent variables, namely the needs, standards and expectations of the elderlies, aspects that are reflected both in *Satisfaction* and in QoL, although not so much in *Functionality*.

The weighted average score achieved for the *Satisfaction* latent variable was 61.2% (see Fig. 3). from which it can be inferred that people aged 65 and over residing in the community, in their homes, are mostly satisfied with the nursing care they delivered (weighted average score greater than 50%). It means that there is a positive outcome on how the individuals evaluated the effects of the nursing care that were delivered, as the individuals health conditions seem to have evolved positively.

Changes in *Functionality* and QoL latent variables produce distinct effects in *Satisfaction*, that is, *Satisfaction* increases with the reduction of functional problems (the correlation coefficient between *Functionality* and *Satisfaction* is −0.74, see Fig. 2) and with the increase in QoL (the correlation coefficient between QoL and *Satisfaction* is 0.95, see Fig. 2), with this effect been more pronounced for the QoL latent variable (the correlation coefficient between QoL and *Satisfaction* presents a greater absolute value −0.95 than the one between *Functionality* and *Satisfaction* −0.74).

6 Conclusions

In this article, an indicator considered as a nursing sensitive outcome, designated as *Satisfaction*, which was theoretically developed by Dubois and colleagues, in their NCPF [7], was operationalized. It was proven that it is possible to obtain this indicator in quantitative terms, from the analysis of the *Functionality* and QoL of individuals. It was concluded that both *Functionality* and QoL are determinants of *Satisfaction*, even though *Satisfaction* manifests itself with greater importance in QoL, rather than in *Functionality*. *Satisfaction* is a definable and measurable dimension, which is why it is suggested that it should be used to assess about the contribution of the nursing professionals in the delivery of healthcare to individuals.

Acknowledgments. This research was funded by FEDER. Programa Interreg VA España-Portugal (POCTEP), grant number 0499_4IE_PLUS_4_E.

List of Acronyms. **SC-ADL(a)**: Self-care – activities of daily living (a); **SC-ADL(b)**: Self-care – activities of daily living (b); **MF**: Mental functions; **COM**: Communication; **SR(a)**: Social relationships (a); **PH**: Physical health; **Psyc**: Psychological **SR(b)**: Social relationships (b); **ENV**: Environment; **Func**: Functionality; **QoL**: Quality of Life; **SAT**: Satisfaction.

References

1. European Observatory on Health Systems and Policies (2018): Health System Review - Portugal (Phase 1 Final Report). World Health Organization
2. World Health Organization (2015): World report on ageing and health. Report, World Health Organization
3. Lopes, M.: Desafios de Inovação em Saúde. Repensar os Modelos de Cuidados. Imprensa da Universidade de Évora (2021)
4. World Health Organization. https://www.who.int/news/item/28-05-2016-world-health-assembly-adopts-framework-on-integrated-people-centred-health-services
5. Kuipers, S.J., Cramm, J.M., Nieboer, A.P.: The importance of patient-centered care and co-creation of care for satisfaction with care and physical and social well-being of patients with multi-morbidity in the primary care setting. BMC Health Serv. Res. **19** (2019). https://doi.org/10.1186/s12913-018-3818-y
6. Larson, E., Sharma, J., Bohren, M.A., Tunçalp, Ö.: When the patient is the expert: measuring patient experience and satisfaction with care. Bull. World Health Organ. **97**, 563–569 (2019). https://doi.org/10.2471/blt.18.225201
7. Dubois, C.-A., D'Amour, D., Pomey, M.-P., Girard, F., Brault, I.: Conceptualizing performance of nursing care as a prerequisite for better measurement: a systematic and interpretive review. BMC Nurs. **12** (2013). https://doi.org/10.1186/1472-6955-12-7
8. Comissão de Ética para a Saúde da Unidade Local de Saúde do Baixo Alentejo. http://www.ulsba.min-saude.pt/2019/02/28/comissao-de-etica-para-a-saude/
9. Goes, M., Lopes, M.J., Oliveira, H., Fonseca, C., Marôco, J.: a nursing care intervention model for elderly people to ascertain general profiles of functionality and self care needs. Sci. Rep. **10** (2020). https://doi.org/10.1038/s41598-020-58596-1
10. Goes, M., Lopes, M., Marôco, J., Oliveira, H., Fonseca, C.: Psychometric properties of the WHOQOL-BREF(PT) in a sample of elderly citizens. Health Qual. Life Outcomes **19** (2021). https://doi.org/10.1186/s12955-021-01783-z
11. Goes, M., et al.: Psychometric qualities of a core set to ascertain the functional profile of Portuguese elderly citizens. In: García-Alonso, J., Fonseca, C. (eds.) IWoG 2019. CCIS, vol. 1185, pp. 314–329. Springer, Cham (2020). https://doi.org/10.1007/978-3-030-41494-8_31
12. Goes, M., et al.: The quality of life of older individuals following the world health organization assessment criteria. Geriatrics **5**, 102 (2020). https://doi.org/10.3390/geriatrics5040102
13. Marôco, J.: Análise de equações estruturais: fundamentos teóricos, software e aplicações (2020). Report Number

Age-Friendly Primary Health Care: A Scoping Review

Idalina Delfina Gomes[1](✉), Liliana Santos Sobreira[1], Liliana Veríssimo da Silva[1], Marina Celly Martins Ribeiro de Souza[2], Gleicy Karina[3], and Rafaella Queiroga Souto[3]

[1] Escola Superior de Enfermagem de Lisboa, 1990-096 Lisboa, Portugal
idgomes@esel.pt
[2] The College of New Jersey, Ewing Township, NJ 08618, USA
[3] Universidade Federal da Paraíba, João Pessoa, PB 58051-900, Brasil

Abstract. *Introduction*: The global increase on the number of older adults leads to an increase in the demand for health services, which needs to adapt their care to the population. This adaptation involves empowerment, knowledge and autonomy, establishment of a partner relationship in the care and decision-making process, so that the quality and dignity of care for the older adults guaranteed. Primary health care should be made available as proximity services, in addition to investing in the continuous improvement of their practices, in which gerontotechnology has an essential contribution.

Objective: To answer the research question "What are the characteristics presented by age-friendly health units in the context of primary health care?".

Method: The scoping review follows the Joanna Briggs Institute (2015) methodology and the PRISMA (Preferred Reporting Items for Systematic Reviews and Meta-Analyses) model.

Results: From the 22 articles analyzed, 7 main themes that characterize this issue resulted: 1. Information, education and communication; 2. Health care management systems; 3. Care management process taking into account most common geriatric syndromes; 4. Physical environment; 5. Transportation network; 6. Keeping older adults in their own context; 7. Health policies.

Conclusions: The characteristics of the age-friendly health centers recommended by the WHO allow bringing older people closer to the health care they need, enabling them to gain in health, well-being, as well as macro advantages in public health. The nurse should work in partnership with the older people, helping them to manage their health process and promoting Care-of-the-Self.

Keywords: Older adults · Age-friendly services · Primary health care · Care-of-the-Self

1 Introduction

The aging of the world population is an inevitable and growing reality, which implies challenges and adaptations of health services. By 2020, the world population aged 60

J. García-Alonso and C. Fonseca (Eds.): IWoG 2021, LNBE, pp. 94–107, 2022.
https://doi.org/10.1007/978-3-030-97524-1_10

and over exceeded 1 billion people, and by 2050 it is expected to reach 2.1 billion [1]. Health policies need to anticipate this trend and prepare health systems to be more adequate, effective, and accessible. They should focus on improving and meeting needs and preferences of older people, adapting health care to this population and providing outreach care, including primary health care, focusing on health promotion, monitoring and prevention of disabling and chronic conditions resulting from aging [2]. These services must be the first access to health care services for the older people. [3, 4].

According to a WHO study, the characteristics of an age-friendly primary health care encompass three dimensions: information, education and communication; health service management systems; and the physical environment [5]. Several authors agree that age-friendly care enables empowerment by increasing older people's knowledge and autonomy so that they become involved and partners in their care process, ensuring the quality and dignity of care. Thus, it is recognized that the lower the barriers to access primary health care are, and the better the needs of people are met, health gains are obtained, and public health spending is substantially reduced. It is essential that these health centers also combine technology with gerontology, i.e., have the fundamentals of gerontotechnology in the context of a multidisciplinary intervention, which acts on the three levels of prevention to improve the quality of life of the older adults [6].

A preliminary search conducted in the JBI Database of Systematic Reviews and Implementation Reports, Cochrane Library, MEDLINE and CINAHL, revealed that there is no Scoping Review (published or in development) on Age-Friendly Primary Health Care. Thus, this review arises from the need to increase knowledge about the Age-Friendly Health Centers (AFHC) in order to contribute to the development of services that provide accessibility to care, health promotion, increased autonomy and involvement of older people in their own health process, promoting the Care-of-the-Self, and ensuring the quality of nursing care provided to older people and their families [7, 8].

2 Methods

2.1 Identifying the Research Question

The research question was formulated according to the Population, Concept and Context (PCC) terminology: What are the characteristics presented at age-friendly health care units in primary health care settings?

The aim of this research is to analyze and map the knowledge produced about the characteristics of age-friendly primary health care, intending to answer the following questions:

- What are the characteristics of age-friendly primary health care centers identified in the studies?
- How do they correspond to the WHO recommendations?

2.2 Research Strategy

The search was conducted on the EBSCOhost and Virtual Health Library platforms, in the databases: Cinahl Complete, Medline Complete, Cochrane Central Register of Controlled Trials and Cochrane Database of Systematic Reviews, MedicLatina, Nursing &

Allied Health Collection: Comprehensive, LILACS and BDENF, with application of temporal filter starting in 2004. The identification, exclusion and eligibility of articles were carried out in different phases, taking into account the previously defined inclusion and exclusion criteria. The search terms defined (Table 1) were grouped using Boolean operators, derived from the indexed language for the search in electronic databases.

The first phase of the search took place on May 8th, 2020, using the indexed language specific to each platform. Then, the results were sorted according to their relevance to the research question. In the last phase, the selected articles were manually analyzed in order to extract the relevant information to the research question.

Table 1. Research terms

		Natural language	Indexed language
Population	Older person Aged 60 or over, as recommended by the WHO and in terms of developed and developing countries	Older person Older adult	Aged; Aged 80 and over Frail Elderly
	Family members/ informal caregivers	Informal caregivers Family caregivers	Caregivers
Context	Primary healthcare		Primary Care Nursing; Primary Health Care; Health Services for the Aged; Community Health Services
Concept	Age-friendly	Age-friendly health care; Age-friendly	

2.3 Inclusion Criteria

In this study, we included the articles involved older adults living in the community and excluded the studies conducted in hospital settings. The search terms, the inclusion and exclusion criteria (Table 2) were defined after reading the studies resulting from an empirical search in the main databases of the ESBCOhost platform on this topic.

2.4 Selection of Articles

The selection of studies was performed by two independent researchers, after analyzing the abstract of each article, keeping in mind the inclusion and exclusion criteria and the research objectives. The selection of articles to be included in this scoping review followed four steps: Identification, Analysis, Eligibility, and Inclusion. In the databases, 56

Table 2. Inclusion and exclusion criteria for the articles identified in the search

Inclusion Criteria				Exclusion criteria
Population	Concept	Context	Publishing Language	
Older people (aged 60 and over) and family caregivers	Age-friendly health services	Primary health care (health centers and community care units)	Articles in Portuguese, English and/or Spanish	- Studies carried out in Hospitals - Articles about activities developed in hospital units

articles were identified, from which 7 articles were excluded, 4 in Mandarin language, 1 systematic review, 1 integrative review, and 1 repeated article. After reading the abstracts and applying the inclusion criteria, 30 articles were selected, but only 22 articles were included in our study (review) after the full text analysis.

2.5 Reviewing Process

The data extracted from the analyzed articles were presented in a table, following the Joanna Briggs Institute [9] methodology for scoping review. The analysis of the relevance of the articles as well as the extraction and synthesis of the data were performed by two independent reviewers.

2.6 Presentation of Data

The data collected from each article presented in Table 3, according to study reference, study population, context, type of study, objectives and WHO recommendations [1].

3 Results

After the analysis of the articles listed in the table above, we grouped the characteristics of the age-friendly health centers (AFHCs) into 7 main themes to characterize them:

1- Information, education, and communication: To guarantee an efficient communication, professionals have the responsibility to gather all the specific technical competences to respond to the needs of the older adults and their families, demonstrating communicational abilities, voluntarism, and availability, not practicing ageism [10–12, 14, 15]. Technological resources are used to expedite the transmission of information, for scheduling appointments and identifying needs [15]. The use of uniforms and badges, by all members of the team, is indispensable, so that all the users know to whom they should go [3]. Information regarding the medication regimen is essential to avoid any errors or pharmacological interactions [16]. Improving the health of the older adults involves health education and promotion of healthy lifestyles, appropriate to their individuality, adopting the partnership model of care.

Table 3. Data extraction grid

Study	- Population - Context of the Study - Type of Study/Article	Objectives of the Study	Characteristics/focus in age-friendly health centers as recommended by the WHO
Woo et al. [3]	-Older people, both sexes (>60 years old) -Community (primary care) -Qualitative	Assessing the adequacy of primary health care to the needs of older people in Hong Kong	Accessibility: easy access; public transportation Signage: suitable for all users Physical environment: suitable for people with different needs and new users Consultation / Information Process: All issues are solved in one interaction. There is no long wait Care management system / fees: reasonable fees Training / knowledge dissemination: through government social media platforms
Pelaez & Rice. [10]	-Older people -Community (primary care) -Qualitative	Define the role of primary health care in promoting healthy aging	Care management system: policies of inclusion of the older adults in the community; combating ageism; flexible retirement projects; continuation of social roles Communication: Health Professionals have specific geriatric knowledge, management, analytical and communication skills Training: Health professionals with specific training in geriatrics
Hoontrakul et al. [11]	-Older people (age > 60 years) -Primary care Case study	Developing age-friendly primary health care in a primary care unit	The basic health unit has reorganized its service to meet the needs of its population, with emphasis on professional culture and attitude, medical biology, and knowledge about aging and care of the older people

(continued)

Table 3. *(continued)*

Study	- Population - Context of the Study - Type of Study/Article	Objectives of the Study	Characteristics/focus in age-friendly health centers as recommended by the WHO
Kuo et al. [12]	-Older people, both genders ($\geq$65 years old) -Community (primary care) -Qualitative	Assessing the quality of outpatient services for older people in Taiwan	Care Management System: Professionalism and availability; Robustness and consistency in operationalizing policies and procedures Communication: Good communication skills of all staff Training: Periodic training of employees Physical space: adequate to the older people
Fulmer & Li. [13]	-Older people, Elderly people with dementia (> 65 years) and family -Health care system in the United States of America (different levels of care) -Qualitative	Identify the characteristics of a more effective, age-friendly health care system to prevent readmissions and avoidable health care expenditures, as well as improve the quality of care	The Age Friendly Health Systems model emphasizes the training of patients and family caregivers and focuses on four key aspects to meet their needs: 1. what is most important to the person (communication skills) 2. mobility 3. medication 4. mental activity
Ssensamba et al. [14]	-Older people, both genders ($\geq$60 years old) -Community (primary care) -Quantitative Descriptive cross-sectional study	Determine the preparedness of Uganda's health care system to meet the needs of geriatric, age-friendly health care	Training: health professionals with special training in geriatrics Physical environment: infrastructure appropriate to the needs of the older people and close to the community; equipment to assist in activities of daily living Care process: Updated health policies, incorporating WHO guidelines; geriatric assessment scales applied
Motsohi et al. [15]	-Older people, both genders (>60 years old) -Community (primary attention) -Qualitative	Evaluation of the experience of older people in two health centers, and the gaps in care provided in the two settings	Communication / Information: Innovative methods to address gaps in information transmission Access: Health services should be reliable, easily accessible, older people should have faster access to health services

(continued)

Table 3. (*continued*)

Study	- Population - Context of the Study - Type of Study/Article	Objectives of the Study	Characteristics/focus in age-friendly health centers as recommended by the WHO
Cheung et al. [16]	- Older people and vulnerable groups -Hospital outpatient consultation and home visits in community settings -Interviews	Assess the difficulties and problems of equity in accessing health services, as well as how health policies can contribute to change the whole community	Involve nurses' representatives in the governmental discussion on health policies Pharmaceutical care: based on the needs of the older person Specialized care: equitable coverage of the country with specialists in different areas
Alhamdan et al. [17]	-Older people, both sexes (>60 years old) -Community (primary attention) -Qualitative Descriptive cross-sectional study	-Assess primary health care provided to older people in Riyadh; -Make it easier for older people to use health centers	Physical environment - accessibility and the structural conditions of the building where they are provided Signage/Information: clear and distinct indications for people with sensory deficits Counseling for healthy lifestyles / Education: specific to the age group and individualized to the needs of each older person
Ricciardi et al. [18]	-Older people/ community -Primary care -Descriptive study	Establish how health and social systems can be sustainable in Europe	The study brings up the need for investment in prevention measures for the control of chronic diseases, since these are responsible for expenses and burdens on local health systems
Petersen et al. [19]	-Older people, both genders (>60 years) -Community -Quantitative	Assess the oral hygiene conditions of older people, including professional use and Care-of-the-Self	Care process: the multidisciplinary team should be involved in the oral health approach to create a complete and detailed oral hygiene care plan;
Lin et al. [20]	Older people, both sexes (≥65 years) Community (primary care) Qualitative	Analyze the impacts of an aging population on Taipei's society	Care Management: Health professionals have a holistic view of the older person, identifying all their needs; Communication between health and social services Training: Development of specific training for health professionals in geriatrics

(*continued*)

Table 3. (*continued*)

Study	- Population - Context of the Study - Type of Study/Article	Objectives of the Study	Characteristics/focus in age-friendly health centers as recommended by the WHO
Liggett et al. [21]	-Older people in the community and in hospital services -Primary care -Descriptive study	Developing an age-friendly system of care to meet the needs of the older population, integrating care after hospital discharge	The integration between all levels of care constitutes a system where the older person goes through "stages" of consultation, from investigation with nurses to care or hospitalization. This is expected to improve care and efficiency, from arrival at the hospital to post-discharge follow-up
Dalmer [22]	-Older people and Family Caregivers -Community setting -Home setting -Ethnographic Study	Assessing whether the work of caring for an older person who stays at home is recognized: "aging at home"	Ageing at home policies, which aim at the importance of older people's choice of where they want to grow old, taking into account access to services and support for their needs. Information is vital, and there is a connection between it and the ability to be a resource
Lee et al. [23]	-Older people, both genders ($\geq$65 years old) -Community -Quantitative Descriptive cross-sectional study	To evaluate the index of community services and health services from the perspective of older people living in Siheung	Care management systems: people should remain in their homes, with home support from all necessary services. Primary health care should provide nursing assessment at the older person's home and intervention to address identified needs
John & Gunter. [24]	-Older population in rural and urban settings, residents in the city of Oregon, USA -Mixed method (quantitative and qualitative)	Finding out how various factors influence, the population's perception of living in an age-friendly community, in rural and urban settings	The "senior-friendly" model is represented as a flower with 8 petals: Transportation; Housing; Social participation; Respect and social inclusion; Civic participation and employment; Communication and information; Community support and health services; Outdoor spaces; and Buildings - all of which are influenced by the physical and social environment and existing services

(*continued*)

Table 3. (*continued*)

Study	- Population - Context of the Study - Type of Study/Article	Objectives of the Study	Characteristics/focus in age-friendly health centers as recommended by the WHO
Doolan-Noble et al. [25]	-Older people, both genders (≥65 years old) -Community (primary care) -Quantitative	Describe the process of funding priorities for healthy aging in New Zealand	Training: The area of age-friendly communities needs more investment if its implementation is to become a social benefit for older people Physical environment: physical accessibility facilitated; availability of transportation to accommodate varying needs
Hancock et al. [26]	-Older people of both genders (>65 years old), family members and caregivers -Community (primary care) -Qualitative	To understand how older people in rural areas maintain their health and well-being, according to the eight domains defined by the WHO, in the town of Wangaratta	Care Management: Equitable distribution of resources Physical Environment: Accessible transportation adapted to restrictions, maintaining autonomy; Accessibility to all areas of public interest Promotion of Care-of-the-Self: Older people are supported in maintaining their independence, cognitive stimulation, and emotional balance
Lehning et al. [27]	-Older people living in Detroit -Community -Systematic review	To examine the association between measures of age-friendly environmental character and self-rated health in a sample of older people in Detroit, Michigan	The study analyses look at the characteristics of the physical environments in which the older adults in Detroit live, and how this influences their self-assessment and perception of their health
Jiang et al. [28]	-Population: 30 older people (65 and older) 30 professionals - Context: 2 rural areas 2 urban areas Method: Qualitative	Identify and prioritize the factors that facilitate behavioral change, such as behavioral settings for nutrition in older people based on the social ecological model	The World Health Organization's Age-Friendly Cities project presents models for communities to promote successful aging in eight domains. This study focuses on the nutritional component of the older population and the role of communities in providing adequate meals for older people

(*continued*)

Table 3. *(continued)*

Study	- Population - Context of the Study - Type of Study/Article	Objectives of the Study	Characteristics/focus in age-friendly health centers as recommended by the WHO
Rahman & Byles. [29]	-Female older adults -Health care centers/residential care homes -Longitudinal study	To examine whether home and community-based care use and characteristics of older people relate to time to admission to Residential Structures for Older People	It is important at a certain point in adult life, particularly in the last years of life, to reside in specific facilities for the older adults (care / nursing homes), which can meet the needs that are not met by community care services for this population
Smith et al. [30]	-Older people, (>60 years old), mostly African-American from the city of Detroit -Age-Friendly Community -Exploratory	Measuring the environmental, social and physical characteristics of an age-friendly community	Age-friendly communities must have: -Access to business and leisure -Social interaction -Scarce neighborhood problems -Community involvement -Transportation -Public services accessible to older adults

2- *Health care management systems:* AFHC offer a complete, multifactorial assessment of the individuals' needs, are responsible for having the resources available to support the development of their activities of daily living, provide all consultations, treatment, and complementary diagnostic tests so that all needs are met in a single visit, and resolve the problems of older people in a timely manner. [3, 12, 14, 17]. There is investment in chronic disease prevention and oral health care, avoiding long-term health system overload and achieving health gains [18, 19]. The articulation between public and private health care and between primary and differentiated health care is effective, and timely communication between all is ensured to improve the service provided to the older people and their families [20, 21].
3- *Care management process considering most common geriatric syndromes:* Nursing care and assistance with basic life activities are provided at the older person's home, avoiding their institutionalization (unless this is their wish). Family members are considered part of the holistic dimension of the older person's well-being and a target of care [22]. Health care professionals should provide health education, geriatric assessment, and an individualized care plan focused on health promotion, disease prevention, maintenance of autonomy and meaningful social interactions [17, 23]. It is important to understand the interaction between the person's characteristics and the context in which they live, as well as how these are involved in their aging process [24].
4- Physical environment: When the AFHC are implemented near the community they serves, facilitates accessibility to the building in which care is provided, reducing the need for travel [14, 25]. Access to the exterior areas and to the interior of the building is facilitated and adapted to people with reduced mobility (parking spaces, access ramps); the circulation areas, waiting rooms, offices and bathrooms have ample structures that

facilitate circulation with wheelchairs or other walking aid devices and/or the presence of a companion, are lit adequately, adapted for a safe circulation; the identification signs of the user circuit are visible, lit adequately, written with high contrast and also available in Braille [3, 11, 14, 17, 26]. In short, the physical space of the AFHC should be adapted to the specific needs of its public [12].

5- *Transportation network:* Age-friendly communities (AFHCs) offer good public transportation options that are adapted to the needs of the older adults, such as the use of oxygen tanks, walking aids, and are affordable, allowing the presence of a companion [3, 17, 25, 26]. Drivers of these services should take into account the population they transport thus adapting their driving style (avoid sudden braking, wait for people to be sat down before starting to drive) [3].

6- *Keeping older adults in their own context:* Maintaining residence in their home, or at least in their community, during the aging process is a factor that increases the quality of life of older people and their families [22, 27]. The use of home support from multidisciplinary teams and volunteer programs that ensure the psychological, cognitive, social, health, and well-being needs are met as well as support structures such as supermarkets, hairdressers, dry cleaners, etc. that allow older adults to maintain their autonomy [23, 24, 28]. However, the older person should be allowed to leave their home if they wish, and the community should provide those answers [29]. Residential care or nursing facilities for the older adults are established in the communities where older adults live, allowing them to remain in a familiar environment [14, 25]. AFHCs offer access to business and leisure, social interaction, good neighborhood, community involvement, transportation networks and public services [30].

7- *Health Policies*: Legislative bodies define policies that enable the active, productive and successful aging of their population, promoting self-sufficiency and independence of each older person, reducing age-related stigma, integrating active older people into the community [10, 14, 19, 22]. Health professionals, through their institutional representatives, contribute to the discussion of health policies and, to the improvement older adults' quality of life [16]. The government is responsible for the equitable distribution of resources and the creation of emergency plans, the definition of social and economic policies to protect older people in their access to financially viable and long-term housing, and the development of flexible retirement plans [10, 23, 26]. Research on aging and AFHCs are stimulated, and the result of these studies should be implemented in practice as soon as possible [19, 25].

4 Discussion

The results of this study are consistent with those defined by the WHO [5] and add further complementary guidelines for the identification of AFHCs. Regarding information, education and communication, there is evidence that shortcomings continue to occur, namely that older people feel that they are not heard. It has been found that health services often do not provide the quality of care expected by citizens [14]. From the point of view of the health care management system, some studies have shown that services are poorly prepared to meet the specific needs of older people, due to a lack of coordination of all actors involved in decision making, from public funding to human resource management, leadership, political decision-making and structural conditions [14]. The emergency and comprehensive assessment systems of older adults do not meet their real needs and should be improved and implemented effectively [23]. The physical environment is widely explored by the literature reviewed, identifying shortcomings such as: insufficient and inadequate public transportation to meet the needs of the older adults, namely, the access to their appointments, treatments and examinations; sidewalks too narrow and busy, constituting an added danger for people with altered mobility [3, 26]. The inequities in the resources available to the rural and urban population are often discussed, making it difficult for older adults to stay at home. Moreover, the level of interaction with the surrounding community varies according to factors such as gender, ethnicity, economic and social status, and level of education [30]. As for the issue of health policies, it is evidenced the responsibility of national and municipal governments to expedite the best practices, offer technical conditions and manage the process of making institutions and cities friendly to the older adults [16].

Throughout this review, we could conclude that this is a topic that raises global interest and that has been discussed since 2002, when the WHO published "Active Ageing: a policy framework". Despite not being a recent theme, studies have indicated that there is still much to be done regarding the primary health care providing to the older adults and their families their real needs. Moreover, a repeated recommendation in many of the articles analyzed here is the dissemination of age-friendly practices in these health care institutions [3, 14, 15, 17].

The contribution of gerontotechnology to improve health responses to the needs of the older adults is implicit in the analyzed articles, demonstrating that many of the means that are already available to health professionals can be better used to respond more effectively to the older population that uses health care services. However, this issue cannot be solved by direct care alone, which is why health professionals must have a voice in policymaking, research, and training [3, 10, 12, 14, 16, 19]. Coordination of all health professionals and administrative staff is needed, as well as political involvement, not only from the Ministry of Health, but from the whole government that should prioritize the issue of age-friendly institutions and communities.

5 Conclusion

The complexity of older adults' health care is a challenge for health workers, and it is increasingly important to constantly update knowledge to improve practices and meet the real needs and expectations of older people and their families. Nurses play a key role and should adapt their interventions to the specific needs of these individuals, namely using gerontotechnology to promote their holistic care and contributing to a sustainable health [6, 31]. In line with the strategy defined by the WHO, a new strategy to provide care to the older adults is necessary and pertinent, in which health promotion and disease management are privileged as opposed to an approach centered on cure. In the approach centered on the older person and their family members living in the community and guided by their life project, nurses should work in partnership with them, helping to manage their health process, contributing to their safety, continuity of care, and active and healthy aging, besides promoting Care-of-the-Self [7, 8].

It is hoped that this scoping review will contribute to knowledge regarding the characteristics of age friendly health centers, to critical analysis in this area, regarding to what is recommended by the WHO, and will allow us to understand the impact of age-friendly health centers on the promotion Care-of-the-Self for the older adults.

References

1. World Health Organization (2020): Decade of healthy ageing: baseline report. Geneve
2. Fonseca, C., De Pinho, G., Lopes, M., Marques, C., Garcia-Alonso, J.: The elderly nursing core set and the cognition of Portuguese older adults: a cross-sectional study. BMC Nurs. **20**(1), 1–8 (2021)
3. Woo, J., Mak, B., Yeung, F.: Age-friendly primary health care: an assessment of current service provision for older adults in Hong Kong. Health Serv. Insights **6**, 69–77 (2013)
4. Abdellatif, T., et al.: Dubai primary health care centers conformation to WHO age-friendly primary healthcare recommendations. Adv. Aging Res. **6**, 83–92 (2017). https://www.scirp.org/pdf/AAR_2017101015355625.pdf
5. World Health Organization (2004): Towards Age-friendly Primary Health Care. Geneve. http://apps.who.int/iris/bitstream/handle/10665/43030/9241592184.pdf;jsessionid=D8ECD3EB64580751EC38DD787ECA9571?sequence=1
6. Graafmans, J.: The history and incubation of gerontechnology. Gerontechnology **1**(1), 3–11 (2016). https://doi.org/10.1891/9780826128898.0001
7. Gomes, I.: To Promote self-care: a partnership between the nurse and the elderly person. The construction of the partnership process in a context of vulnerability and dependency. New scholarly editions, Saarbrucken/Deutsche (2016)
8. Gomes, I.: Partnership of care in the promotion of the care-of-the-self: an implementation guide with elderly people. In: García-Alonso, J., Fonseca, C. (eds.) Gerontechnology III. IWoG 2020. Lecture Notes in Bioengineering. Springer, Cham (2021). https://doi.org/10.1007/978-3-030-72567-9_32
9. Peters, M., Godfrey, C., McInerney, P., Khalil, H., Parker, D.: The Joanna Briggs Institute Reviewers' Manual 2015 - Methodology for JBI Scoping Reviews. The Joanna Briggs Institute (2015). https://nursing.lsuhsc.edu/JBI/docs/ReviewersManuals/Scoping-.pdf
10. Pelaez, M., Rice, M.: Primary health care and aging: edited proceedings of the consultative group meeting on geriatric training in primary health care. Calif. J. Health Promot. **2**(3), 99–108 (2004). https://doi.org/10.32398/cjhp.v2i3.884
11. Hoontrakul, D., Sritanyarat, W., Nuntaboot, K., Premgamone, A.: Development of age-friendly primary health care: case study of one primary care unit. Thai J. Nurs. Res. **12**(2), 131–141 (2008)
12. Kuo, R., Wu, Y., Hsu, T., Chen, L.: Improving outpatient services for elderly patients in Taiwan: a qualitative study. Arch. Gerontol. Geriatr. **53**(2), e209–e217 (2011). https://doi.org/10.1016/j.archger.2010.09.013
13. Fulmer, T., Li, N.: Age-friendly health systems for older adults with dementia. J. Nurse Pract. **14**(3), 160–165 (2018). https://doi.org/10.1016/j.nurpra.2017.09.001
14. Ssensamba, J., Mukuru, M., Nakafeero, M., Ssenyonga, R., Kiwanuka, S.: Health systems readiness to provide geriatric friendly care services in Uganda: a cross-sectional study. BMC Geriatr. **19**(256), 1–13 (2019). https://doi.org/10.1186/s12877-019-1272-2
15. Motsohi, T., Namane, M., Anele, A., Abbas, M., Kalula, S.: Older persons' experience with health care at two primary level clinics in Cape Town, South Africa: a qualitative assessment. BJGP Open **4**(3), 1–9 (2020). https://doi.org/10.3399/bjgpopen20X101048

16. Cheung, B., Felfeli, T., Sorouri, K., Zewude, R.: The national seniors strategy: an opportunity for sustaining a healthy future for the aging population. Univ. Toronto Med. J. **93**(1), 18–21 (2015). ISSN: 1913–5440
17. Alhamdan, A., Alshammari, S., Al-Amoud, M., et al.: Evaluation of health care services provided for older adults in primary health care centers and its internal environment: a step towards age-friendly health centers. Saudi Med. J. **36**(9), 1091–1096 (2015). https://doi.org/10.15537/smj.2015.9.11789
18. Ricciardi, W., Specchia, M., Marino, M.: Health of the elderlies and healthy aging: a challenge for Europe. Active Ageing Healthy Living **1**(1), 1–9 (2014). https://doi.org/10.3233/978-1-61499-425-1-1
19. Petersen, P., Kandelman, D., Arpin, S., Ogawa, H.: Global oral health of older people - call for public health action. Community Dent. Health **27**(2), 257–268 (2010). https://doi.org/10.1922/CDH
20. Lin, M., Chou, M., Liang, C., Peng, L., Chen, L.: Population aging and its impacts: strategies of the health-care system in Taipei. Ageing Res. Rev. **9**(SUPPL.), S23–S27 (2010). https://doi.org/10.1016/j.arr.2010.07.004
21. Liggett, A., McKoy, M., Bradley, S., O'Brien, K., Dobschuetz, D., Lindquist, L.: Creating an age-friendly health system: lessons learned for the post-acute care setting. Jamda **21**, B17–B18 (2020).https://doi.org/10.1016/j.jamda.2020.01.053
22. Dalmer, N.: A logic of choice: problematizing the documentary reality of Canadian aging in place policies. J. Aging Stud. **48**(1), 40–49 (2019). https://doi.org/10.1016/j.jaging.2019.01.002
23. Lee, C., Cho, B., Cho, Y., Park, Y.: Older adults' perceptions of age-friendliness with an emphasis on community supports and health services in a city in South Korea. J. Korean Acad. Community Health Nurs. **30**(2), 234–242 (2019). https://doi.org/10.12799/jkachn.2019.30.2.234
24. John, D., Gunter, K.: EngAGE in community: using mixed methods to mobilize older people to elucidate the age-friendly attributes of urban and rural places. J. Appl. Gerontol. **35**(10), 1–26 (2015). https://doi.org/10.1177/0733464814566679
25. Doolan-Noble, F., Mehta, P., Waters, D., Baxter, G.: Supporting ageing well research: findings from a research priority setting exercise. Australas. J. Ageing **38**(2), 136–143 (2018). https://doi.org/10.1111/ajag.12615
26. Hancock, S., Winterton, R., Wilding, C., Blackberry, I.: Understanding ageing well in Australian rural and regional settings: applying an age-friendly lens. Aust. J. Rural Health **27**(4), 298–303 (2018)
27. Lehning, A., Smith, R., Dunkle, R.: Age-friendly environments and self-rated health: an exploration of Detroit elders. Res. Aging **36**(1), 1–9 (2014). https://doi.org/10.1177/0164027512469214
28. Jiang, Q., Cohen, N., Marra, M., Woolf, K., Gilbride, J., Francis, S.: Community priorities for healthy eating in older adults. J. Nutrition Gerontol. Geriatr. **36**(2–3), 75–91 (2017). https://doi.org/10.1080/21551197.2017.1365039
29. Rahman, M., Byles, J.: Older women's patterns of home and community care use and transition to residential aged care: an Australian cohort study. Maturitas **131**(1), 28–33 (2020). https://doi.org/10.1016/j.maturitas.2019.10.004
30. Smith, R., Lehning, A., Dunkle, R.: Conceptualizing age-friendly community characteristics in a sample of urban elders: an exploratory factor analysis. J. Gerontol. Soc. Work **56**(2), 90–111 (2013). https://doi.org/10.1117/12.2549369
31. Goes, M., Lopes, M., Oliveira, H., Fonseca, C., Marôco, J.: A nursing care intervention model for elderly people to ascertain general profiles of functionality and selfcare needs. Sci. Rep. **10**(1), 1–11 (2020)

Preparing the Return Home of a Person After a Hip Arthroplasty - Capacitation for a Safe Transition

Célia Nicolau[1], Mário Ciríaco[1], Bruno Ferreira[2], Rogério Ferreira[3], Cristina Lavareda Baixinho[4,5], and Luís de Sousa[5(✉)]

[1] Hospital of Litoral Alentejo, Santiago do Cacém, Portugal
[2] Beatriz Ângelo Hospital, Loures, Portugal
[3] Polytechnic Institute of Beja, Beja, Portugal
[4] Nursing School of Lisbon, Nursing Research, Innovation and Development Centre of Lisbon (CIDNUR), Center for Innovative Care and Health Technology (ciTechcare), Leiria, Portugal
[5] Comprehensive Health Research Centre (CHRC), University of Évora, Evora, Portugal
lmms@uevora.pt

Abstract. With a person's natural aging, the prevalence of degenerative diseases increases, including the inflammation or trauma of the acetabulofemoral articulation, case in which the hip arthroplasty is the most successful response. In this context, rehabilitation nursing makes it possible to empower and capacitate the person and their family, increasing their functional capacity, diminishing their dependence for self-care, and contributing for a safe transition home. The objective od this study is to evaluate the gains in health from a program of nursing rehabilitation interventions to prepare the return home of people who underwent hip arthroplasty. The multiple-case study methodology was used, based on Orem's Nursing Theory and Meleis's Transition Theory. The participants were people who had undergone hip arthroplasty due to fractures or arthrosis and accepted participating in the rehabilitation program after it was explained to them. A rehabilitation nursing intervention was implemented with them, and the training results for the person's self-care were evaluated. The knowledge they acquired was also assessed. The evaluation carried out at admission, after surgery and on the day of discharge showed improvements in the functionality of the person, also indicating that they acquired knowledge about their situation, showing gains in health that are related to the rehabilitation nursing care. There was an improvement in functionality, capacity and in empowering the people who underwent a hip arthroplasty and their families.

Keywords: Rehabilitation nursing · Empowering · Hip arthroplasty · Continuity of patient care

1 Introduction

The phenomenon of aging brings with it numerous anatomical and physiological which contribute to the increase in the prevalence of chronic diseases and, consequently, to the

J. García-Alonso and C. Fonseca (Eds.): IWoG 2021, LNBE, pp. 108–120, 2022.
https://doi.org/10.1007/978-3-030-97524-1_11

increase of people in a situation of dependence. The alterations that most contribute to this increase affect the vestibular, visual, cardiovascular, musculoskeletal, skeletal, and central nervous systems, which, besides causing a greater risk of falling and functional disability, also constitute one of the most common causes of chronic pain and fatigue [1, 2].

Similarly, the joint structures and cartilage wear and tear caused by degenerative diseases, such as arthrosis, is the main cause of incapacity among elderly, affecting vital joints for functionality, such as those in the hand, knee, hip, spine, and foot [3].

Fractures in the proximal femur, which are generally consequences of falls, also contribute to the loss of independence in mobility and functional disability in the various activities of daily life (ADL), with high morbidity and mortality levels [4].

These orthopedic pathologies are the main causes of significant impairments in joint function. In this context, hip arthroplasty emerges as an important surgical intervention with the potential for functional recovery of people with such problems, contributing to the improvement of pain, mobility and autonomy, and functional independence in performing ADL, thus allowing for an improve in quality of life [1].

To minimize this dependency and functional disability, it is extremely important to early identify the real needs of the person in a health/disease situation, so as to develop an effective rehabilitation intervention. Family involvement allows for the continuity of a set of planned-care actions, initiated and maintained during hospitalization, thus promoting the adaptation to the new reality of care [5].

The Specialist Nurse in Rehabilitation Nursing (SNRN) is the key element in the rehabilitation process, having the relevant competences, and being present during the hospitalization and reinsertion into home and community, being able to assess the person and the family's abilities, as well as their economic and time availability, so as to help make the best decisions and ensure continuity of care [4]. On the other hand, the development of advanced nursing care is a challenge to the development of the competences of master's degree nurses' skills to plan, implement, and evaluate care, dealing with complex health-disease transitions and in different clinical practice environments.

Thus, nurses should ensure that the person and family leave the hospital well prepared and supported, enabling a good articulation and communication between professionals, caregivers, and health services [6].

The objective of this multiple case study was to evaluate the gains in health from a program of nursing rehabilitation interventions to prepare the return home of people who underwent hip arthroplasty.

2 Methodology

The methodological strategy used was the case study, consisting of a more detailed examination of a phenomenon related to an individual, family or group. This detailed examination may be of a single situation at a given moment or of its evolution over a period, in which case the objective is to increase the knowledge or studying the changes produced through time in an individual or group [7]. The case study can be classified into single-case or multiple-case study. In the latter, there is the involved of more cases and presents as an advantage providing a more robust study [8]. Here, we chose to include eight cases, which has the advantage of generating a more consistent study with regard to the evidence found. The stages for the development of this type of study are: Stage 1 - Definition and elaboration of the project; Stage 2 - Data collection and analysis; Stage 3 - Analyzing and concluding [8].

Stage 1 defined the purpose of the study and how data would be collected, defining the scales that will be used. Based on the question "What is the effect of a rehabilitation nursing intervention program on the empowerment and capacitation of a person who underwent a hip arthroplasty for a safe return home?", the scales used were: Mini-Mental State Examination (MMSE), Function Independence Measure Scale (FIM), Medical Research Council Scale (MRC), Timed Up and Go test, and Numerical Pain Rating Scale, and goniometry assessment, in addition to the list to verify the knowledge acquired.

An informal interview was carried out with the person and their caregiver at the moment of admission, sociodemographic data and the health/disease conditions were collected, on a spreadsheet elaborated for that purpose, as well as the consultation data from clinical files.

A checklist of the topics addressed in the educational intervention was applied to assess the gains in knowledge. The checklist included 16 items and the knowledge acquired in respiratory and motor functional reeducation was evaluated. In terms of respiratory functional reeducation, the knowledge about exercises of awareness and control of breathing, abdomen-diaphragm breathing, costal reeducation, and directed and assisted cough. Regarding motor functional reeducation, the knowledge of position in bed, exercises to be performed lying down, getting up from bed, sitting down and getting up from chair, using the shower/bath and toilet, gait training with walking aid and crutches, going up and down stairs, getting in and out of a car and prevention of prosthesis dislocation were assessed. This was applied on admission, on the day after surgery and on the day of discharge as well as the remaining assessment tools.

On Stage 2, data was collected, and an individual report was elaborated for each of the eight participants.

On Stage 3 the cases were analyzed individually, and later, an analysis was performed with cross-referencing of the data in total [8].

The nursing foci defined were: the ability of performing ADLs, body balance, muscle strength, pain, and articular amplitude, all individually assessed.

The participants were selected according to the following criteria: having been submitted to hip arthroplasty from March to May 2021, regardless the etiology and accepting to participate in the rehabilitation program after receiving adequate explanations.

The sample only included eight people, due to the pandemic and the gradual resuming of scheduled surgeries. The rehabilitation program was shown to the participants, and the informed consent form was delivered and signed by the person and the main investigator, each of whom kept a copy, in accordance with ethical principles.

To evaluate the cognitive function at the time of admission, the Mini-Mental State Examination (MMSE) was also, and the score for exclusion was calculated considering their educational level, as proposed by Morgado et al. [9].

For this study several data collection instruments were used: Mini-Mental State Examination (MMSE), Function Independence Measure Scale (FIM), Medical Research

Council Scale (MRC), TUG (Timed Up and Go) test, Numerical Pain Rating Scale, and Goniometry.

An informal interview and a consultation of the clinical process of each person were also used for data collection.

To evaluate the cognitive function we used the Mini-Mental State Examination Test, which consists of 2 parts, with a total score of 30 points [9]. The scores proposed by Morgado et al. [9] were used, since they take into consideration the educational level. Patients who had from 0 to 2 years formal education were included when score $\geq$22; from 3 to 6 years, when $\geq$24; and those with more than 7 years of formal education, when the score was $\geq$27 [9].

The ability to perform ADLs was assessed using the Function Independence Measure Scale (FIM), which evaluates the level of functional independence of the person where each item receives a score from 1 to 7 and the total score varies from 18 to 126. The lower the score, the greater the dependence, and the highest the score, the greater the independence [10].

Muscle strength was evaluated using the Medical Research Council Scale (MRC), which quantifies strength between 0 and 5 [10]. The Timed Up and Go test (TUG) was used to assess mobility, balance, capacity of walking/stability when walking, and the risk for falling by measuring the time of performance of the test, in seconds.

A time equal to 10' or less indicates a good performance for healthy adults and a low risk for falls; time between 10.1' to 20' indicates a normal performance for frail elderly and those with some disability, but who are independent for most ADLs, indicating some risk for fall; time between 21' to 29' requires a mandatory functional assessment and a specific approach on falls risk, as they present a moderate falls risk; a time equal or greater than 30' indicates a high risk of falls [10].

Pain was assessed using the Numerical Pain Rating Scale. This is a ruler divided in 11 equal parts, each numbered from 0 to 10, corresponding 0 to "no pain" and 10 to "maximum pain", being the pain of maximum intensity imaginable [11].

A goniometer was used to assess the articulation range, as it is an instrument used to measure the flexion and extension range of articulation movements from the segments of the articulation [10].

Sociodemographic data collection was performed, namely age, gender, marital status, family unit/caregiver, educational level, personal/surgical history, profession/occupation, surgery to be performed, as well as vital signs evaluation. The knowledge of the participants was evaluated using a checklist elaborated with this goal in mind and filled in by the participant, according with the surgery the patient would go through and with the necessary post-operative care.

The scales were applied in three different moments: admission, day after the surgery, and day of discharge, adapting the rehabilitation interventions according to person's needs.

To carry out the analysis, the Excel® spreadsheet were imported into the software Statistical Package for the Social Sciences (SPSS), version 24.0 using descriptive and inferential statistical techniques. For descriptive statistics, central tendency and dispersion measures were used (mean and standard deviation, median and interquartile range) and absolute (n) and relative (%) frequencies. For inferential statistics the Wilcoxon

Signed Ranks test was used to compare the continuous variables at the three moments of evaluation. A significance level adopted was 95% ($p \leq 0.05$).

Each person was identified with a number, and the instrument to record the assessment and interventions had no information to identify the person in the sample.

All participants were informed about the interventions and objectives of the study so they could provide a free and informed consent. In all stages of the study, the anonymity of the participants was ensured, and their choices and interests were respected.

The application of the project was approved by the Ethics Committee of the Hospital, and its application was authorized.

3 Results

From the sample comprised mostly males, with a mean age of 72.13, a minimum of 57 and a maximum of 89 years old (Table 1).

Table 1. Sociodemographic and health characterization of the sample

Participants	Case 1	Case 2	Case 3	Case 4	Case 5	Case 6	Case 7	Case 8
Gender	Male	Male	Male	Female	Female	Female	Male	Male
Age	75	76	57	76	66	89	79	59
Marital status	Married	Widower	Divorced	Married	Married	Widow	Married	Single
Educational level	5th grade	5th grade	5th grade	High school	Illiterate	Illiterate	5th grade	3rd grade
Occupation	Retired	Retired	Truck driver	Retired	Farmer	Retired	Retired	Farmer driver
Personal history	BPH, HH	AH, RL, BPH	AH, diabetes	AH	Obesity	AH	AH, RL, diabetes,	AH,gout, cataract
Caregiver	Spouse and son	Daughter	Alone	Husband	Husband	Lives in a home	Spouse and son	Mother
MMSE	24	28	30	27	22	22	28	22

Legend: AH - Arterial Hypertension, BPH - Benign Prostatic Hyperplasia, HH – Hiatus Hernia; MMSE - Mini-Mental State Examination, RL – Renal Lithiasis.
Source: the author.

Most of the participants were married and had high school education, although they found writing very difficult being that 62.5% have education up to 5th grade and 25% are illiterate. The background of the patients was varied although most had hypertension.

The mean Mini Mental State Examination scores were 25.38, with a standard deviation of 3.249, a minimum of 22, and a maximum of 30. About 62.5% of the sample is male. Half of the sample (50%) is married, 12.5% is single, 12.5% is divorced, and 25% is widow/widower, regarding occupation, 62.5% of the sample are retired, 25% are heavy trucks drivers or agricultural machinery, and 12.% are agricultural workers.

The caregivers of 25% of the sample were their husbands/wives; 25% also mention a son; 25% have no informal caregiver, one of whom lives in a home, while another lives alone; 12.5% indicate a son or daughter as the only caregiver, and in one case (12.5%), the mother was (Table 1).

Table 2. Central tendency and dispersion measures of the variables at the three moments of the application of Wilcoxon's test

Measures	Preoperative (t1)		Immediate postoperative - 24 h (t2)		Day of discharge (t3)	
	M (SD)	Me (IQR)	M (SD)	Me (IQR)	M (SD)	Me (IQR)
Functional Independence Measure (18–126)	119.88 (8.39)	122 (8)	78.38 (7.78)	76.5 (10.25)	102.38 (7.78)	107 (19)
Timed Up and Go Test	24.84 (13.75)	20.18 (23.34)	–	–	75.75 (35.32)	58 (63)
Pain (0–10)	7.63 (1.77)	7.50 (3.25)	3.25 (1.28)	3.50 (1.75)	0.88 (0.64)	1.00 (0.75)
Acetabulofemoral articulation flexion strength (0–5)	2.86 (1.77)	4.00 (3.00)	2.88 (1.13)	3.00 (2.00)	3.75 (0.463)	4.00 (0.75)
Acetabulofemoral articulation flexion range	55.0 (10.80)	57.50 (20)	36.25 (7.906)	40.00 (8.75)	54.38 (7.76)	55.00 (10.00)
Knee articulation flexion range	120.0 (20.0)	130.00 (30.00)	78.13 (14.62)	80.00 (20.00)	116.25 (9.54)	117.50 (17.5)
Checklist of knowledge acquired (0–16)	2 (5.26)	0 (0.75)	9.50 (2.92)	9 (2)	15.9 (0.35)	16 (0)

Legend: M-Mean; Me – Median, SD - standard deviation; IQR - interquartile range.
Source: the author.

The functionality, as measured by the FIM scale, showed a decrease in the immediate post-operation period ($Z = -2.525$; $p = 0.012$), going back up at the time of discharge ($Z = -2.525$; $p = 0.012$); however, most members of the sample showed, at the time of discharge, values that were lower than those from the moment of hospitalization ($Z = -2.525$; $p = 0.012$).

The mean values of the TUG test in the pre-operative were inferior to the mean value at the moment of discharge, but the differences found were not significant ($Z = -1.841$; $p = 0.066$).

The mean self-reported pain in the pre-operative was 7.63 (1.77); in the post-op it decreased ($Z = -2.536$; $p = 0.011$), and at discharge was even lower ($Z = -2.539$; $p = 0.011$).

The muscle strength improved significantly from the immediate post-operative to the discharge ($Z = -2.121$; $p = 0.034$); the same can be said for the acetabulofemoral articulation range ($Z = -2.546$; $p = 0.011$) and the knee articulation flexion range ($Z = -2.527$; $p = 0.012$).

Before the surgery, people who were to undergo the hip arthroplasty had little knowledge. After the operation they had better knowledge, and at discharge, they had most of the knowledge in the checklist. There was a large improvement from the pre-operative to the post-operative ($Z = -2.530$; $p = 0.011$) and from the post-operative to the discharge ($Z = -2.388$; $p = 0.017$) (Table 2).

4 Discussion

Analazing the previous results, we can see a sample mostly composed by males (62.5% - 5 participants), with a mean age of 72.13 years old, with 50% being aged between 70–79 years, staying in line with the existing literature, according to which both arthrosis and fractures increase in incidence between 70 to 79 years old [12, 13].

Several comorbidities were also found, and arterial hypertension was common to 75% of the sample.

The total hip replacement with a prothesis was carried out for 87.5% of the sample participants, while 12.5% had a hemiarthroplasty. 50% were doing the surgery due to a prior arthrosis, while 50% due to falls fractures. Regarding the incidence per gender, although some authors indicate that the incidence of arthrosis is greater among females [14], most members of our sample were males.

The 37.5% of females are aged between 66 to 89 years old and are undergoing surgery due to fractures caused by falls, corroborating the literature which indicates that fractures in the higher extremity of the femur are more common among women and have an increased incidence after 60 years old, being more frequent from 70 to 79 years old [12].

In five cases of our sample, the length of hospital stay was five days, with admission on the first day, surgery on the second, and three post-operation days, with daily sessions of training for the ADLs and gait exercises using walking aids. In two cases, the patients were discharged in the fourth day, and in the only case where there was a complication due to which the person had to go back to the operating room, the hospitalization lasted for seven days. These periods of hospital stay are in accordance with current rehabilitation programs, such as the Enhanced Recovery After Surgery (ERAS) Protocols [15].

Some studies have proven the benefit of the ERAS protocol in people undergoing arthroplasty, this protocol is based on interventions that reduce post-traumatic psychological trauma and stress by fostering rapid recovery [15, 16]. According to Zhu et al. [17], this protocol contributes to a reduction in hospitalization times, reintervention rates and dependence on analgesics, thus contributing to improve patient satisfaction and reduce costs, based on preoperative education reducing anxiety; pre-hospital optimization with reduction of risk factors such as alcohol, tobacco, anemia, nutritional status; antimicrobial and antithrombotic prophylaxis; standardization of an anesthetic process; prevention of perioperative blood loss and normothermia; efficient postoperative analgesia, early mobilization after surgery and standard-based discharge, including elements such as ability to dress independently, sit down and stand up from bed/chair/toilet, take care of personal hygiene and to walk with the walking aid [18].

On the other hand, the shortening of hospitalization times hinders the intervention of the rehabilitation nurse, since, in order to facilitate the acquisition of knowledge, it was necessary to divide the information into several interventions, taking into account advanced ages, stressful situations and people's availability, using the expository method with demonstrative intervention. There was a training exercise whenever possible, using a pre and postoperative guide in which, besides the written text, there were images to facilitate the apprehension of knowledge and skills. This educational intervention was appropriate to the real needs of the person, enabling their reintegration into the family and allowing them to carry out their activities and functions. [19].

As a result, it can be considered that 62.5% of our sample had nearly four days in the rehabilitation nursing intervention program, while 37% participated on five days of intervention. Whenever necessary, the continuity of rehabilitation nursing care was ensured by the specialist nurses from the orthopedics department. This should be ensured to minimize disabilities secondary to the surgery and to promote the knowledge and capabilities of the person and their relatives, so they can adapt to their new situation. The safe transition home should be safely and with the assurance that the person and their family will have all the necessary help in the difficulties experienced [20].

The evaluation of the results of all cases showed that most of the items assessed improved between assessments, being independent in carrying out their ADLs, although two of them needed crutches to walk, of these only two had knowledge about the important post-surgery aspects, one had had a hip arthroplasty and the other had the support of her son who had the necessary knowledge.

On the day of admission, the emphasized of the educational intervention was on the particularities of the surgery, as well as the immediate pre and post operative moments. On the postoperative and after the patient stood for the first time, their education and their ADL training were carried out, as well as transfers and the gait training with a walking aid, whenever possible.

Through the analysis of data obtained from the FIM, it was found that, although in none of the cases was a total recovery in carrying out the ADLs, the dependency decreased in all cases. At the time of discharge, 75% of patients had complete independence, with a score between 104 to 111 out of 126. The remaining 25% had a modified dependence requiring assistance up to 25% of the tasks, requiring help only to dress the lower body and wear footwear. Given the pandemic restrictions, it was not possible to finish the training to go up and down stairs, which I consider a limitation; despite the obvious evolution, the levels of autonomy and independence in the performance of ADLs were not reached in all participants on admission, and this is in agreement with the literature, with months being necessary to acquire the pre-surgery functionality [19].

All individuals received a guidebook with instructions and illustrations, assuming that even those who could not read would have some help to clarify their doubts.

Saraiva et al., [21] showed that people undergoing hip arthroplasty and received preoperative education and rehabilitation had a clear recovery of functional independence after surgery. Preoperative rehabilitation plays an essential role for a quick and efficient functional recovery based on the level of independence in performing ADLs.

This study allowed us to note that the educational intervention of rehabilitation, contributed to training the person as early as possible, increasing their functional potential and independence, facilitating their integration into the family and social contexts, using the leaflets as enlighteners for the family person. Educational support is one of the support mechanisms mentioned by Orem to improve self-care, in addition to acting or doing for the other, guiding and counselling, providing physical and psychological support, and keeping an environment conducive to personal development [22].

Regarding pain, there were significant improvements in all cases, and on discharge, pain was between 0 and 1 for 87.5% of the sample; the oldest participant was only reporting a level 2 pain. In our sample, 87.5% of cases were submitted to surgery under a spine block anesthesia (SBA), while 12.5% (1 case) a general anesthesia (GA) was used.

The efficient control of pain allows for early mobilization, which should start as soon as possible. Many studies advocate for mobilization on surgery day, leading to a fast functional recovery, preventing thromboembolic complications [23, 24].

Regarding muscle strength, in half of the cases (50%) there was an improvement; in three of them (37.5%), the strength evaluation had the same result on the day of admission and discharge. In a single case, the evaluation decreased from level 5 to 4, according to the MRC scale. The intervention of the SNRN, with the adequate and individualized isometric and isotonic exercises, prevents immobility complication.

Although there is a positive evolution, the TUG test showed that all participants, on discharge, had a high risk for fall. In two cases, the test lasted for more than 3 min. These two cases result from fractures from fall; one of them, related to a fall of an 89-year-old person. The test was carried out with the support of crutches in 87.5% of cases; in one case (12.5%), a walking frame was used. According to Scheffers-Barnhoon, et al. [25], the fear of falling negatively influences functional recovery after hip fracture, arguing Ko, et al. [26] that it is necessary to teach and encourage fall prevention behaviors, since fractures are presented as debilitating consequences combined with marked declines in health, long-term complications and increases in dependence and disability [27]. Many studies prove that elderly who have fallen impose to themselves physical activity restrictions, due to the fear of a new fall, facing Post-fall Syndrome which is considered to be a risk factor for mobility reduction, affecting the capacity to carry out ADLs, diminish the perception of health state, and quality of life [28].

For the fear to be quantifiable, it must be reported by the elderly or assessed, and its non-assessment avoids preventive measures from being taken against the risk of falls. In the clinical context, fear of falling should be evaluated systematically, using scales adapted and validated to guarantee the reliability and validity of the results [28]. Cognitive changes, confusion, reduced visual and hearing acuity, changes in mobility and functionality, appropriate footwear, changes related to medication and environmental conditions are part of the screening programs in hospital settings [12].

According to literature, the educational component addressing the specific interventions of each situation should also be included, as well as the delivery of information leaflets and, if possible, audiovisual support to reinforce all the information provided and facilitate their learning [12].

A program with these characteristics allows, when applying a list of verification of the knowledge, to check what were the gains achieved from the training of the person, thus contributing to increase their quality of life, since it has a positive influence on the functionality of the person.

As previously mentioned, Orem's Theory and Meleis' Theory of Transitions are of vital importance in guiding the practice of nursing care and rehabilitation care. Under the light of Orem's Theory, it is possible to understand the limitations of the person, thus determining the actual need for nursing care, as to guarantee that self care is carried out [29]. The dependency of the person undergoing hip arthroplasty begins with the chronic disease (arthrosis) or trauma (fracture), passing through the surgery. Their functional capacity interferes with the performance of activities that are part of daily life, making third-party intervention necessary. at this point, the rehabilitation nurse determines the need for care, establishing strategies for empowering the person to perform self-care independently.

According to Meleis's [30], this process should be considered as a transition, bearing in mind the individuality, depending on previous experiences and family support. The nurse's role is to identify and help to manage the acceptance process, developing interventions that lead to independence for self-care, promoting, as a result, a safe health-illness transition, being demonstrated by process indicators, identifying the person's evolution towards health and well-being, verifying family interaction, friends and health professionals, being contextualized in the situation and developing confidence and strategies to overcome the situation, and result indexes, allowing the definition of whether the transition was healthy and safe for the person, through the evaluation of the development of new competencies and attitudes to manage the new situation (mastering it), or through the reformulation of the person's identity, the integration of new knowledge, and behavioral change [30–33].

One limitation of this project is the sample size, since the reduced number of participants is not representative of the universe of people who undergo hip arthroplasty.

As a suggestion, we recommend carrying out research with larger samples that can be more representative of the universe and corroborate the data found, which can value the work and impact that the SNRN interventions on capacitation have on the functionality and, consequently, on the life of the people.

Future studies should also explore the evolution of the functionality and gait capacity in the first 3 months after the return home. It is also important to explore SNRN interventions that include the whole period of transitional care, with the SNRN care continuing in the community.

5 Conclusions

In the eight cases of this study there was improvement from the immediate postoperative to the moment of discharge in terms of functionality, capacity of gait, pain control, increased range of articulations and of knowledge, to guarantee the continuity of care.

Lately there has been an increase in chronic and incapacitating diseases, and, frequently, people and their families do not know how to adapt to new realities. Therefore, the intervention of the SNRN is an important milestone in the early detection of the real needs of the person, as well as for their capacity to develop abilities to help them overcoming health/disease transitions. The findings of our study indicate that educational interventions in the pre and postoperative stages of hip arthroplasty, allow to empower and capacitate people in such a way that their autonomy and independence for self-care are recovered, leading to a safe transition as they return home.

References

1. Cruz, A., Carvalho e Sá, M., Conceição, V., Castro, J., Baixinho, C., Sousa, L.: A Pessoa com Doença Músculo Esquelética. In: Marques-Vieira, C., Sousa, L., Baixinho, C. (eds.) Cuidados De Enfermagem À Pessoa com Doença Aguda, pp. 761–785. Sabooks Lusodidacta (2021)
2. Esquenazi, D., Silva, S., Guimarães, M.: Aspectos fisiopatológicos do envelhecimento humano e quedas em idosos. Revista HUPE **13**(2), 11–20 (2014). https://www.arca.fiocruz.br/bitstream/icict/10944/2/sandra_silvaetal_IOC_2014.pdf
3. Direção Geral da Saúde. Programa Nacional Contra as Doenças Reumáticas. (2005). https://www.dgs.pt/areas-em-destaque/plano-nacional-de-saude/programas-nacionais/programa-nacional-contra-as-doencas-reumaticas-pdf.aspx
4. Martins, R., Mesquita, M.: Fraturas da extremidade superior do fémur em Idosos. Millenium **50**, 239–252 (2016)
5. Baixinho, C.L., Sousa, L., Ferreira, Ó.R.: Transitional care in times of COVID 19: opportunities for e-health interventions. In: García-Alonso, J., Fonseca, C. (eds.) IWoG 2020. LNB, pp. 336–344. Springer, Cham (2021). https://doi.org/10.1007/978-3-030-72567-9_31
6. Paniagua, D., Ribeiro, M., Correia, A., Cunha, C., Baixinho, C., Ferreira, Ó.: Project K: training for hospital-community safe transition. Rev. Bras. Enferm. **71**(5), 2396–2403 (2018). https://doi.org/10.1590/0034-7167-2018-0190
7. Fortin, M.-F.: Fundamentos e etapas do processo de investigação. Lusodidacta (2009)
8. Silva, L., Mercês, N.: Multiple case study applied in nursing research: a case report. Rev. Bras. Enferm. **71**(3), 1263–1267 (2018). https://doi.org/10.1590/0034-7167-2017-0066
9. Morgado, J., Rocha, C., Maruta, C., Guerreiro, M., Martins, I.: Novos valores normativos do mini-mental state examination. Sinapse **9**(2), 10–16 (2009)
10. Ordem Dos Enfermeiros. Enfermagem de Reabilitação, Instrumentos de recolha de dados para a documentação dos Cuidados Especializados em Enfermagem de Reabilitação (2016). https://www.ordemenfermeiros.pt/arquivo/colegios/Documents/2017/InstRecolhaDadosDocumentacaoCuidEnfReabilitacao_Final_2017.pdf
11. Direção Geral da Saúde. A Dor como 5° sinal vital. Registo sistemático da Intensidade da Dor (2003). https://nocs.pt/registo-sistematico-intensidade-dor/
12. Sousa, L., Carvalho, M.: Pessoa com fratura da extremidade superior do fémur. In: Marques-Vieira, C., Sousa, L. (eds.), Cuidados de Enfermagem de Reabilitação á pessoa ao longo da vida, pp. 421–428. Lusodidacta (2017)
13. Sousa, L., Carvalho, M.: Pessoa com Osteoartrose na Anca e Joelho em Contexto de Internamento e Ortopedia. In: Marques-Vieira, C., Sousa, L. (eds.), Cuidados de Enfermagem de Reabilitação á pessoa ao longo da vida, pp. 405–417. Lusodidacta (2017)
14. Lespasio, M., et al.: Hip osterarthrosis: a primer. Perm. J. **22** (2018). https://doi.org/10.7812/TPP/17-084
15. Christelis, N., et al.: An enhanced recovery after surgery program for hip and knee arthroplasty. MJA **202**(7), 363–369 (2015). https://doi.org/10.5694/mja14.00601
16. Ripollés-Melchor, J., et al.: Association between use of enhanced recovery after surgery protocol and postoperative complications in total hip and knee arthroplasty in the postoperative outcomes within enhanced recovery after surgery protocol in elective total hip and knee

arthroplasty study (Power2). JAMA Surgery **155**(4) (2020). https://doi.org/10.1001/jamasurg.2019.6024

17. Zhu, S., Qian, W., Jiang, C., Ye, C., Chen, X.: Enhanced recovery after surgery for hip and knee arthroplasty: a systematic review and meta-analysis. Postgrad. Med. J. **93**, 736–742 (2017). https://doi.org/10.1136/postgradmedj-2017-134991
18. Wainwright, T., et al.: Consensus statement for perioperative care in total hip replacement and total knee replacement surgery: enhanced Recovery After Surgery (ERAS) Society recommendations. Acta Orthop. **91**(1), 3–19 (2020). https://doi.org/10.1080/17453674.2019.1683790
19. Martins, M., Fernandes, C.: Percurso das necessidades em Cuidados de Enfermagem nos Clientes submetidos a Artroplastia da Anca. Referência – Revista de Enfermagem **II** (11), 79–91 (2009). http://comum.rcaap.pt/handle/10400.26/33473
20. Ferreira, E., et al.: Active Life: a project for a safe hospital-community transition after arthroplasty. Rev. Bras. Enferm. **72**, 147–153 (2019). https://doi.org/10.1590/0034-7167-2018-0615
21. Saraiva, P., Anunciação, S., Pontinha, C., Neves, I., Batista, A., Monteiro, G.: Ganhos em independência funcional como promotor da qualidade de vida. Millenium, Ciências da vida e da saúde **2**(12), 225–231 (2020). 10.293527/mil0205e.00297
22. Petronilho, F.: Autocuidado, conceito central da enfermagem. Coimbra: Formasau (2012)
23. Götz, J., et al.: Implementing fast-track in total hip arthroplasty: rapid mobilization with low need for pain medication and low pain values: retrospective analysis of 102 consecutive patients. Zeitschrift fur Rheumatologie (2021). https://doi.org/10.1007/s00393-021-00978-5
24. Hua-ping, S.: An analysis for the application of rapid rehabilitation surgery concept in the nursing satisfaction of the perioperative period of the elderly's hip arthroplasty. Med. Res. **2**(1), 21–25 (2020). https://orcid.org/0000-0002-4487-5920
25. Scheffers- Bamhoom, M., et al.: A multi-component cognitive behavioural intervention for the treatment of fear of falling after hip fracture (FIT-HIP): protocol of a randomised controlled trial. BMC Geriatrics **17**(71) (2017). https://doi.org/10.1186/s12877-017-0465-9
26. Ko, Y., et al.: Older adults with hip arthroplasty: an individualized transitional care program. Rehabil. Nurs. **44**(4), 203–212 (2017). https://doi.org/10.1097/rnj.0000000000000120
27. Baixinho, C.L., Dixe, M.A., Madeira, C., Alves, S., Henriques, M.A.: Falls in institutionalized elderly with and without cognitive decline: a study of some factors. Dement. Neuropsychol. **13**(1), 116–121 (2019). https://doi.org/10.1590/1980-57642018dn13-01001
28. Marques-Vieira, C.M.A., Sousa, L.M.M.D., Baixinho, C.R.S.L., Reis, M.G.M.D., Pérez-Rivas, F.J., Sousa, L.M.R.D.: Validação da Falls Efficacy Scale Internacional 7 itens em idosos portugueses residentes na comunidade. Texto & Contexto-Enfermagem **30** (2021). https://doi.org/10.1590/1980-265X-TCE-2019-0243
29. Fernandes, S., Silva, A., Barbas, L., Ferreira, R., Fonseca, C., Fernandes, M.A.: Theoretical contributions from Orem to self-care in rehabilitation nursing. In: García-Alonso, J., Fonseca, C. (eds.) IWoG 2019. CCIS, vol. 1185, pp. 163–173. Springer, Cham (2020). https://doi.org/10.1007/978-3-030-41494-8_16
30. Meleis, A.: Transitions Theory- Middle Range and Situation Specific Theories in Nursing Research and Practice. Springer Publishing Company, Heidelberg (2010)
31. Ferreira, B.A.S., Gomes, T.J.B., Baixinho, C.L., Ferreira, Ó.M.R.: Transitional care to caregivers of dependent older people: an integrative literature review. Rev. Bras. Enferm. **73**(Suppl 3), e20200394 (2020). https://doi.org/10.1590/0034-7167-2020-0394

32. Sousa, L., Martins, M., Novo, A.: Rehabilitation nursing in person's empowerment and training in health-disease transition processes. Revista Portuguesa de Enfermagem de Reabilitação **3**(1), 64–69 (2020). https://doi.org/10.33194/rper.2020.v3.n1.8.5763
33. Baixinho, C.L., Presado, M.H., Ribeiro, J.: Qualitative research and the transformation of public health. Cien Saude Colet. **24**(5), 1583 (2019). https://doi.org/10.1590/1413-81232018245.05962019

Technology and Care for the Elderly in Rural Areas and Its Incorporation into Public Policies

L. López-Lago Ortiz(✉), B. Muñoz González, and M. A. Serrano Alfonso

University of Extremadura, Cáceres, Spain
luislopezlago@unex.es

Abstract. The significant aging of rural areas has highlighted the need to find increasingly efficient care systems for the elderly. In this context, technological devices for care emerge strongly as a feasible solution to maintain the well-being of the elderly. In this article, we address the perspective of mayors and councilors of rural municipalities in Extremadura (Spain) characterized by a high level of socio-aging on the technological devices that can be incorporated into the care services for the aging in their localities. Fieldwork was carried out in 10 municipalities where 14 mayors and councilors were interviewed and direct observation of the operation of care services. The results show the lack of knowledge of this type of technology on the part of political leaders, the low level of implementation in municipal resources, the main obstacles to its adoption, and the high expectations and interest in introducing it in the services of their municipalities. The article highlights the need for institutional support to develop programs to facilitate the technologization of care in the rural world.

Keywords: Care · Technology · Rural areas · Aging · Public policies

1 Introduction

Both Spain and Portugal share demographic structures characterized by significant aging. Both countries rank second and fourth in the United Nations list with the highest aging rates worldwide [1]. Moreover, demographic projections, with the gradual incorporation of the baby boom generations into the over-65 age group and the progressive and sustained increase in life expectancy, draw a scenario that will consolidate this trend towards a very long-lived society [2–4].

This phenomenon is accentuated in rural areas, where there is hardly any generational replacement due to low fertility rates, youth emigration, and the unattractiveness of the immigrant population, the latter two phenomena being linked to precarious job prospects and the lack of opportunities [5]. Extremadura, the Spanish region where the research was carried out, is a clear example of this situation. The aging rate had increased from 49.28% in 1980 to 147.42% in 2021. Furthermore, in the last five years, the annual increase in this rate has exceeded two points per year [6].

This generalized aging of Western societies threatens the sustainability of welfare systems. The investment required for health and care systems geared to an increasingly aging population puts pressure on public financing systems [7]. In order to meet

J. García-Alonso and C. Fonseca (Eds.): IWoG 2021, LNBE, pp. 121–130, 2022.
https://doi.org/10.1007/978-3-030-97524-1_12

these challenges, public administrations have been gradually incorporating technological developments in policies for the care of the elderly (e-Health, telecare, sensors, wearables, communication technologies, etc.) [8]. Interest on the part of policymakers has increased due to the COVID-19 pandemic since technologies have been a fundamental element to counteract the loneliness and isolation of the elderly at this time [9, 10].

In Spain, the system of care for the elderly is mainly decentralized, with the autonomous community and municipal levels playing a significant role [11]. As a result, the perspective, sensitivity, and knowledge of local political representatives (mayors and councilors) about technology and care for the elderly have a decisive influence on the activities and actions to be developed in each municipality.

The purpose of this article is threefold: (a) to identify the knowledge that municipal policymakers have about the different technologies involved in the care of the elderly, (b) to identify the expectations (obstacles and possibilities) that could be derived from this knowledge, and (c) to examine their possible incorporation into municipal public policies on care that are developed in rural areas undergoing an accelerated aging process. The research is part of the Project "International Institute for Research and Innovation on Ageing (4IE+)" in its Public Policies on Aging line, which aims to define strategies and political actions with an impact on aging based on scientific evidence in the regions of Alentejo (Portugal) and Extremadura (Spain) [12].

2 Methodology

Qualitative research was carried out in 10 rural localities of the autonomous community of Extremadura (Spain), all of them with a population of fewer than 2,000 inhabitants and characterized by a high rate of over-aging. A balance has been sought between the localities of the two provinces that make up the region, with 5 of these being in the province of Cáceres and 5 in Badajoz. A total of 14 interviews have been carried out between May and July 2021, 7 of them to mayors and the other 7 to councilors responsible for aging policies. Likewise, there is also a balance between the political parties to which the interviewees belong, 7 are from the *Partido Socialista Obrero Español* and 7 from the *Partido Popular*. Concerning gender, there is parity among the interviewees since 8 are women, and 6 are men. The choice of the qualitative method, with semi-structured interviews, responds to the will of the research team that the fieldwork should also be a dialogic and participatory process; where not only concrete quantitative data is provided, but also a dense and deep knowledge about the imaginaries and representations of technology in the group of municipal political representatives [13–15].

With this objective, in the interviews, we asked a series of questions about aging technologies and the use of devices by the elderly, and their possible incorporation into the care policies of the municipalities studied. These questions formed a specific block within the semi-structured interview of the research on public policies on aging in rural municipalities of Extremadura during COVID-19. This block began by explaining the use of communication technologies by the elderly during confinement to reduce loneliness and isolation [16, 17]. Afterward, questions were asked about the existence of technological devices in the local care services. Then a taxonomy of care technologies was presented following the criteria of the European Parliamentary Technology Assessment, focusing on its three main categories: e-Health, Ambient Assisted Living (AAL), and Robotic technology [18], where they were asked about their knowledge, their existence in the local elderly care programs, the obstacles to their adoption, the expectations generated by these devices and the availability that they would have as municipalities to introduce them in the care services and resources (Table 1).

Table 1. Questions on technology for the care of the elderly. Source: Own elaboration.

Block of questions on care technologies for the elderly		
Technologies	Devices/ technological developments	Types of questions
Communication technologies widely used in pandemics	• Smartphones • Tablets • Instant messaging applications • Video-call software	Do you know [technology name]? Does your local elderly care service use this technology? What barriers might such technology face to adoption by seniors? What barriers might such technology face to adoption by seniors? Would you be willing to promote the introduction of this technology in your local elderly care resources and services?
e-Health	• Teleassistance • Health wearables • Software y apps m-health (smartphones) • Software e-health (computers)	
AAL. Ambient Assisted Living	• Assisted cleaning machines • Smart homes, domotics, sensors inside home • Voice assistants • Technologies for housework • Smart pillboxes • Apps and software autonomy • Exoskeletons y exosuits	
Robotic technology	• Robots with different degrees of anthropomorphization	

All the interviews were transcribed and reviewed by members of the research team and analyzed with ATLAS.ti software (Scientific Software Development GmbH, v.8.4.24.0 for Windows). The resulting empirical material was analyzed employing inductive analysis. Seven analytical categories emerged that allow a deeper understanding of the reality of the implementation of care technologies and their possibilities for incorporation into public policies in very aged rural municipalities. Firstly, knowledge of the technologies, with which to evaluate the capacity of the councilors to re-known the care devices. Secondly, the existence of the technologies in the municipalities, which allows an approach to the reality of their current implementation. Next, there are the barriers that the councilors consider to exist in their localities, which would constitute the obstacles to the technologization of care for the elderly. In fourth and fifth place are the expectations raised by these devices and the possibilities of introducing them into the services of the local councils. Lastly, the gender and age categories allow us to appreciate some differences in the imaginaries about the technologization of care that exist among the councilors, whether they are men or women, or whether they belong to different generations.

3 Results

3.1 Technology Knowledge

Mayors and councilors recognize that their knowledge of the technologies used in the care of the elderly is low. According to the councilors, this lack of knowledge is due to factors such as age, lack of contact with technology for professional reasons, and lack of interest. Thus, the recognized primary devices are not specific devices developed for care but for general ones. Thus, we find that all the interviewees are familiar with smartphones and tablets and their use for communication with the elderly during the pandemic, mainly through video calling and instant messaging applications. Likewise, many of the aldermen have identified devices such as anthropomorphic robots, cleaning and cooking robots, or voice assistants, but they re-aware that they had not thought of them as elements that could be used for care or improvement quality of life of the elderly. On the other hand, the only elements that have been recognized in a personalized way as care devices for the elderly are telecare terminals.

3.2 Existence of Technologies in the Resources

Concerning the technologies available in the resources and services of the municipalities, the responses are limited to identifying, on the one hand, the t-assistance devices, and on the other, those that facilitate communication for the elderly. The former is widely used in all the municipal assistance services analyzed. The municipalities play a central role in their management since through the municipal social services, the users are decided when the service is subsidized, although there is also the possibility of private contracting on a personal basis. When the service is part of public programs, the execution in all localities is carried out by the Red Cross, and its financing is through the Cáceres and Badajoz provincial councils or the municipalities themselves. Regarding the devices that facilitate communication, in all the municipalities where there are residences for the elderly, tablets and smartphones were used to make video calls to the families.

At the beginning of the confinement, smartphones were used by the workers of the residences. Subsequently, through a specific program, the provincial governments of Cáceres and Badajoz provided the residences with tablets that facilitated communication through videoconferencing. Moreover, in the case of one of the residences, the telephone company with which they have a contract also supplied them with two tablets for use by the elderly residents.

3.3 Obstacles to the Incorporation and Introduction of Technologies

The municipal councilors identify three main obstacles to implementing these devices: the generalized rejection of technology by the elderly, the lack of technological literacy, and the deficiencies in infrastructure for Internet connection in rural areas. The first of these barriers, the rejection of the elderly, related to technophobia or the fear that the use of technologies produces in them, which link to situations of stress and stress.

Concerning the second barrier, almost all political leaders indicated that the elderly have little digital literacy in their localities. At the same time, they indicated that instant messaging applications are becoming more common, encouraging the use of devices. On the other hand, in six of the ten localities studied, mayors and councilors report that digital literacy actions were carried out before the pandemic, mainly introductory computer courses, access to and use of the Internet, and courses on how to use cell phones. The success of this training is uneven, with a high level of participation in some areas, while in others, it has been shallow. The explanation for this disparity could lie in the unequal levels of public participation between localities so that in some of them, there is a solid associative fabric that favors participation in activities. In contrast, in others, the associationism of the elderly is non-existent, and there is hardly any participation of this group in courses and training. Although to confirm this hypothesis, it would be necessary to carry out fieldwork among the beneficiaries of this type of course.

Finally, concerning the third barrier analyzed, infrastructure, most of the mayors and councilors stated that in their localities, the infrastructure related to the Internet is precarious, there is no optical fiber, and several of them have reported common connection problems.

3.4 Expectations on Care Technologies

The municipal councilors are very optimistic about the potential of care technologies for the well-being of the elderly. They generally assume that technologies will continue to be implemented among the elderly, albeit with some difficulty, and that this will improve sociability and help reduce loneliness and isolation. Some policymakers appreciate the possibilities of the medical use of smartphones and tablets, although they insist on the importance of personal care, especially for the medical culture of the elderly. Likewise, those devices related to personal autonomy in the home of the elderly, such as cleaning robots, kitchen robots, voice assistants, or home automation sensors, arouse much interest in the aldermen and consider that they will improve the quality of life of the elderly, allowing them to stay in their homes as long as possible. However, in general, they agree that these devices will not replace caregivers and support staff but will gradually take over some of their tasks, facilitating their work on the one hand and contributing to the independence of users on the other.

3.5 Introduction of Technologies in Resources and Services

Regarding the possibility of introducing care technologies in the resources and services for elderly care in the municipalities, mayors and councilors show a high level of interest. In addition to extending telecare services, they emphasize the value of introducing these devices mainly in nursing homes, day centers, and home care services. In this regard, the technologies that arouse the most interest are voice assistants, kitchen, cleaning and companion robots, assisted toileting machines, digital pill dispensers, and intelligent sensors for use in the home.

However, they encounter a significant obstacle: their high cost. A good number of councilors point out that the purchase and general maintenance of these devices are unaffordable for the modest economies of rural municipalities. They would depend on public aid or participation in programs of other higher-ranking administrations to introduce these devices.

3.6 Gender and Age in the Interpretation of Technologies

Men and women have similar knowledge of the technologies. Equally, all identified telecare, although, in the case of women, they showed more excellent knowledge describing

Table 2. Results of the questions in the block on technologies of care for the elderly. Source: Own elaboration.

In	S	A	K	E	O	Ex.	I	Abbreviations	Keys
E01	♀	61	↓	↓	T	↑	↑	In: Interviewed	♀Female ♂Male
E02	♂	65	↓	↓	TLD	↑	↔		
E03	♀	62	↓	↓	TD	↑	↑	S: Sex	↑ · Extensive knowledge: identification of more than 10 devices
E04	♀	30	↔	↓	TLD	↑	↑	A: Age	· Existence of more than 10 types of devices in municipal resources
E05	♂	61	↓	↓	TLD	↔	↔	K: Knowledge	· Elevated expectations on care technologies
E06	♂	45	↓	↓	TLD	↑	↑		· Significant interest in introducing care technologies in municipal services
E07	♀	50	↔	↓	T	↑	↑	E: Existence	
E08	♀	40	↔	↓	TD	↑	↑	O: Obstacles	↔ · Average knowledge: identification of 6 to 10 devices
E09	♀	40	↔	↓	LD	↑	↑	Ex: Expectation	· Existence of between 6 and 10 types of devices in municipal resources
E10	♂	57	↓	↓	TLD	↑	↔		· Average expectations on care technologies
E11	♂	31	↔	↓	TD	↔	↔	I: Introduction	· Average interest in introducing care technologies in municipal services
E12	♂	56	↓	↓	TLD	↔	↑		
E13	♀	47	↔	↓	T	↑	↑	T: Technophobia	↓ · Low knowledge: identification of between 1 and 5 devices
E14	♀	62	↓	↓	T	↑	↑	L: Low literacy	· Existence of between 1 and 5 types of devices in municipal resources
								D: Deficient infrastructures	· Low expectations on care technologies · Low interest in introducing care technologies in municipal services

how the service works and their close relationship with users. Likewise, women showed more significant knowledge of technologies related to everyday activities, identifying kitchen or cleaning robots with commercial brands. Women also identified other care devices, such as electronic pill dispensers or assisted toilet machines.

In terms of obstacles, men are generally more pessimistic than women. This also translates into less confidence in introducing the devices in the resources and services of the municipalities. Likewise, women are more optimistic in terms of expectations, showing greater confidence in the impact of technologies on the well-being of the elderly, and are also significantly more inclined to introduce them into municipal resources.

Concerning age, there is a more excellent knowledge of the devices and greater expectations and willingness to introduce technologies in municipal services among respondents under 50 years of age. However, there is no significant variation by age in the perception of the barriers for older people in adopting technological devices (Table 2).

4 Discussion

The low awareness of care technologies by municipal decision-makers seems to coincide with the low penetration of specialized technological devices in rural areas [19], except for those telecare services that are widely spread throughout the country [20]. In addition, while there is a technology adoption gap between the rural and urban worlds, there is also a gap between the urban and rural areas [21]. The so-called care technologies, especially the so-called E-Healthcare, have become promising tools for improving the well-being of the elderly, on which there is an extensive scientific production [22]. However, there is a disconnect between research centers and the reality of those who ultimately decide to introduce devices in municipal services, as evidenced in the fieldwork. This is despite the initiatives of European, national and regional institutions (Smart Rural 21 [23], España Digital 2025 [24], SOTEX [25]) whose objective is the technologization of rural environments.

On the other hand, the barriers described by mayors and councilors to adopt technologies aimed at the elderly in rural areas coincide with those described in the scientific literature: technophobia, low levels of technological literacy, and deficient infrastructures [26]. In the case of technological rejection on the elderly, this is accentuated in those users or potential users with less academic training and work histories that have not been related to technology [27, 28]. In the same sense, we found that low educational levels and the development of jobs with little technology are related to lower digital literacy [29].

To combat the low levels of technological literacy, since the beginning of the 21st century, there has been a strong institutional commitment to improve the digital competencies of citizens living in rural areas [30]. In the case of Extremadura, the Technological Literacy Plan developed by the Asociación de Universidades Populares de Extremadura (AUPEX) has placed particular emphasis on the training of the elderly [31]. However, as Depatie [32] points out, for an adequate relationship between the elderly and technology, it is necessary to go beyond the classic concept of literacy, and training in technological matters must be aimed at creating a new type of relationship with technological devices, facilitating their entry into the daily life of the elderly.

About infrastructure, the main problem reported by the residents is poor access to the network/connections. This connectivity problem directly affects the activity of some of the care devices that are being developed and hinders their implementation in rural areas [33]. Extremadura has the worst broadband coverage at the national level, with almost 10% of the Extremaduran population still without an Internet connection of at least 30 Mbps. Moreover, the rural areas of this region are the first focus of disconnection [34]. Although the state and regional authorities, aware of this situation, have opted to implement broadband through an ambitious plan to provide this type of coverage to 92.5% of Extremadura's territory by 2023 [35].

On the other hand, institutional support is essential in digital literacy and in improving infrastructure and connectivity. The depopulation of rural areas makes them economically unprofitable for private initiatives, and the municipal authorities are aware of this circumstance. For this reason, they insist in their testimonies on the idea that the introduction of care technologies in municipal services requires solid institutional support. Thus, as Goyal & Dixit [36] stated, the success of the technologization of care will go hand in hand with public policies and programs that promote active aging and care.

5 Conclusions

The perspective of municipal politicians is essential for introducing care technologies in the services and resources for the aging of the municipalities of sparsely populated rural municipalities since they play a crucial role in decision-making on the public policies developed in their localities. The existing disconnection between the areas of technological production (universities, research centers, companies, etc.) and the rural world leads to a non-acceptable lack of knowledge about the devices among mayors and councilors. To solve this problem, it is proposed that there should be specific programs from the universities, with the support of regional and provincial institutions, to bring the advances in care technology closer to these councilors. During this research, the presentation of devices to political leaders has been very well received, raising very positive expectations and an evident willingness to introduce these technologies if the opportunity arises. For the latter, several types of problems identified by policymakers need to be solved. Firstly, technophobia and the lack of technological literacy among the elderly. To this end, programs must be developed for technological awareness and training, pedagogically adapted to the elderly, with an eminently personalized character, including the possibility of individual training at home, given the vulnerability of this group to Covid-19. Secondly, for the use of many of these technologies, there must be a notable improvement in the infrastructure for Internet connection in the rural areas of Extremadura. Finally, given the budgetary limitations of these municipalities, the introduction of this type of technological device must be facilitated by programs of other administrations with more significant economic capacity.

Finally, to facilitate the introduction of care technologies in the resources and services of municipalities in the rural world, it is recommended to carry out a more significant ethnographic type of research than the one presented here, which includes caregivers and elderly beneficiaries of care programs research subjects.

Acknowledgment. This work was supported by the 4IE+ project (0499-4IE PLUS 4 E) funded by the Interreg V-A España-Portugal (POCTEP) 2014–2020 program.

References

1. United Nations (2017): World Population Ageing. New York
2. Palazón Ferrando, S.: Los desafíos del progresivo envejecimiento de la población de España. In: Sempere Souvannavong, J.D., Cutillas Orgilés, E. (eds.) La población en España. 40 años de cambio (1975–2015), pp. 209–228. Universidad de Alicante, Alicante (2017)
3. Valente Rosa, M.J.: O envelheciemnto da sociedade portuguesa. Fundaçao Manuel Dos Santos, Lisboa (2012)
4. Nieto Calmaestra, J.A., Capote Lama, A.: Geografía del envejecimiento en España y Portugal. Ería Rev. Cuatrimest Geogr. **40**, 107–122 (2020)
5. Scharf, T., Walsh, K., O'Shea, E.: Ageing in rural places. In: Shucksmith, M., Brown, D. (ed.) Routledge International Handbook of Rural Studies. Routledge, London (2016)
6. Spanish National Statistics Institute (INE): Instituto Nacional de Estadística (2020) Índice de Envejecimiento Por Comunidad Autónoma. https://www.ine.es/jaxiT3/Datos.htm?t=1452#!tabs-tabla. Accessed 29 July 2020
7. Rodríguez Cabrero, G.: Longevidad y dependencia. La nueva contingencia del siglo XXI. Ekon Rev. vasca Econ. **96**, 140–169 (2019)
8. López-Lago Ortiz, L., Arroyo Chacón, S., Cipriano Crespo, C., Luengo Polo, J., Muñoz González, B.: Technology in the face of the challenges of the long-term care system for the elderly in spain. In: García-Alonso, J., Fonseca, C. (eds.) Gerontechnology III. IWoG 2020. Lecture Notes in Bioengineering. Springer, Cham (2021). https://doi.org/10.1007/978-3-030-72567-9_34
9. Flores Tena, M.J.: Las redes sociales se incrementan en las personas mayores durante el Covid-19. Fam Rev Ciencias y Orientación Fam **58**, 161–171 (2020). https://doi.org/10.36576/summa.131289
10. Chimento-Díaz, S., et al.: Have people over 64 used technological devices during COVID-19? In: García-Alonso, J., Fonseca, C. (eds.) Gerontechnology III. IWoG 2020. Lecture Notes in Bioengineering, pp. 168–176. Springer, Cham (2021). https://doi.org/10.1007/978-3-030-72567-9_17
11. Huete-García, A., Chaverri-Carvajal, A., Morales-Romo, N.: El Sistema Para La Autonomía Y Atención a La Dependencia En España (Saad): Memoria De Debilidades Desde Su Implantación. Prism Soc. **32**, 25–44 (2021)
12. López-Lago Ortiz, L., Rivero Jiménez, B., Fonseca, C., et al.: Instituto Internacional de Investigación e Innovación del Envejecimiento (4IE): Experiencia de un proyecto de investigación interdisciplinar entre España y Portugal. Iberografías **16**, 313–324 (2020)
13. Crabtree, A., Rouncefield, M., Tolmie, P.: Doing Design Ethnography. Springer, London (2009)
14. Crabtree, A., Rodden, T.: Ethnography and design. In: Proceedings of the International Workshop on Interpretive Approaches to Information Systems and Computing Research, pp. 70–74. Association of Information Systems., London (2002)
15. Botin, L., Bertelesen, P., Nohr, C.: Techno-Anthropology in Health Informatics. IOS Press, Amsterdam (2015)
16. Bertić, Ž, Telebuh, M.: Self-assessment of social and family loneliness in elderly during COVID-19 pandemic in relation to current level and type of communication intensity. Coll. Antropol. **44**, 209–217 (2020). https://doi.org/10.5671/ca.44.4.3

17. López-Hernádez, D.: Covid-19: Mayores conectados para evitar el aislamiento y la soledad. Conversat (2020)
18. EPTA (2019): Technologies in care for older people. Stockholm
19. OECD [Organisation for Economic Cooperation & Developmen] (2020): Rural regions of the future: Seizing technological change. In: Rural Well-being Geogr. oppotunities. https://www.oecd-ilibrary.org/sites/ae6bf9cd-en/index.html?itemId=/content/component/ae6bf9cd-en#chapter-d1e19840. Accessed 1 Oct 2021
20. IMSERSO (2016): Servicio de teleasistencia en España. Perfil de personas usuarias. 31 diciembre 2016. Madrid
21. Giner Pérez, J.M., Tolosa Bailén, C.: La brecha digital en España: factores explicativos. In: XXXIV. Reunión de Estudios Regionales. Asociación Española de Ciencia Regional, Baeza (2008)
22. Bebea-González, I., et al.: Management framework for sustainable rural e-healthcare provision. In: Proceedings of the IADIS International Conference e-Society, pp. 157–164 (2011)
23. E40 Group (2019): Smart Rural 21. https://www.smartrural21.eu/smart-rural-21-project/. Accessed 4 Oct 2021
24. Ministerio de Asuntos Económicos y Tranformación Digital (2020): España Digital 2025. Madrid
25. Direccción General Agenda Digital Junta de Extremadura (2020) Smart Office para el Territorio de Extremadura–SOTEX. http://smartcity.juntaex.es/oficina/que-es. Accessed 27 Apr 2021
26. Morales Romo, N.: The challenge of the digital divide and elderly in spanish rural areas. the case of castile and león. Fonseca J. Commun. **13**, 165–185 (2016)
27. Nimrod, G.: Technophobia among older internet users. Educ. Gerontol. **44**, 148–162 (2018). https://doi.org/10.1080/03601277.2018.1428145
28. Di Giacomo, D., Guerra, F., Perilli, E., Ranieri, J.: Technophobia as emerging risk factor in aging: Investigation on computer anxiety dimension. Heal Psychol. Res. **8** (2020).https://doi.org/10.4081/hpr.2020.8207
29. Hülür, G., Macdonald, B.: Rethinking social relationships in old age: digitalization and the social lives of older adults. Am. Psychol. **75**, 554–566 (2020). https://doi.org/10.1037/amp0000604
30. Cabrera Cabrera, P.J., et al.: Nuevas Tecnologías y exclusión social. Un estudio sobre las posibilidades de las TIC. Universidad Pontificia Comillas., Madrid (2005)
31. Equipo Técnico de la Asociación de Universidades Populares de Extremadura: El plan de alfabetización tecnológica y software libre de Extremadura. Una estrategia libre para un proyecto de libertad. Tabanque Rev Pedagógica, vol. 19, pp. 71–82 (2005)
32. Depatie, A.: Rural Older Adult Readiness to Adopt Mobile Health Technology: A Descriptive Study. University of California Davis (2013)
33. Conde-Caballero, D., Rivero-Jiménez, B., Cipriano-Crespo, C., et al.: Treatment adherence in chronic conditions during ageing: uses, functionalities, and cultural adaptation of the assistant on care and health offline (acho) in rural areas. J. Pers. Med. **11**, 1–18 (2021). https://doi.org/10.3390/jpm11030173
34. Ministerio de Asuntos Económicos y Transformación Digital (2020): Informe de cobertura de banda ancha en España. Madrid
35. Ministerio de Política Territorial (2021): Extremadura contará en 2023 con cobertura de banda ancha de nueva generación en el 92,5% de su territorio. https://www.mptfp.gob.es/va/portal/delegaciones_gobierno/delegaciones/extremadura/actualidad/notas_de_prensa/notas/2021/06/08-06-2021-01.html. Accessed 7 Oct 2021
36. Goyal, V.C., Dixit, U.: Technology Interventions for Elderly People. Help India-R&D Jl, vol. 14 (2008)

Solutions for Active Aging, Social Integration and Self-Care

Teleconsultation Script for Intervention on Frail Older Person to Promote the Care-of-the-Self: A Gerontotechnology Tool in a Pandemic Context

Idalina Delfina Gomes[1](✉), Liliana Santos Sobreira[1], Hermínia Daniela Teixeira da Cruz[1], Isabel Almeida[1], Marina Celly Martins Ribeiro de Souza[2], and Rafaella Queiroga Souto[3]

[1] Escola Superior de Enfermagem de Lisboa, 1990-096 Lisboa, Portugal
idgomes@esel.pt

[2] The College of New Jersey, Ewing Township, NJ 08618, USA

[3] Universidade Federal da Paraíba, João Pessoa, PB 58051-900, Brazil

Abstract. *Introduction:* The nursing care management of frail older people in the context of the SARS-CoV-2 pandemic requires the development of innovative actions. Those new interventions aim to meet the older population needs thru continuity of care, preventing previously existing health conditions from deteriorating and promoting their quality of life. Thus, the conception of the nursing teleconsultation (TC) is seen as an innovative answer to the ever-increasing frailty problem, in the sphere of gerontotechnology and the current pandemic challenges.

Methods: This paper shows an action-research methodology. There were 8 participants, of which 5 were nurses of the health care centre (USFX) and 3 frail older people that were identified using the Tilburg Index. The instruments used were the face-to-face consultation flowchart and the nursing guide to direct the intervention. All the ethical and deontological principles were respected throughout the study.

Result: The nursing teleconsultation was developed based on a script of a nursing theoretical model that has been recognized as an important tool to promote the care of older frail people by continuing to promote the Care-of-the-Self in the pandemic circumstance.

Conclusion: The TC implementation is a nursing intervention that is effective on assessing and controlling frailty on older people, besides being a way of promoting adherence to the therapy plan, preventing complications of frail conditions and fighting loneliness that many older people are exposed every day. The material resources are available in the health care centres, what makes the TC implementation easier to achieve.

Keywords: Care-of-the-Self · Older person · Frailty · Teleconsultation

1 Introduction

The aging population it is a growing reality globally, especially in Portugal which is currently the third most aged country amongst the European Union [1]. In 2020 the

J. García-Alonso and C. Fonseca (Eds.): IWoG 2021, LNBE, pp. 133–145, 2022.
https://doi.org/10.1007/978-3-030-97524-1_13

aging index of Portugal was 165,5 which corresponds to 2,3 Million people aged 65 or over [2]. This demographic change increases the amount of people who live with chronic diseases and are dependent on their daily activities, what does impact them on several domains such as: the ability to perform at their usual physical level, keep their social and psychological wellbeing and sustain safety. All those changes can lead to the fragility syndrome that has its consequences in their quality of life. Frailty is a geriatric syndrome that has been gathering more attention in the recent years, both nationally and internationally, and requires a quick public health response that promotes the maximum functionality of the older person [3].

The literature in geriatrics and gerontology has shown the importance of fragility syndrome in older people as given that every single old person is at risk of developing frailty, and it is related with the fall risk, incapability, hospital admission and death [3, 4]. In this sense, it is essential that nurses are able to identify people at risk of developing frailty and start an intervention as soon as possible to minimize the risks and maximize the potentials of each individual. Considering that one of the nursing missions is the promotion of independence, functionality and health of older people and their families, nurses must take the prevention, diagnosis, and management of frailty as a priority in their daily practice [5].

The current pandemic context brought another challenge to the nursing practice to the older population, especially to the most fragile people, due to the lockdown imposed to slow down the spread of SARS-CoV-2, those people were unable to reach out the services they needed in the community, including healthcare services. Simultaneously, older people find it more difficult to adapt to new circumstances, such as using new technologies to communicate at distance with families, friends, and professionals to breakdown their isolation and loneliness (problems that they had already been facing prior to the pandemic, which has become worse). When facing this reality, nurses are driven to provide an answer to the specific needs and difficulties that population has faced [6, 7].

The nursing practice management in a crisis context, as this pandemic, must include the development of new answers to the challenges that older frail people encounter, promoting a successful aging process and avoiding the deterioration of conditions already imbedded.

The gerontotechnology is an important tool that can work as a cornerstone for healthy ageing promotion, as it allows intervention in controlling and monitoring chronic diseases, preventing diseases across all four intervention levels, and adopting lifestyles that promote health. One of the strategies mentioned in the literature to achieve healthy aging is the establishment of the triangle older person/technology/environment, connecting the corners through the adaptation of technology to the specific context in order to ensure the satisfaction of the older people' needs [8].

The development of a nursing teleconsultation (TC) was seen as a gerontotechnologic answer that aims to address the growing concern of frailty syndrome, in a pandemic context, using already available resources (telephone). The TC allows the reduction of the distance between the primary health care services to the older people, without exposing them to a contamination, due to the increased risk that this age group has to develop COVID-19. Despite the need of lockdown and physical distancing, older people also need interactions with other people to prevent and control their frailty, which is one of the factors responsible for the comorbidities increase during this period.

Therefore, the goal of this paper is to propose a nursing teleconsultation systematized intervention guide to the older person and family according to the partnership model to promote of Care-of-the-Self [9, 10]. The following section of this paper presents a review of frailty concept, nursing teleconsultation and the partnership model to promote the Care-of-the-Self [9, 10]. Section 3 presents the approaches taken to develop the guide. Results and discussion are presented in Sect. 4 and the Conclusion is presented in Sect. 5.

2 Nursing Teleconsultation for Frail Older Person: Partnership Intervention Model to Promote the Care-of-the-Self

It is essential to implement a multidimensional frailty assessment in order to establish the most suitable nursing intervention with the older person, identifying this problematic as soon as possible, acting in partnership with her/him, providing the most suitable care for one's needs [11]. Defining frailty is a subject that still has not gathered complete consensus amongst the authors, nevertheless, it is important to recognize that there are multiple views to provide holistic care to a human being in nursing interventions. There are several models and theories that explain frailty and its impacts on the older person. In this paper we are exploring the models proposed by Fried [12] and Gobbens [13]. The model developed by Fried is known as the biological model with the frailty phenotype that can be measured through five components: non-intentional weight loss (>4,5 kg or 5% of the total weight in a year); tiredness and low resistance to small intensity activity; low physical activity; reduced walking speed (seconds/4,5 m) according to gender and height; e muscular strength (20% below average) [12]. Gobbens presents an integral model that understands the older person as a holistic being which is affected by frailty in all aspects of their lives regardless of the specific domain that frailty may be identified. In this holistic approach the frailty can affect the physical, psychological, and social life domains [13]. Therefore, the nursing intervention must be done in these three domains to avoid fragmentation of care and disrespect by the holistic model.

The concept of frailty is dynamic, since this process can be reverted, therefore the nursing intervention must be directed in supporting older people doing the shift from a frail state to a non-frail one [14]. It is also essential that we apply a holistic and multidimensional approach, where all dimensions are seen with same level of importance (and not where the physical aspect is perceived as the most important) and the interaction amongst all of them are understood and integrated in the nursing practice by establish a partnership with the older person/family that values their life project to promote the Care-of-the-Self [9, 10].

The partnership model adopted in this TC allows the establishment of a trustworthy relationship between the nurse and the older person, diagnose the nursing problems the person lives with, plan and implement a nursing intervention in a compromised environment that permits achieving a continuous improvement practice. In order to be effective on this clinical practice, the nurse must have specific knowledge, based on the most recent scientific evidence [15]. Also, the older person and family should feel supported in the care process, along with increasing their trust, knowledge, and abilities, helping them in decision making, so that they will have better health outcomes. This model is structured into five phases: Reveal Oneself; Get Involved; Train/Enable; Commit; Ensure the Care-of-the-Self/Ensure the Care-of-the-Other [9, 10].

The Reveal Oneself phase occurs when the older person and the nurse are presenting themselves to each other, establishing the boundaries of the relationship they are building together. The nurse needs to understand the way of living of the older person and what brings meaning to the older person's life. On the Get Involved phase both partakers establish a safe environment, with time and space, to develop and embed the therapeutic relationship. The next phase is Train/Enable at which nurse and older person/family negotiate a joint action; the nurse trains the older person on developing abilities to decide what the goals to be achieved are by converting potential skills in real ones; the enabling happens when the older person lacks the autonomy to make their own decisions, the nurse takes that responsibility, enabling the family member who cares for the older person, to continue the care necessary for their continuum of care. On the Commit phase there are gathered efforts to achieve the goals agreed. The last phase can be seen in two perspectives: Ensure the Care-of-the-Other when the older person is not autonomous on decision making regarding their life project, the nurse ensures that a family member makes that decision on their behalf, or if that is not possible, the nurse ensures the resources for care are continued by other means. Although, whenever possible, the core goal of this model is to promote the Care-of-the-Self, which happens when the older person takes responsibility over their own life project, controlling what actions to take and what objectives to achieve [9, 10].

A teleconsultation is defined by an intervention made by a healthcare professional, using information technology with the aims of assessing, planning, and implementing a care plan. By using the TC, healthcare professionals and people who need care are closer to each other, optimizing the resources available and avoiding unnecessary commutes [16]. When implementing this consultation nurses must follow all the ethical and deontological principles inherent to the profession, such as the principle of beneficence and non-maleficence, as well as discuss and obtain the informed written consent prior to the TC. All records must be kept in the personal record of each TC completed, so that continuity of care is warranted, and the TC should take around thirty minutes. However, the TC is not always appropriate for all situations and when necessary, a face-to-face consultation must take place, so that a physical assessment can be performed. Likewise, prior to the TC, a face-to-face consultation should occur as a first contact between the nurse and the older person [7].

3 Methods

This paper presents the results of an action-research intervention that aims to solve a practical problem and requires the commitment of all participants on implementing an intervention plan for frailty prevention in the older person, following the partnership model to promote the Care-of-the-Self [9, 10]. The participants of this project were 5 working on the health centre and 8 frail older people aged $\geq$65 years, after identification with Tilburg Index (this index assesses the wellbeing of older people in three domains:

physical, psychological and social, each section shows several questions with multiple answers options or just yes or no, each answer has a specific punctuation and, in the end, if the score is $\geq$6, that indicates a frail person). This index operationalizes the integral frailty model and it has been validated to the Portuguese context [17].

In this project, all the ethical and deontological requirements were followed, so confidentiality, anonymity and data protection rules were strictly complied with. All participants were asked to give written consent after explaining the purpose of the project. The draft of this TC was adapted from "A Script for Nursing Intervention on Elderly People with Chronic Pain by Telephone Consultation" [10], along with the orientations from the World Health Organization [18]. Then the draft was submitted to the expertise's analyses and the pre-test with three older people during a home care visit. The next step was the improvement of the draft to the script final version that is better suited to respond the older population and their families' communication needs and moreover is improved to establish a trustworthy relationship.

As already mentioned, it was necessary to complete a face-to-face consultation prior to the nursing intervention with the TC [7, 18]. Thus, we developed a pre-TC script, which main goal was to complete a multidimensional assessment of the older person. This assessment was essential to identify nursing diagnosis and evaluate the cognitive, affective, social, financial, spiritual and environmental context of the older person [19] and to understand their life projects [9, 20], so by appreciating the complexity of the person and all his/her spheres, nurses will be able to provide care with better outcomes, improving the older person's satisfaction with her care and general health [20].

4 Results and Data Discussion

The nurse executes the consultation according to the flowchart on image 1, which is organized into four steps. In the first step the nurse performs the 10 min comprehensive screening [18], in which is possible to assess, with a short number of questions, dimensions such as memory, functional capacity, urinary continence, psychosocial aspects, falls, nutrition, hearing and vision, medication and caregiver burden. The second step is about assessing the issues identified in the first screening, using assessment tools like Mini Mental Statement Examination, Mini Nutritional Assessment, Geriatric Depression Scale, Modified Barthel Index, Lawton & Brody Scale, Fluid chart, Downton scale, Snellen-type eye test, Tilburg Frailty Indicator, Assessment adherence to therapy, and Zarit Burden Interview Scale. The third step is to establish the nursing diagnosis for the older frail person (falls risk/compromised physical mobility/unbalanced diet/deteriorated memory/loneliness threat/depression/social withdrawal/low self-esteem/unsuccessful health management risk/ineffective medication management) and accordingly establish the required nursing intervention to prevent and control frailty. The fourth and last step is the follow up that occurs in TC (Fig. 1).

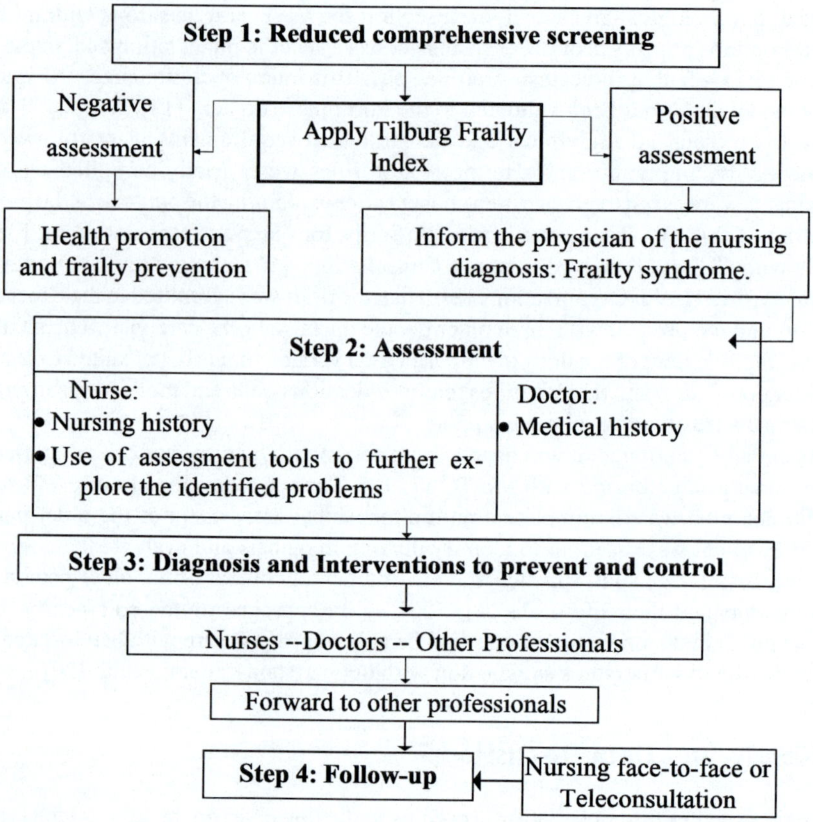

Fig. 1. Intervention flowchart for nursing consultation to prevent and control frailty on the older people [18]

4.1 Face-to-Face Consultation

A face-to-face consultation with the older person and family can either occur in the health care centre or in the person's home. When initiating this consultation, the nurses should introduce themselves, explaining the reason of the consultation (two stages – face-to-face and TC), clarifying that whenever needed, the face-to-face consultation will take place, express the advantages of the TC in avoiding wasting resources in commuting. The nurse should inform the order person about the TC and all the scales and indexes that intends to apply and the reasons for them, if the person agrees to participate, obtains the written informed consent. This first consultation allows the establishment and/or strengthening of the therapeutic trustworthy relationship between the nurse and the older person/family.

5 Teleconsultation (TC)

The nursing TC intervention plan is divided into four stages that include the five phases of the partnership model [9, 10]. The analysis from the nursing practice showed the need of organizing the TC in a guide that could be followed and replicated to support older frail people. This guide is presented below.

- **Stage 1 - Preparation of TC**

The objectives of this stage are the following:

- To provide an appropriate framework for effective TC;
- To get to know the patient, its health/illness, and context, including the surrounding context.

Step 1 – Preparation of the elements for the TC
• Confirm that there is a written and signed consent form; • Confirm that all required scales and indexes are ready and available; • Review the individual nursing and medical record of the older person; • Ensure that there is a calm and protected environment, without interruptions or distractions for the development of the TC; • Safeguard the privacy and confidentiality of the older person and family.

- **Stage 2 - Start of TC**

The objectives of this stage are the following:

- To build a trusting relationship in a short time;
- To create the best conditions for proceeding with TC;
- To optimize the time for the TC;
- To meet the person and family, their environment and understands what is significant for them as well as revealing oneself.

Step 1 – Reveal Oneself
• Introduce oneself, reminding the name, institution where is calling from and the reason for the call; • Clarify if the person has any question from the face-to-face consultation; • Question how the person has been in the last couple of weeks.

Other questions for the nurse proceeding with the TC are the following:
Is there anything from our last consultation that you would like to discuss?
How have you been in the last couple of weeks?
In the last couple of weeks, have you felt any change in your health?

Step 2 - Engagement

- To deepen the knowledge about the older person identity, his/her values and culture;
- To get information regarding his/her ability to Care-for-the-Self and to practice his/her autonomy.

Other questions for the nurse proceeding with the TC are the following:
Are you able to describe a typical day of yours?
What are the things you like to do the most?
What is the most important thing of your day?

- **Stage 3 - Development of TC**

The objectives of Stage 3 are the following:

- To perceive the current problem (evaluate, guide, empower, …);
- To give time to the person present and explain its/their main problem(s);
- To evaluate the problem, adherence and management of therapy, functionality, and capacity to take Care-of- the-Self;
- To validate the problem;
- To capacitate or enable the patient and family in identifying the problem and strategies for solving it.

Step 1- Get Involved

- Show availability to listen to the older person concerns;
- Assume the responsibility to assist the older person to continue their life path;
- Reinforce the partnership model and a non-judgmental posture throughout the nursing process;
- Continues the geriatric assessment according to the results of the triage questions using the tools marked in **A** - (A) Mini Mental Statement Examination; Mini Nutritional Assessment Geriatric Depression Scale; Modified Barthel Index; Lawton & Brody Scale; Fluid chart; Downton scale; Snellen-type eye test; Tilburg Frailty Indicator; Assessment adherence to therapy and Zarit Burden Interview Scale.

Examples of questions for the nurse proceeding with the TC are the following:
Could you tell me what do you need help within your daily routine?
How do your difficulties impact on your daily life?
How can I help you with your problem?

Step 2- Train / Enable / Commit

- Confirm the nursing diagnosis from the older person individual records;
- Question the older person / family if he / she perceives any problem in their lives;
- If the person identifies more than one problem, ask him/her which problem is the most relevant and why.
- Negotiate an intervention in partnership according to the older person's values;
- Assess their autonomy on executing activities of daily living:
    - Identify the number of visits to Emergency Department in the past year;
    - Establish the number of falls in the past year;
    - Assess loneliness, depression and quality of life;
    - Evaluate the caregiver burden;
    - Value the self-perception of health;
    - Assess the physical and socioeconomic environment of the older person.
- Establish a shared view with the older person for the nursing intervention to promote the Care-of-the-Self, such as:
    - Prevent frailty;
    - Promote adequate nutritional status and vitamin D intake;
    - Medication review to avoid polymedication and promote medication compliance;
    - Promote physical exercise and leisure activities;
    - Prevent falls;
    - Engage the older person in educational and prevention programs;
    - Refer to other professionals when needed;
- Assist the person and family to take forward the decision made;
- Reinforce that the nurse is a resource on the team to support the life path of the older person.

Examples of questions for this step are the following:

- *Among all the problems you told me, which one worries you the most?*
- *How would you like to resolve this problem?*
- *What goals would you like to achieve regarding this concern?*
- *Since our last encounter, is there anything that you can do better?*
- *Have you been taking all your prescribed medications? Can you explain to me how you have been taken them and what are the tablets for?*

Step 3- Validation of strategies and commitments
• Validate strategies and commitments; • Ensure the progression of the older person life´s path; • Assist the older person and family to keep their commitments; • Reiterate the decision made in partnership. Examples of questions for this step are the following: - *If I understood, what you told me is that you and your family are going to…* - *Would you mind to repeat the information I gave you?*

- **Stage 4 - Conclusion of TC**

Step 1- Assessing the older person and family' ability to assume the Care-of-the-Self and the Care-of-the-Other
• Foresee complications; • Assess if the person is able to keep her / his autonomy and Independence to promote frailty; • Assess if the family member / carer is able to assume the Care-of-the-Other; • Reinforce his / her availability as partner in the care process. Examples of questions for this step are the following: -*Can you describe what did we agree in this consultation?* -*You can always reach me to clarify any question or report any problem by contacting the health centre.* -*Are you (family member) confident with the care you are providing to your relative?*

Step 2- Conclusion of the CT
• Double check if there is any further question; • Confirm the importance of the TC; • Schedule the next TC; • Close the TC in a friendly manner; • Record all the necessary information. Other questions for this step are the following: - *Do you have any further questions for me?* - *Was this TC important to you? Why was that?*

The objectives of Stage 4 are the following:

- To evaluate the importance of TC;
- To schedule the next TC;
- To optimize the time for the next TC;
- To make records of the conversation and underline the topics/issues which need to be addressed in the next TC;
- To keep the trustworthy relationship;
- To ensure the continuity of care.

Each one of those stages and steps have different goals and programmed interventions and are presented in a sequential manner to make it more comprehensible and logical, although in a real-life context, they can happen simultaneously.

After the nursing intervention by TC, we made a questionnaire to the older people and their families, as well as to the nurses regarding their opinion about the TC. The evaluation given by the older people and their families was documented on their personal clinical records (SClínico®). All participants reported that they felt less lonely, and that this intervention had been a very important health resource in a pandemic context. They also highlighted the advantages of this safe nursing intervention that did not pose any risk to them. Two older people reported that they usually spent the day alone, so the TC was a very valuable resource to fight loneliness and isolation. This consultation was also important to promote adherence to the therapeutic plan, particularly when reinforcing the same intervention face-to-face and in the TC, and to prevent complications of frail conditions, such as falls or polymedication, through the holist assessment and interventions established in partnership for the Care-of-the-Self. The nursing team, likewise, expressed that the TC is an important tool to provide continuous care to frail older people, without the risk of complications due to SARS-CoV-2.

6 Conclusion

The healthcare professionals have an essential role in promoting healthy active aging and quality of life, so it is critical to raise awareness, call up the community resources, develop public health politics and increase their civil participation [21]. The telenursing, using information and communication technology in care practice, allows the interaction between nurses and people who need care at an immense distance, with interventions such as telemonitoring, telerehabilitation, teletracking and teleconsultation, within the nursing competences domain [7]. The implementation of the TC is not only an effective nursing intervention for assessing and controlling frailty in older people but also a very good way of combatting the isolation and loneliness. The material resources needed to execute the TC are available in the health care centres and older people commonly have at least one telephone at home, making it easier to implement the TC.

This project was carried out in the middle of a global health crisis, but due to the advantages previously mentioned, we consider that the TC should be kept as a nursing resource for the future, as the health gains for older people and their families overtake by far the investment required and it represents one step closer in our communities to become age friendly. If the needs of the older population are met and our communities are projected with their capabilities in mind, they will feel more integrated, will be more adapted, will need healthcare less often and it will be possible to prevent or even revert the frailty syndrome, promoting in partnership with the older people and their families the Care-of-the-Self.

The TC based on the script presented on this paper is an important tool to ensure continued care to the older frail people. Hence, for future works it is recommended the use of this script in other healthcare centers as well as its adaptation for other problematics such as older people with chronic diseases.

References

1. Eurostat. Healthy life years statistics - statistics explained. Published (2020). https://ec.europa.eu/eurostat/statistics-explained/index.php/Healthy_life_years_statistics#Healthy_life_years_at_age_65
2. Pordata – Base de Dados Portugal Contemporâneo. Números de Portugal – Quadro Resumo (2020). https://www.pordata.pt/Portugal/Quadro+Resumo/Portugal-254136
3. Llano, P., Lange, C., Sequeira, C., Jardim, V., Castro, D., Santos, F.: Factors associated with frailty syndrome in the rural elderly. Rev. Bras. Enferm. **72**(Suppl. 2), 14–21 (2019). https://doi.org/10.1590/0034-7167-2017-007
4. Hoogendijk, E., Afilalo, J., Ensrud, K., Kowal, P., Onder, G., Fried, L.: Frailty: implications for clinical practice and public health. Lancet **394**(10206), 1365–1375 (2019). https://doi.org/10.1016/S0140-6736(19)31786-6. PMID: 31609228
5. dos Enfermeiros, O.: Lei n° 156/2015 - Estatuto da Ordem dos Enfermeiros e REPE. Diário da República **1**(181), 8059–8105 (2015). https://www.ordemenfermeiros.pt/media/5154/repe_estatuto2016_versao03-05-17.pdf
6. Fonseca, C., Pinho, L., Lopes, M., Marques, M., Garcia-Alonso, J.: The elderly nursing core set and the cognition of Portuguese older adults: a cross-sectional study. BMC Nurs. **20**(1), 1–8 (2021). https://doi.org/10.1186/s12912-021-00623-1
7. dos Enfermeiros, O.: Parecer do Conselho de Enfermagem no 53/2021. Ordem Dos Enfermeiros **1**(1), 1–11 (2021)
8. Graafmans, J.: The history and incubation of gerontechnology. Gerontechnology **1**(1), 3–11 (2016). https://doi.org/10.1891/9780826128898.0001
9. Gomes, I.: Partnership of care in the promotion of the care-of-the-self: an implementation guide with elderly people. In: García-Alonso, J., Fonseca, C. (eds.) Gerontechnology III. IWoG 2020. Lecture Notes in Bioengineering, pp. 345–356. Springer, Cham. https://doi.org/10.1007/978-3-030-72567-9-32
10. Gomes, I., Mela, M., Guerreiro, D., Lopes, M., Gomes, B.: A script for nursing intervention on elderly people with chronic pain by telephone consultation. Gerontechnology 213–218 (2020). https://doi.org/10.1007/978-3-319-69892-2_1087-1
11. Craig, L.: The role of the registered nurse in supporting frailty in care homes. Br. J. Nurs. **28**(13), 833–837 (2019). https://doi.org/10.12968/bjon.2019.28.13.833
12. Fried, L., et al.: Frailty in older adults: evidence for a phenotype. J. Gerontol.-Ser. A, Biol. Sci. Med. Sci. **56**(3), 146–157 (2001). https://doi.org/10.1093/gerona/56.3.m146
13. Gobbens, R., Luijkx, K., Wijnen-Sponselee, M., Schols, J.: Towards an integral conceptual model of frailty. J. Nutr. Health Aging **14**(3), 175–181 (2010). https://doi.org/10.1007/s12603-010-0045-6
14. Wleklik, et al.: Multidimensional approach to frailty. Front. Psychol. **564**(11), 1–11 (2020). https://doi.org/10.3389/fpsyg.2020.00564
15. Uchmanowicz, I., Jankowska-Polańska, B., Wleklik, M., Lisiak, M., Gobbens, R.: Frailty syndrome: nursing interventions. SAGE Open Nurs. **4**, 1–11 (2018). https://doi.org/10.1177/2377960818759449
16. Serviços Partilhados do Ministério da Saúde. Centro Nacional de TeleSaúde. PENTS – Plano Estratégico Nacional Para a TeleSaúde 2019–2022 (2019)
17. Coelho, T., Santos, R., Paúl, C., Gobbens, R., Fernandes, L.: Portuguese version of the tilburg frailty indicator: transcultural adaptation and psychometric validation. Geriatr Gerontol Int **15**(8), 951–960 (2015). https://doi.org/10.1111/ggi.12373
18. World Health Organization: Age-friendly Primary Health Care Centres Toolkit WHO Library Cataloguing-in-Publication Data. World Health Organization, ed., Geneva (2008)

19. Sousa et al.: Avaliação Geriátrica Global em Medicina Interna: Um Modelo Mais Adequado na Avaliação dos Doentes Idosos Internados. Medicina Interna **26**(1), 40 46 (2019). https://doi.org/10.24950/rspmi/original/214/1/2019
20. Goe, M., Lopes, M., Oliveira, H., Fonseca, C., Marôco, J.: A nursing care intervention model for elderly people to ascertain general profiles of functionality and self care needs. Sci. Rep. **10**(1), 1–11 (2020). https://doi.org/10.1038/s41598-020-58596-1
21. World Health Organization: Decade of healthy ageing: baseline report, Geneve (2020)

Rehabilitation Nursing in the Person with Self-care Deficit Due to Neurological Changes - Systematic Literature Review

André Gordo[1], José Garcia[1], Rúben Galheto[1](✉), Celso Silva[2], and Isabel Nunes[3]

[1] São João de Deus School of Nursing, University of Évora, Évora, Portugal
rubengalheto@hotmail.com
[2] North Alentejo Local Health Unit, Portalegre, Portugal
[3] UCC de Odivelas, ACES Loures-Odivelas, Santo António dos Cavaleiros, Portugal

Abstract. Background: Population aging is progressively a characteristic universal phenomenon. During the life cycle, the risk of chronic diseases and dependence increases, with a general decline in the individual's intrinsic capacity. Neurological disease is increasingly prevalent, with a social and economic impact, associated with high mortality, with adverse consequences at various levels such as cognitive, behavioral and motor, and a growing demand for health care. The Rehabilitation Nursing Specialist Nurse [RNSN] has a relevant role in the self-care of the person with neurological disorders, in his/her family and in the community. Objective: To investigate the sensible gains from rehabilitation nursing interventions that promote self-care in people aged 65 and older with neurological disorders. Methodology: Systematic Literature Review. The search for studies was performed using databases [Academic Search Complete, Business Source Complete, CINAHL Plus with Full Text, ERIC, Library, Information Science & Technology Abstracts, MedicLatina, MEDLINE with Full Text, Psychology and Behavioral Sciences Collection, Regional Business News, SPORTDiscus with Full Text], with the following descriptors extracted from the Medical Subjects Heading vocabulary [MeSH]: [[outcome] or [intervention] or [education]] AND [[nursing] or [nursing care] or [nursing interventions]] AND [[neurology] or [neurological assessment] or [neurological rehabilitation]. The search was conducted in the month of September 2021, using the chronological frieze 2015–2021, with the linguistic limiter of articles in English and Portuguese language. Results: A total of nine studies were obtained, with a description of three dimensions that mirror appreciable gains in RNSN care for the person with neurological disorders. Conclusion: Interventions and outcomes were identified in the cognitive, social and functional dimensions of the RNSN in self-care to people with neurological pathology: The Nurse Rehabilitation Specialist has an essential role in the intervention to people with self-care deficit with neurological pathology. Interventions and outcomes were identified in the cognitive, self-care literacy and functional domains with a view to maximizing functional capacity.

Keywords: Nursing · Rehabilitation · Neurology · Self-care

J. García-Alonso and C. Fonseca (Eds.): IWoG 2021, LNBE, pp. 146–157, 2022.
https://doi.org/10.1007/978-3-030-97524-1_14

1 Introduction

Population aging is now a characteristic universal phenomenon, both at the European level and in developing countries [1]. This phenomenon has given rise to sudden demographic changes in populations worldwide; caused by the abrupt increase in a short period of time [1, 2].

With increasing age, numerous physiological changes develop, with increased risk of developing chronic diseases and dependence on others, with a general decline in the individual's intrinsic capacity [2]. Concomitantly, population aging may lead to an increase in the proportion and number of people in need of long-term care in all countries at different levels of development [1, 2]. Aging with health, autonomy and greater functional capacity is today a challenge with individual and collective responsibility, with direct impact on the economic development of countries, with the need for adaptation of society [2, 3].

Neurological disease is increasingly prevalent, with a social and economic impact, especially in developed countries, where the trend tends to increase as a consequence of population aging and socioeconomic development index [4, 5]. According to Deuschl et al. [5], neurological diseases have become the leading cause of disability in the world and the second cause of death, behind cardiovascular diseases. Diseases of the nervous system are associated with high mortality, with adverse consequences at various levels such as cognitive, behavioral and motor, accompanied by high disability rates and an increasing demand for health care [6].

Thus, ensuring the maximization of self-care, enabling the continuity of their personal development and their active role in societies through five essential domains: ability to meet basic needs; ability to learn, develop and make informed decisions; ability to move around; ability to make and maintain relationships; ability to contribute to their families and communities [1–33]. That said, it is urgent to create intervention programs, which enable and ensure self-care, through strategies related to stimulation and motor and cognitive rehabilitation [7].

It should be noted that the central idea of the Self-Care Deficit Theory arises from the need for nursing care associated with the subjectivity of maturity regarding the limitations of health-related actions. The limitations that derive from this assumption lead to a lack of ability to self-care oneself and/or one's dependents [8, 9]. Orem [10] assumes that any person is capable of self-care, since they have skills, knowledge and experiences acquired throughout life, but these can be affected by factors that influence education and life experiences that allow learning, exposure to cultural influences and use of daily living resources, which may interfere with/decrease their ability to self-care adequately [9]. Roughly speaking, the general essence of the general theory of self-care deficit determines the need for Nursing intervention when the needs and demands in terms of self-care are greater than the person's own capacity to develop this care [9].

The professional practice of nurses in Portugal is governed by the therapeutic and interpersonal relationship with humanistic personal characteristics, guides its professional practice through a systemic and systematic approach, identifying needs, identifying problems, performing interventions based on the principles of risk prevention, early detection of problems and minimizing complications [11].

There is evidence of the contribution and evolution in the number of specialist nurses in Rehabilitation in Portugal, to the provision and quality of care, focused on self-care, well-being and functional rehabilitation [12, 13], as well as evidenced gains in recovering functionality and contributions to autonomy [14].

The Rehabilitation Nurse Specialist has the broad general goals of improving function, promoting independence and maximizing the person's satisfaction. As Rehabilitation is a multidisciplinary specialty, the RNSN has the unique vision to design, implement and monitor differentiated nursing plans based on individual problems and potentials. Coupled with these increased competencies, these professionals are able to increase knowledge through new discoveries through research of practice, evidence-based practice, through observation and evaluation of sensitive outcomes [15].

2 Methodology

The methodological design of the Joanna Briggs Institute [JBI] and the PICOD model [Patient/Problem, Intervention, Comparison, Outcome, Design] were used as research strategies during the systematic review (Table 1).

Table 1. PICOD research question

P	People aged 65 and older	Keywords: Nursing; Rehabilitation; Neurology; Self-care
I	Rehabilitation nursing interventions	
C	Does not apply	
O	Promotion of self-care	
D	Fully published quantitative studies	

Thus, the PICOD research question was formulated: "**What are the sensible gains from self-care-promoting RN interventions in the person aged 65 and older with neurological changes?.** The search for studies was performed using the EBSCO Host Web database, with the following descriptors extracted from the Medical Subjects Heading [MeSH] vocabulary: [[outcome] or [intervention] or [education]] AND [[nursing] or [nursing care] or [nursing interventions]] AND [[neurology] or [neurological assessment] or [neurological rehabilitation]. The search was conducted in the month of September 2021, using the chronological frieze 2015–2021, with the linguistic limiter of articles in English and Portuguese language. As can be seen (Fig. 1), a total of 6897 articles were identified. After screening for articles published in the chronological range of the last 5 years, written in Portuguese or English, not duplicated and peer-reviewed, a total of 2614 articles resulted. Next, articles whose abstracts displayed the words [outcome] and [rehabilitation] were searched, resulting in 130 articles. Subsequently, the inclusion criteria were applied: including people aged 65 and over with neurological pathology, quantitative studies related to the topic in question, correlating EEER interventions in the promotion of self-care. As exclusion criteria: studies with a qualitative approach and without framing the theme's relevance.

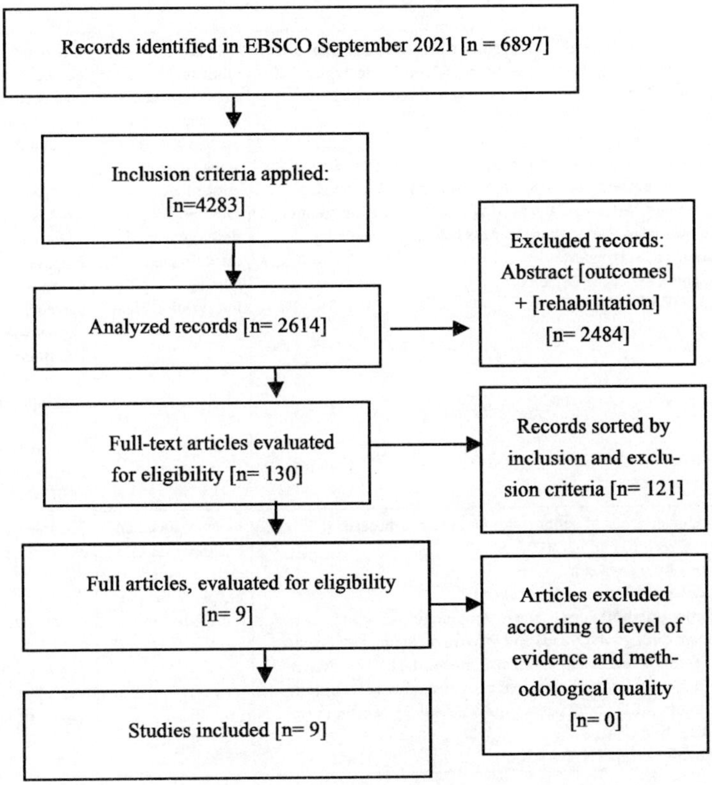

Fig. 1. Research methodology developed using the Prism 2009 flow diagram

Results

A total of 9 studies were included, which present a high level of evidence, where we highlight the existence of 3 randomized controlled studies and 2 pre-test post-test studies. Most studies aim at a set of RNSN interventions in the care of stroke patients with self-care deficit, focusing on the enhancement of functional capacity and maximum quality of life (Table 2).

Table 2. Description of summary results

Art.	Title/Source/Authors/Methodology/Participants/Description/Level of evidence	Objectives	Results/Conclusions
16	**Title** – Research on the Head and Neck MRA Image to Explore the Comprehensive Effect on the Recovery of Neurological Function and Rehabilitation Nursing of Patients with Acute Stroke **Origin-** China [2020] **Authors** – Xiao et al. **Methodology** – Observational study without control group **Description methodology** - An initial head and neck imaging evaluation was performed, the nursing rehabilitation intervention program was started, and then, 15 days later, a new imaging evaluation was performed **Participants** – 294 participants **LEVEL OF EVIDENCE – 3.e**	To study the clinical value of the combined imaging assessment of acute ischemic stroke before and after the development of a rehabilitation nursing intervention plan	The rehabilitation nursing intervention plan consisted of interpersonal communication, improving behavioral disturbances with stimulation of cognitive and sensory function, motor training focusing on balance, sitting/standing and gait training Rehabilitation nursing can improve neurological and cognitive conditions, improving the quality of life of the person
17	**Title** – Unmet needs of people with Parkinson´s disease **Origin** - Czech Republic [2021] **Authors** – Kozakova et al. **Methodology** – Cross-sectional study **Description methodology** - The methodology comprised a needs assessment through the Needs and Provision Complexity Scale [which assesses health and social sector needs], Barthel Index and the SCH-E scale [in order to assess activities of daily living] **Participants** – 183 participants from 4 neurology centers in the Czech Republic **LEVEL OF EVIDENCE** – 4.b	Identify social and health needs as well as social factors in people with Parkinson's Disease [PD]	The role of nurses in caring for people with PD is characterized by the identification of needs, individualizing and humanizing the care to each person, actively influencing the quality of life

(*continued*)

Table 2. (*continued*)

Art.	Title/Source/Authors/Methodology/Participants/Description/Level of evidence	Objectives	Results/Conclusions
18	**Title** – Implementation and feasibility of the stroke nursing guideline in the care of patients with stroke: a mixed methods study **Origin** - Iceland [2017] **Authors** – Bjartmarz et al. **Methodology** – Pre-test – post-test **Description methodology** - An explorative method was used, with pre-test and post-test measures. The quantitative part explored the electronic data recorded by nurses, retrospective of 78 participants. In the qualitative part, nurses were interviewed about the usefulness of the guideline for stroke patients and their experiences in implementing it **Participants** – 78 participants and 33 nurses **LEVEL OF EVIDENCE** – 2.d	To investigate and evaluate the implementation and feasibility of using a nursing guideline for stroke with a focus on mobility, depression, pain, falls, education and discharge planning	This study showed an improvement in 23 categories after the implementation of the guideline, with significant improvements in the promotion of activities of daily living and mobility, through the assessment of functional status, ADL training and development of interventions focused on the education of both people and relatives
19	**Title** – Digitally enabled aged care and neurological rehabilitation to enhance outcomes with Activity and MObility UsiNg Technology [AMOUNT] in Australia: A randomised controlled trial **Origin** - Australia [2019] **Authors** – Hasset. L et al. **Methodology** – Randomized controlled trial **Description methodology** - Clinical trial conducted in 3 Australian hospitals, where 2 groups with adults with mobility limitations and under neurological rehabilitation program were selected **Participants** – 300 participants **LEVEL OF EVIDENCE** – 1.c	To test the effectiveness of using digital assistive devices to improve mobility and physical activity in people with neurological deficits, rehabilitation potential, and mobility limitations	This study showed that there was an improvement in mobility in the intervention group relative to the control group. The use of digital media in the hospital environment and later at home presented itself as an important tool in increasing mobility and reducing sedentary lifestyles
20	**Title** – Effectiveness of mirror therapy on improvement of motor functions of affected upper limb among stroke patients **Origin** - India [2020] **Authors** – Navdeep et al. **Methodology** – Quasi-experimental study **Description methodology** - Quantitative approach, with non-probability sampling technique in order to select 60 participants with stroke and with motor impairment at the level of the upper limbs. The analysis was done by means of descriptive and inferential statistics **Participants** – 60 participants **LEVEL OF EVIDENCE** – 2.c	To investigate the effectiveness of mirror therapy in improving upper limb motor functions in stroke patients	Mirror therapy is a relatively widely used approach to rehabilitation in different neurological disorders including stroke. It has been shown that the functional organization of the motor system can be modulated by movement of the ipsilateral limb and passive observation of movement of the contralateral limb

(*continued*)

Table 2. (*continued*)

Art.	Title/Source/Authors/Methodology/Participants/Description/Level of evidence	Objectives	Results/Conclusions
21	**Title –** Access to post - stroke physical rehabilitation after acute reperfusion therapy– the neglected link in ischemic stroke management: a retrospective cohort study **Origin –** Romania [2021] **Authors –** Alexandru et al. **Methodology –** Cohort study **Description methodology -** Application of a structured questionnaire by telephone about access to post-stroke rehabilitation and what outcomes emerged post-rehabilitation **Participants –** 109 participants **LEVEL OF EVIDENCE – 3c**	Determine the access and how rehabilitation care is described for people with ischemic stroke who have undergone thrombolysis and/or thrombectomy	Of the 35 [32.1%] who had access to rehabilitation care while still in the hospital, 29 benefited from faster discharge criteria
22	**Title –** Effectiveness of Early Rehabilitation Combined With Virtual Reality Training on Muscle Strength, Mood State, and Functional Status in Patients With Acute Stroke: A Randomized Controlled Trial **Origin:** USA [2020] **Authors:** Lin et al. **Methodology:** Randomized controlled trial **Description methodology:** 152 people with ischemic stroke. Both groups received rehabilitation care, but the experimental group received rehabilitation care with virtual reality **Participants –** 145 participants **LEVEL OF EVIDENCE:** 1.c	To investigate the effectiveness of virtual reality training in improving muscle strength, mood [depression and anxiety] and functional status in people after stroke	Both groups showed gains in all dimensions evaluated At the end of the intervention, the experimental group showed greater gains in upper limb hemibody strength, comparative decrease in depression and degrees of anxiety
23	**Title –** Nursing staffs self-perceived outcome from a rehabilitation 24/7 educational program – a mixed-methods study in stroke care **Origin:** Denmark [2018] **Authors:** Loft et al. **Methodology:** Pre-test and post-test **Description methodology:** Collection of information in the form of a questionnaire [N = 33] and a semi-structured interview [N = 10] with nurses **LEVEL OF EVIDENCE:** 2.d	To determine nurses' self-perception of their ability, opportunity and motivation to practice with a rehabilitation approach after participating in a rehabilitation training program after stroke	The nurses consider that the training program had a positive influence on their professional identity and skills. At the end of the program, they were able to better understand their interdisciplinary role and improve communication between colleagues, better understanding the importance of a rehabilitative approach and the need to better prepare and plan for this approach

(*continued*)

Table 2. (*continued*)

Art.	Title/Source/Authors/Methodology/Participants/Description/Level of evidence	Objectives	Results/Conclusions
24	**Title –** Effects of motor imagery training on lower limb motor function of patients with chronic stroke: A pilot single-blind randomized controlled trial **Origin:** China [2021] **Authors:** Yin et al. **Methodology:** Randomized controlled trial **Description methodology:** A group of 32 randomly selected people were divided into 2 groups [experimental and control] **Participants:** 32 participants **LEVEL OF EVIDENCE:** 1.c	To demonstrate the importance of motor rehabilitation by imagining movements in the results of rehabilitation nursing intervention in the person with stroke	After 6 weeks both groups showed functional gains The experimental group showed quantifiable gains in gait and balance, quantified by the Functional Independence

3 Discussion

In this systematic review of literature, it was possible to evidence gains resulting from the EEER intervention directed to people aged 65 and older with neurological pathology reflected in three domains [cognitive, social and functional] with different outcomes: cognitive [16, 18, 22, 24]; literacy and self-care [17–22, 24]; and functional [16–21, 24] (Table 3).

Table 3. Outcomes of rehabilitation nursing

Field of intervention	Outcomes
Cognitive	Improved attention span, reasoning ability [16, 18, 22, 24]
	Lower level of anxiety and depression [16, 18, 22]
Literacy and self-care	Education for family members [18]
	Adequacy of care according to human needs [17, 22]
	Less sedentary lifestyle [19, 21, 24]
	Increased quality of life of the person [1617, 20]
Functional	Increased mobility [16–22, 24]
	Gains in performing ADLs [16, 18, 20–22, 24]
	Increased muscle strength and balance [16, 20, 22, 24]

Cognitive Domain

In the cognitive domain, appreciable gains from the RNSN intervention in improving cognitive function are highlighted [16, 18, 22, 24]. The RNSN intervention plan, based on interpersonal communication, sought to clarify and inform about the health status, in order to gain trust and establish a helping relationship between the RNSN-person [16, 18, 22]. It was also considered essential to ensure improvement at the cognitive level, the implementation of training exercises in reasoning and attention span [16, 18, 22]. The systematic review developed by Rogers et al. [25], corroborates the need for stimulation of cognitive function in attention, memory and executive functions, respectively, which show more significant improvements, highlighting the need to focus the practice on activities of daily living. Another of the interventions that are included in this domain is the reduction of symptoms of depression and anxiety of people and family members regarding the disease/disability process. A decrease in the appearance of these symptoms was noted after the implementation of the RNSN rehabilitation plan [16, 18, 22]. According to Medeiros et al. [26] cognitive rehabilitation should be considered the cornerstone in the intervention in stages of post-stroke depression. In addition, several studies demonstrate the importance of cognitive functions in selfcare [27, 28].

Literacy and Self-care Domain

In terms of the social dimension, the RNSN intervention in people with neurological pathological changes urges the adequacy of nursing care, taking into account the individual needs of each person, their core-family context, within a community [17]. The present study pointed to the lack of response regarding the rehabilitation needs of the population. Thus, the RNSN must identify the needs, individualizing and humanizing the care to each person, being able to actively influence the improvement of the quality of life not only of the person but also of the family members [16, 17]. In general, the RNSN intervention seeks to relate to the achievement of the person's inclusion in society, developing an adaptive process, enhancing their functional capabilities [8].

Functional Domain

In this dimension, there is strong evidence that RNSN is able to promote in the person an increase in global mobility, through consistent motor training with balance training [16, 22, 24], sit-up training [16, 24] and gait training [16, 19, 24]; improvement in mobility of the affected limb [22, 24]; gains in participation in ADLs [17, 21, 24]. Simultaneously, it seeks to decrease or eliminate complications by changing modifiable factors. It develops intervention programs aimed at reducing sedentariness, enabling the development of several outdoor activities. Note that these outcomes enhance the quality of life of each person.

Virtual reality has proven to be a useful tool in improving mobility and reducing sedentary lifestyles in elderly people with neurological deficits and mobility limitations [19]. Similar results were found by Lee et al. [29] by using virtual reality in a rehabilitation program, where he observed improvements in muscle strength and muscle strengthening, with better performance in performing activities of daily living, and therefore, improved mobility and quality of life. These rehabilitation programs directed towards muscle strengthening, static and dynamic balance, with a focus on mobility and ADLs, can contribute to significant results in empowering the person for self-care and performing exercise safely [19, 29–31]. The teaching of adaptive techniques to improve self-care aims to improve the quality of life and the maximum functionality [31].

In the review by Matos and Simões [31], they named the decisive role of the RNSN in the interdisciplinary team for the design, implementation, evaluation and reformulation of motor training programs. They concluded that motor functional re-education programs should integrate cognitive and physical psychological dimensions, dependence and ADL development, personal care and mobility management, goals and expectations, and ensure, guide and supervise program adherence and continuation. This role reveals the importance of the RNSN, which, through health education and empowerment of the person/family/caregiver, enhances the improvement of functional re-education. In a quantitative, exploratory, descriptive and retrospective study by Sá et al. [32] explained the importance of the continuity of rehabilitation care, even after discharge, allowing for an early detection of complications, aiming at maximizing the functional potential and social integration. In this process, in order to achieve gains, it is essential to meet the individual goals of the person [33].

4 Conclusion

This SLR contributes to the evolution of specialized nursing in rehabilitation in people with neurological disorders through the analysis and comparison of several articles to determine the state of the art. During this review, a large amount of information was found on the person affected by stroke, but there are many gaps and a lack of research on the person with other neurological disorders. This indicates that the work of RNSN is not yet finished and there is still a long way to go. Even so, based on the results, it was possible to find that the person who receives care from the RNSN has privileged access to multidimensional rehabilitation: cognitive, with improved attention and reasoning and lower levels of anxiety and depression; social, with greater participation of family members/caregivers, adequacy of care to individual needs, decrease in sedentariness and consequent social reintegration; and at the functional level, with greater mobility, gains in performing ADLs, greater muscle strength and balance, empowering the person and ensuring maximum functional capacity.

References

1. World Health Organization [WHO]: Decade of healthy ageing 2020–2030 (2019). https://www.who.int/docs/default-source/documents/decade-of-health-ageing/decade-ageing-proposal-en.pdf?Status=Temp&sfvrsn=b0a7b5b1_12. Accessed 25 Sept 2021
2. World Health Organization [WHO]: Integrated care for older people - guidelines on community-level interventions to manage declines in intrinsic capacity (2017). https://apps.who.int/iris/bitstream/handle/10665/258981/9789241550109-eng.pdf?sequence=1&isAllowed=y. Accessed 26 Sept 2021
3. Direção Geral de Saúde [DGS]: Estratégia Nacional para o Envelhecimento Ativo e Saudável (2017). https://www.sns.gov.pt/wp-content/uploads/2017/07/ENEAS.pdf. Accessed 19 Out 2021
4. Teixeira, L., Araújo, R.: Teleneurologia: Situação atual, oportunidades e desafios para Portugal. Sinapse **20**(1) (2020)
5. Deuschl, G., Beghi, E., Fazekas, F., Varga, T., Christoforidi, K., Sipido, E.: The burden of neurological diseases in Europe: an analysis for the global burden of disease study 2017. Lancet Pub. Health **5**, 551–567 (2020). https://doi.org/10.1016/S2468-2667[20]30190-0
6. Rede de Referenciação Hospitalar: Neurologia (2016). https://www.sns.gov.pt/wp-content/uploads/2017/05/RRH-Neurologia-Para-CP.pdf. Accessed 28 Sept 2021

7. Imaginário, C., Rocha, M., Machado, P., Antunes, C., Martins, T.: Functional capacity and self-care profiles of older people in senior care homes. Scand. J. Caring Sci. **34**(1), 69–77 (2020). https://doi.org/10.1111/scs.12706
8. Petronilho, F., Machado, M.: Teorias de Enfermagem e Autocuidado: Contributos para a Construção do Cuidado de Reabilitação. In: Sousa, L., Marques-Vieira, C. (eds.) Cuidados de Enfermagem de Reabilitação à pessoa ao longo da vida, pp. 3–23. Loures, Lusodidata (2017)
9. Queirós, P., Vidinha, T., Filho, A.: Autocuidado: o contributo teórico de Orem para a disciplina e profissão de Enfermagem. Revista de Enfermagem Referência **3**, 155–164 (2014). https://doi.org/10.12707/RIV14081
10. Orem, D.: Nursing: Concepts of Practice. Mosby, Maryland Heights (2001)
11. Ordem dos Enfermeiros [OE] Divulgar - Regulamento do Perfil das Competências do Enfermeiro de Cuidados Gerais. Lisboa: Ordem dos Enfermeiros (2012)
12. Ordem dos Enfermeiros: Anuário Estatistico (2020). https://www.ordemenfermeiros.pt/estat%C3%ADstica-de-enfermeiros. Accessed 23 Sept 2021
13. Martins, M., Ribeiro, O., Silva, V.: O Contributo Dos Enfermeiros Especialistas Em Enfermagem De Reabilitação Para A Qualidade Dos Cuidados. Revista Portuguesa Enfermagem de Reabilitação **1**, 22–29 (2018). https://doi.org/10.33194/rper.2018.v1.n1.04.4386
14. Santos, J.T., Campos, C.M., Martins, M.M.: A pessoa com AVC em processo de reabilitação: Ganhos com a intervenção dis Enfermeiros de reabilitação. Revista Portuguesa de Enfermagem de Reabilitação **3**(2), 36–43 (2020). https://doi.org/10.33194/rper.2020.v3.n2.6.5799
15. Ordem dos Enfermeiros. Regulamento das Competências Específicas do Enfermeiro Especialista em Enfermagem de Reabilitação (2019) https://dre.pt/application/conteudo/122216893. Accessed 30 Sept 2021
16. Xiao, J., Li, J., Yang, Q., Liu, M.: Research on the head and neck MRA image to explore the comprehensive effect on the recovery of neurological function and rehabilitation nursing of patients with acute stroke. World Neurosurg. **149**, 420–427 (2020). https://doi.org/10.1016/j.wneu.2020.10.135
17. Chaudhuri, K.R., Bhidayasiri, R., Laard, T.: Unmet needs in Parkinson's disease: new horizons in a changing landscape. Parkinsonism Relat. Disord. **33**, 52–58 (2016). https://doi.org/10.1016/j.parkreldis.2016.11.018
18. Bjartmarz, I., Jónsdóttir, H., Hafsteinsdóttir, T.B.: Implementation and feasibility of the stroke nursing guideline in the care of patients with stroke: a mixed methods study. BMC Nurs. **72** (2017). https://doi.org/10.1186/s12912-017-0262-y
19. Hassett, L., et al.: Digitally enabled aged care and neurological rehabilitation to enhance outcomes with activity and MObility UsiNg technology [AMOUNT] in Australia: a randomised controlled trial. PLoS Med. **17**(2), 1–24 (2021). https://doi.org/10.1371/journal.pmed.1003029
20. Navdeep, S.K., Gurbir, K., Rawat, H.C.L.: Sulena: Effectiveness of mirror therapy on improvement of motor functions of affected upper limb among stroke patients. Baba Farid Univ. Nurs. J. **19**(2), 20–28 (2020). https://doi.org/10.7897/2230-8407.099210
21. Alexandru, R.R., Oana, T.E., Bogdan, C., Iulian, E., Cristina, G., Cristina, T.: Access to post - stroke physical rehabilitation after acute reperfusion therapy-the neglected link in ischemic stroke management: a retrospective cohort study. Balneo Res. J. **12**(1), 46–52 (2021). https://doi.org/10.12680/balneo.2021.418
22. Lin, R.-C., et al.: Effectiveness of early rehabilitation combined with virtual reality training on muscle strength, mood state, and functional status in patients with acute stroke: a randomized controlled trial. Worldviews Evid.-Based Nurs. **17**(2), 158–167 (2020). https://doi.org/10.1111/wvn.12429

23. Loft, M.I., et al.: Nursing staffs self-perceived outcome from a rehabilitation 24/7 educational programme - a mixed-methods study in stroke care. BMC Nurs. **17**, 17 (2018). https://doi.org/10.1186/s12912-018-0285-z
24. Yin, X.-J., Wang, Y.-J., Ding, X.-D., Shi, T.-M.: Effects of motor imagery training on lower limb motor function of patients with chronic stroke: a pilot single-blind randomized controlled trial. Int. J. Nurs. Pract. e12933 (2021). https://doi.org/10.1111/ijn.12933
25. Rogers, J.M., Foord, R., Stolwyk, R.J., Wong, D., Wilson, P.H.: General and domain-specific effectiveness of cognitive remediation after stroke: systematic literature review and meta-analysis. Neuropsychol. Rev. **28**(3), 285–309 (2018). https://doi.org/10.1007/s11065-018-9378-4
26. Medeiros, G., Roy, D., Kontos, N., Beach, S.: Post-stroke depression: a 2020 updated review. Gen. Hosp. Psychiatry **66**, 70–80 (2020). https://doi.org/10.1016/j.genhosppsych.2020.06.011
27. Fonseca, C., Pinho, L.G., Lopes, M.J., Marques, M.C., Garcia-Alonso, J.: The elderly nursing core set and the cognition of Portuguese older adults: a cross-sectional study. BMC Nurs. **20**(1) (2021). https://doi.org/10.1186/s12912-021-00623-1
28. Lopes, M.J., et al.: Functioning and cognition of Portuguese older adults attending in residential homes and day centers: a comparative study. Int. J. Environ. Res. Pub. Health. Spec. Issue: Ageing Health: Funct. Psychol. Perspect. **18**, 7030 (2021). https://doi.org/10.3390/ijerph18137030
29. Han, S.L., Yo, J.P., Sun, W.P.: The effects of virtual reality training on function in chronic stroke patients: a systematic review and meta-analysis. BioMed. Res. Int. (2019). https://doi.org/10.1155/2019/7595639
30. Magalhaões, R.P., Barbeiro, S.R., Taveira, V., Magalhães, B., Ferreira, G.: Jogos usados na Reabilitação após Acidente vascular cerebral: scoping review. Revista Portuguesa Enfermagem de Reabilitação **3**, 27–41 (2020). https://doi.org/10.33194/rper.2020.v3.n1.4.5740
31. Matos, M., Simões, J.: Enfermagem de Reabilitação na Transição da Pessoa com alteração motora por AVC: Revisão Sistemática de Literatura. Revista Portuguesa de Enfermagem de Reabilitação **3**, 10–19 (2020). https://doi.org/10.33194/rper.2020.v3.n2.2.5770
32. Sá, N., Oliveira, A., Silva, A., Brandão, S.: Consulta de Enfermagem de Reabilitação ao doente pós event cerebrovascular: que desvios encontrados ao plano delineado à alta pelo Enfermeiro de Reabilitação?. Revista Portuguesa de Enfermagem de Reabilitação **3**, 5–13 (2020). https://doi.org/10.33194/10.33194/rper.2020.v3.n1.1.4579
33. Silva, A., et al.: Promotion of functional independence in the deficit of self-care in the elderly person with stroke in home context and technology. In: García-Alonso, J., Fonseca, C. (eds.) IWoG 2020. LNB, pp. 291–302. Springer, Cham (2021). https://doi.org/10.1007/978-3-030-72567-9_27

Sensitive Indicators for Rehabilitation Nursing Care in Older Persons with Mobility Impairment Through a Rehabilitation Program: A Systematic Literature Review

Mauro José Lopes[1](✉), Celso Silva[2], Isabel Nunes[3], Eduardo Pimenta[4], and Vanda Seromenho[4]

[1] School of Health of the Polytechnic Institute of Beja, Beja, Portugal
maurolopes22@gmail.com
[2] North Alentejo Local Health Unit, Portalegre, Portugal
[3] UCC de Odivelas, ACES Loures-Odivelas, Santo António dos Cavaleiros, Portugal
[4] Local Health Unit of the Alentejo Coast, E.P.E., Santiago do Cacém, Portugal

Abstract. Mobility impairment has deleterious effects at various levels, affecting the functional capacity of people, being more evident in the elderly population. The approach to the elderly person subject to mobility restriction should include a rehabilitation program that integrates early mobilization and the RNSN will be an important professional for this goal to be achieved. It is of interest to know the sensitive indicators for RN care, which allow measuring the gains in health, in terms of functionality and quality of life. Objective: To identify the indicators sensitive to RN care, at the level of functionality, in the elderly with mobility impairment, inserted in rehabilitation programs. Methodology: Performed SLR through the EBSCO Host platform, including the databases: Academic Search Complete; Business Source Complete; CINAHL Plus with full text; ERIC; Library, Information Science & Technology Abstracts; MedicLatina; MEDLINE with full text; Psychology and Behavioral Sciences Collection; Regional Business News; SPORTDiscus with full text, using the PICO method. Results: A total of 37 indicators sensitive to RN care are identified, with the outcome dimension producing the greatest number of indicators, supporting the importance of results in achieving health gains. Conclusions: In order to achieve health gains, the interventions of the RNSN should be guided by specific indicators. Thirty-seven indicators sensitive to Nursing Rehabilitation care were identified, dominating indicators within the outcome dimension, highlighting the importance of the results achieved in the translation of health gains. We highlight indicators that aim at maximizing the functional capacities of people, through rehabilitation programs, promoting muscle movement and walking, as a way to prevent or counteract the harmful effects of immobility.

Keywords: Rehabilitation nursing · Sensitive indicators for rehabilitation nursing care · Mobility · Elderly

J. García-Alonso and C. Fonseca (Eds.): IWoG 2021, LNBE, pp. 158–170, 2022.
https://doi.org/10.1007/978-3-030-97524-1_15

1 Introduction

Aging may be characterized by the complex interaction between the processes of cellular aging and multi-organ system, with environmental, physical, psychological, and social factors, leading to biological changes that deteriorate the person's defense and homeostasis mechanisms. As a consequence, the disease process is more frequent, and some pathologies predominate and coexist simultaneously, precipitating an exponential increase of multi-morbidities, since this phenomenon is associated with increased average life expectancy [1].

Supporting this trend, the World Health Organization (WHO) [2] marks an increase in life expectancy from 66.5 years to 72 years, for the period between 2000 and 2016, and for the same period and as for healthy life expectancy, it marks an increase from 58.5 years to 63.3 years. In Portugal, there has been an increase in average life expectancy at birth from 67.1 years in 1970 to 80.9 years in 2018, and life expectancy at age 65 corresponding to the same period, increases from 13.5 years to 19.6 years [3].

In 2019, the elderly population in Portugal was around 2,262,325 representing 22% of the general population, whereas in 1971 the proportion was 9.7%. The ageing rate in Portugal has also been increasing, from 101.6% in 2001 to 161.3% in 2019 [3].

According to EUROSTAT [4], healthy life expectancy at age 65 in Portugal was 7.3 years in 2018, noting also that, according to PORDATA [3], the total dependency ratio in Portugal in the year 2019 was 55.3%, with 34.2% relating to the elderly dependency ratio. Portugal can be portrayed as a country that has a low birth rate, an aging population, and multiple chronic pathology [5], and in the short and long term, the increase in the number of these chronic diseases implies an increase in the prevalence of functional disability [6].

Functional limitations and declining physical and mental well-being increase with age, and few lifestyle interventions are available to prevent adverse events in frail or pre-frail elderly [7].

According to Fonseca and Lopes [8], international organizations such as the WHO, the United Nations (UN) and the European Commission (EC) advocate a restructuring of health systems, not only aimed at the disease, but also focusing on issues such as functionality, promoting its sustainability by increasing the activity of people aged 65 and over, promoting active aging, since, with the global trend towards population aging, health care consumption and associated costs tend to increase in the future [7].

Høy et al. (2007) cited by Fonseca [8], point to self-care as a health resource, since intervening in it increases functional status and decreases health care costs.

Orem, through his theory of self-care deficit, conceptualizes that everyone has the potential for self-care, with skills and experience throughout life. However, when the demands of self-care are greater than the ability to perform them, they need support, either from caregivers (family, friends, neighbors), or from health professionals, namely nurses [9].

It seems essential to us, agreeing with Petronilho and Machado [9], given the aging population and the high prevalence of chronic diseases, we must move towards the production of knowledge, through intervention models that address sustainable responses, adapting to the needs of self-care, from a perspective of functionality and promoting the autonomy of people.

Most adults preserve their ability to mobilize until they are allowed to, that is, until it is restricted, compromised, or causes pain, realizing that movement is essential for the person to interact with the environment, and problems resulting from immobility are readily apparent in the person's health [10] and believing that the major goal for most people, and more specifically for the elderly population, is to maintain their independence and live at home as long as possible [7].

Periods of acute inactivity, or bed rest associated with hospitalization or illness, pose a real threat to muscle tissue and functional capacity. Even for people who ambulated before the disease process, immobility is common during hospitalization. Particularly in the elderly, physical inactivity during hospitalization is almost accepted as part of the hospitalization experience, but leads to markedly negative outcomes, including a reduced ability to perform activities of daily living (ADLs), an increased incidence of readmissions, and increased length of stay [11], as well as admissions to convalescent units and long-term care facilities [12].

Immobility and functional limitation represent enormous challenges and can promote processes of increased pain, incontinence, balance changes, as well as depressive syndromes, disorientation, and irritability [10], leading health professionals, with emphasis on the Rehabilitation Nursing Specialist Nurse (RNSN), to permanently seek strategies that help optimize the functional abilities of people, particularly the elderly [13].

The functional mobility may be altered, due to a physical or clinical situation, derived from certain pathologies, surgeries or injuries, with possible repercussions at the respiratory, cardiovascular, gastrointestinal, musculoskeletal, genitourinary, metabolic, cutaneous, neurological levels, among others [14, 15].

Inactivity and loss of innervation promote a decline in muscle mass, strength, and endurance, and can lead to neuromuscular, pulmonary, cognitive, and quality of life complications that can endure over time [15].

Supported by scientific and technological advances, it is promoted that the restriction of mobility, as an adjunct to the therapeutic process, is prescribed less and less frequently, since the negative effects of immobility are now recognized. The early recovery, after a prolonged disease situation, is essential to try to revert the harmful picture of organic alterations, potentiated by immobility/inactivity, being particularly more important in the elderly population, which is itself more vulnerable to the effects of mobility alterations [14].

With the evolution of scientific knowledge, an earlier mobilization is now possible, decreasing the risks associated with mobility alterations/immobility syndrome, which can, by themselves, have more serious consequences than the pathology that originated them [14], aiming at progressive mobility, minimizing its loss and optimizing autonomy, being important in terms of gains in functional capacity, independence of the person and improvement in quality of life [15].

Even in people admitted to Intensive Care Units (ICUs) who, due to multiple etiologies, including medication-associated effects, electrolyte changes, and systemic dysfunctions, are more limited in mobility and where bed rest was often used as a therapeutic modality, we have witnessed a paradigm shift, with the promotion of early mobilization, as a way to avoid complications associated with immobility and avoid more or less permanent disabilities in people, when they return home, and also showing results, with improvement in some indicators, such as, length of stay either in ICU or hospital, time needed to wean from mechanical ventilation, incidence of delirium and also in terms of readmission rates [11, 16].

Early mobilization plays an important role, too, for a successful hospital-to-home transition process [11].

Hoeman [10] points to benefits in the person's overall health status, namely in age-related changes in muscle function, in the practice of both aerobic and strength training exercises. Benefits are also pointed to load exercises, both in terms of strength, postural stability, and the ability to be alert.

Regular exercise, appropriate to the patient's situation and functional goals are beneficial, and before the person is clinically stabilized, the goal is to prevent contractures or atrophy, as well as to avoid joint pain or injury, maintain muscle tone, strength, and function. The exercise should also be adapted in order to conserve energy and avoid fatigue [10].

For Dirkes and Kozlowski [11], the nurse plays an important role in promoting early mobilization, even in people hospitalized in critical care units, a view also shared by Cerqueira and Grilo [17], who argue that the RNSN working in an ICU has a key role in the design and implementation of rehabilitation programs, in order to minimize the consequences of immobility, including respiratory, motor and functional, and Hoeman [10], believes that the RNSN helps patients develop their potential, optimizing function and advocating for patients to achieve maximum autonomy and independence, outlining appropriate goals together with the person that promote quality of life and satisfaction. For Hoeman [10], therapeutic interventions for mobility and self-care are a cornerstone of rehabilitation nursing care, and maintaining mobility is of utmost importance to avoid complications associated with immobility and for the efficient performance of ADL and instrumental activities of daily living (IADL).

Therefore, an adjusted planning of nursing care, including interventions directed to the maintenance of mobility, promoting self-care, is a fundamental contribution to avoid these complications [14].

The care we provide must be adapted throughout the life cycle, and there are certain specificities associated with old age that must be taken into account and where rehabilitation nursing plays a key role, not only by producing scientific evidence for the development of specific care plans, but also in their execution [13].

Supporting the analysis about the importance of the RNSN intervention, at the level of self-care and ADL, we point out that it is written in the Regulation of the specific skills of the RNSN, (Regulation no. 392/2019 of May 3) [18], as some of its competence units, that this professional "designs intervention plans with the purpose of promoting adaptive capacities, aiming at self-control and self-care in health/illness and/or disability transition processes" and "designs and implements ADL training program aiming at adapting to mobility limitations and maximizing autonomy and quality of life" [18] (p. 13567).

The RNSN develops its practice based on evidence, oriented to results, responding to people's specific needs and to new demands in terms of care, using sensitive indicators for Rehabilitation Nursing (RN) care, in order to assess health gains, both in terms of empowerment, autonomy and quality of life [18, 19].

Assuming that the approach to the elderly person subject to mobility restriction, in different contexts, should include a rehabilitation program that integrates early mobilization and that the RNSN is an important professional for this goal to be achieved, it is of interest to know the sensitive indicators of RN care, which allows assessing the health gains in terms of functionality and quality of life, through a Systematic Literature Review (SLR), formulating the following question: "What are the sensitive indicators of RN care in terms of functionality, in the elderly person with mobility impairment, through a rehabilitation program?" following the PICO methodology.

2 Methodology

SLR seeks to aggregate evidence that meets pre-defined eligibility criteria in order to answer a particular research question, trying to minimize any bias by making use of systematic, explicit, and reproducible methods [20].

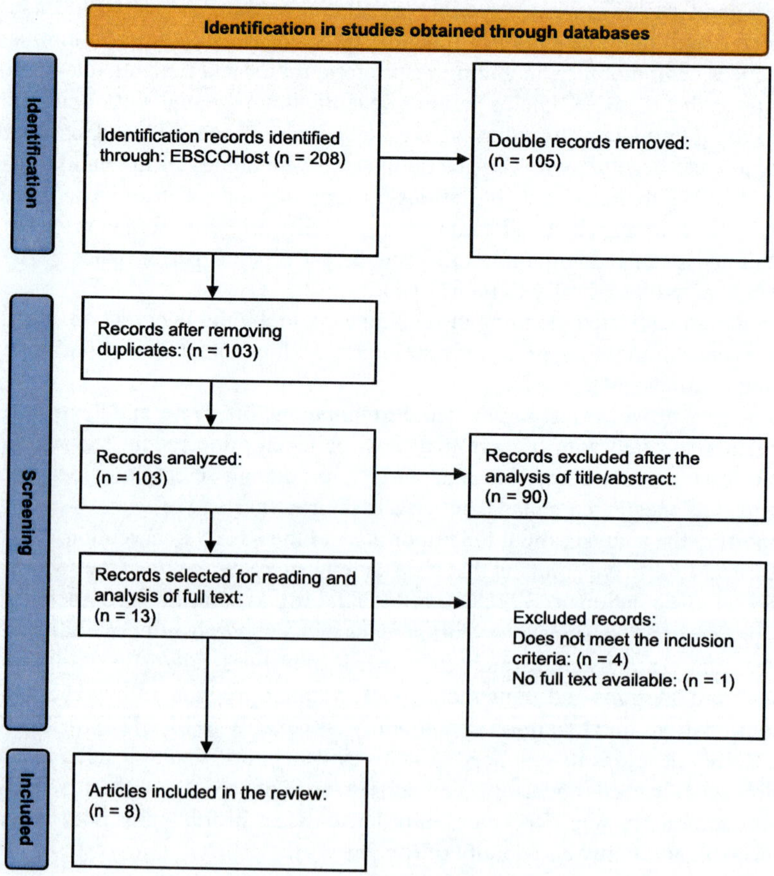

Fig. 1. Research methodology, PRISMA type [23]

In building this SLR, we followed the guidelines of the Joanna Briggs Institute (JBI) and, using the PICO method (P - Participants; I - Intervention; C - Context/Control; O - Outcomes), we defined inclusion criteria that allowed us to select the appropriate studies according to the research question formulated, as shown below: P - People aged 65 years or older, with mobility impairment; I - Submitted to a Rehabilitation program; C - At the level of functionality; O - Sensitive indicators to Rehabilitation Nursing.

A search was carried out on the EBSCO Host - Research Databases platform, in January 2021, selecting all available databases: Academic Search Complete; Business Source Complete; CINAHL Plus with full text; ERIC; Library, Information Science & Technology Abstracts; MedicLatina; MEDLINE with full text; Psychology and Behavioral Sciences Collection; Regional Business News; SPORTDiscus with full text, using the validated descriptors, either by MeSH (Medical Subject Heading) or by CINAHL Subject Headings: "nursing", "nursing interventions", "nursing care", "outcomes", "nursing outcomes", "education", "physical mobility", "elderly", "geriatrics" and "self-care", using the Booleans "AND" and "OR" and respecting the search inclusion criteria: full text available, in the English language, for publications dated between the year 2015 and 2020.

The search resulted in a total of 208 articles, which, after eliminating duplicate results, derives in 103 records for title and abstract analysis. After reading the titles/abstracts, 90 records are eliminated for not fitting the theme of the study, resulting in 13 articles for full-text analysis. From the full-text analysis, four articles were excluded for not meeting the inclusion criteria and one for not providing access to the full text, resulting in a total of eight articles to be included in this review.

Articles were submitted to JBI Critical Appraisal Tools evaluation of methodological quality and levels of evidence [21, 22], meeting more than 50% of the proposed quality criteria. All articles were analyzed by two authors.

In a systematized way, the flow chart in Fig. 1 details the research path:

3 Results and Discussion

From the search carried out, the articles identified in Table 1 appear as the result:

The idea of quality in health care is brought to us by the Donabedian theory, which proposes three essential components - structure, process, and outcome - that are interconnected and evolve sequentially, in the sense that the quality of the structure promotes quality to the process and, in turn, the quality of the process adds quality to the outcome. «Structure» is understood as the physical space, material, human and organizational resources where health care takes place; «process» can be understood as the sum of care actions and interpersonal relationships and «outcome» is what emerges from the care provided [24].

Table 1. Identification of the analyzed articles

Authors/Title Participants	Objectives	Methodology/level of evidence
Dirkes and Kozlowski (2019): **Early Mobility in the Intensive Care Unit: Evidence, Barriers, and Future Directions**	- Study the aspects of care that can affect expected patient outcomes; - Address the effects of immobility, as well as the challenges to achieving mobility and the tools currently available to help overcome them	Expert Opinion 5.c
Imhof et al. (2015): **Effects of Mobility-Enhancing Nursing Intervention in Patients with MS and Stroke: Randomised Controlled Trial** Patients older than 18 years, admitted to a Swiss clinic, diag-nosed with multiple sclerosis, stroke or brain injury: 61 in the intervention group and 65 in the control group	- To investigate the effect of a new nursing intervention (nursing intervention to improve mobility) designed to improve rehabilitation outcomes	Randomised Controlled Trial 1.c
Liang et al. (2019): **Effects of Multidisciplinary Team-Based Nurse-led Transitional Care on Clinical Outcomes and Quality of Life in Patients With Ankylosing Spondylitis** Adults admitted to the Rheuma-tology Department of a Chinese hospital with a confirmed diagnosis of ankylosing spondylitis: 49 in the intervention group and 46 in the control group	- To investigate the impact of transitional care, by a nurse-led multidisciplinary team, on the clinical outcomes and quality of life of patients with ankylosing spondylitis	Randomised Controlled Trial 1.c
Young et al. (2018): **Identifying Barriers to nurse - Facilitated Patient Mobility in The Intensive Care Unit** Two nurses and one nursing technician from a North American Medical Intensive Care Unit	- To report on a project design, implementation and results of an approach to identify and understand lack of time as a barrier to promoting mobility by nurses in an Intensive Care Unit	Observational study without a control group 3.e

(*continued*)

Table 1. (*continued*)

Authors/Title Participants	Objectives	Methodology/level of evidence
Augustine et al. (2020): **Implementation of Post-Acute Rehabilitation at Home: A Skilled Nursing Facility-Substitutive Model** Patients over 18 years of age, admitted to a US hospital, able to progress to convalescent units: 267 patients	- To describe and evaluate the services and functional out-comes, as well as, identify the factors associated with the provision of a 30-day post-acute rehabilitation care package consisting of medical and social services provided through a Home Rehabilitation program	Observational study without a control group 3.e
Lowthian et al. (2016): **Predicting functional decline in older emergency patients--the Safe Elderly Emergency Discharge (SEED) project** Patients aged $\geq$ 65 years, dis-charged home from the Emergency Department of an Australian hospital: 959 patients	- To profile the trajectory and risk factors for functional decline, in elderly people, in the 30 days following discharge from the Emergency Department	Prospective cohort study 3.b
Crotty et al. (2019): **Should we provide outreach rehabilitation to very old people living in Nursing Care Facilities after a hip fracture? A randomised controlled trial** People aged $\geq$ 70 years who underwent hip surgery and main-tained gait prior to surgery: 119 in the intervention group and 121 in the control group	- To determine whether a four-week postoperative rehabilitation program, performed in nursing facilities, for elderly people undergoing post hip fracture surgery would improve quality of life and mobility compared to traditional postoperative care	Randomised Controlled Trial 1.c
Van Lieshout et al. (2018): **The Effectiveness of a Proactive Multicomponent Intervention Program on Disability in Independently Living Older People: A Randomized Controlled Trial** People aged $\geq$ 65 years, living independently in a Dutch semi-rural community: 139 in the intervention group and 142 in the control group	- To test the effectiveness of an interdisciplinary multidimensional intervention program to prevent disability in older people in the community	Randomised Controlled Trial 1.c

Thus, based on this perspective, we found sensitive indicators for RN care, with the purpose of promoting the intervention of the RNSN, in order to obtain health gains, promoting the continuous improvement of the quality of care provided to people [25].

In Table 2, we analyze the sensitive indicators of RN care to the elderly person with mobility impairment, at the level of functionality, in a rehabilitation program, which stand out from the selected articles.

Table 2. Sensitive indicators for RN care identified (adapted from NO) [25]

Type	Indicator (ID[a])
Structure	- Percentage of clients for whom a scale was applied to assess **body balance** [26]; - Percentage of clients who used muscle strength assessment equipment (dynamometer) **(muscle movement)** [27]; - Hours of rehabilitation nursing care per client per day of hospitalization **(organization of rehabilitation nursing care)** [28]
Process	- Number of partnerships/cooperation protocols established with entities in the community, aimed at promoting a safe environment **(health promotion)** [29]; - Percentage of clients to whom a rehabilitation plan and/or program was applied to maximize functional abilities **(health promotion)** [7, 12, 26, 27, 29, 30]; - Percentage of clients with potential to improve knowledge about **walking** adaptation technique [12, 26]; - Percentage of clients with potential to improve **walking** ability [12, 26]; - Percentage of clients with potential to improve knowledge about **walking with a walking aid** [29]; - Percentage of clients with potential to improve knowledge about adaptation technique for **standing up** [12, 26]; - Percentage of clients with potential to improve ability to use adaptation technique **to stand up** [12, 26]; - Percentage of clients with potential to improve knowledge about adaptation technique **to position themselves** [12]; - Percentage of clients with potential to improve ability to use adaptation technique **to position themselves** [12]; - Percentage of clients with potential to improve knowledge on adaptation technique **to transfer themselves** [12]; - Percentage of clients with potential to improve ability to use adaptation technique **to transfer themselves** [12]; - Percentage of clients with potential to improve knowledge of **body balance** technique [26]; - Percentage of clients with potential to improve ability to use **body balance** technique [26]; - Percentage of clients with potential to improve knowledge about exercise habits **(activity intolerance)** [7]; - Percentage of clients with potential to improve knowledge of muscle and joint exercise techniques **(muscle movement)** [11, 26, 27, 30]; - Percentage of clients with potential to improve ability to perform muscle and joint exercise techniques **(muscle movement)** [11, 26, 27, 30]

(*continued*)

Table 2. (*continued*)

Type	Indicator (ID[a])
Outcome	- Gains in knowledge about **walking** adaptation technique [12, 26]; - Gains in **walking** ability [12, 26]; - Gains in knowledge about home adaptation for **walking with a walking aid** [29]; - Resolution rate of compromised **standing up** [12, 26]; - Gains in knowledge about adaptation technique for **standing up** [12, 26]; - Gains in ability to use adaptation technique for **standing up** [12, 26]; - Gains in knowledge about adaptation technique for **taking a position** [12]; - Gains in ability to use adaptation technique for **taking a position** [12]; - Gains in knowledge about adaptation technique for **transfer** [12]; - Gains in ability to use adaptation technique for **transfer** [12]; - Rate of resolution of compromised **body balance** [26]; - Gains in knowledge about **body balance** technique [26]; - Gains in ability to use **body balance** technique [26]; - Activity intolerance resolution rate **(intolerance to the activity)** [7]; - Gains in knowledge about exercise habits **(intolerance to the activity)** [7]; - Gains in improved muscle movement **(muscle movement)** [11, , 26–28, 30]; - Gains in knowledge about muscle and joint exercise techniques **(muscle movement)** [11, 26, 27, 30]; - Gains in ability to perform muscle and joint exercise techniques **(muscle movement)** [11, 26, 27, 30]

[a]The Identity Cards (ID) of the indicators defined by NO, are highlighted in bold

It was possible to identify 37 indicators that stand out from the theme under study.

In the "structure" dimension, indicators referring to the use of scales and equipment, both for the evaluation of body balance and muscle movement, and also in the scope of the organization of RN care, stand out, regarding the time available for nurses to develop their care, also standing out in the work of Young et al. [28], other barriers that influence the intervention of these professionals.

In the dimension «process», stands out, largely, the indicator «Percentage of clients for whom a rehabilitation plan and/or program was applied to maximize functional abilities» within the scope of health promotion, followed by indicators for muscle movement, standing, and walking, respectively, «Percentage of clients with potential to improve knowledge of muscle and joint exercise techniques», «Percentage of clients with potential to improve ability to perform muscle and joint exercise techniques»; «Percentage of clients with potential to improve knowledge about adaptation technique for standing up», «Percentage of clients with potential to improve ability to use adaptation technique to stand up»; «Percentage of clients with potential to improve knowledge about walking adaptation technique»; «Percentage of clients with potential to improve walking ability».

In the dimension «outcome», the emphasis is on indicators related to muscle movement, «Gains in improved muscle movement», «Gains in knowledge about muscle and joint exercise techniques» and «Gains in ability to perform muscle and joint exercise techniques», followed by those related to walking «Gains in knowledge about walking adaptation technique» and «Gains in walking ability».

The outcome dimension is the one that produces the largest number of indicators in this review, meeting the importance of results, which translate into health gains, through sensitive indicators to RN care and since this is not a watertight system, it also demonstrates the importance of proper planning and intervention in care.

In line with what has been previously explained, the indicators related to the application of a rehabilitation program to maximize the functional capacities of people and those that are directly related to muscle movement and walking stand out, confirming that one should counteract the adverse effects caused by immobility, especially to a more fragile group such as the elderly, through structured rehabilitation programs that include joint mobilization interventions with muscle strengthening, in order to maximize the person's functionality, promoting mobility and gait.

4 Conclusions

Aiming at excellence of care, and to obtain health gains, the RNSN's interventions must be evidence-based and guided by specific indicators for its intervention.

From the studies analyzed, we were able to identify 37 indicators sensitive to RN care, for the intervention with the elderly person with mobility impairment, through a rehabilitation program.

Indicators within the "outcome" dimension dominate, highlighting the importance of the results achieved in the translation of health gains through the RN intervention. It is also highlighted indicators that aim to maximize the functional capacities of people, through rehabilitation programs, promoting muscle movement and walking, to prevent or counteract the deleterious effects of immobility.

More studies are needed, in the promotion of sensitive indicators of RN care, especially in the dimension «structure», having been the one that was least developed throughout this work.

References

1. Faria, M., Ramalho, J., Nunes, A., Fernandes, A. (coords.): Visões sobre o envelhecimento. IPBeja Editorial, Beja (2020)
2. World Health Organization: World health statistics 2021: monitoring health for the SDGs, sustainable development goals ISBN. World Health Organization (2021). https://www.who.int/publications/i/item/world-health-statistics-2019-monitoring-health-for-the-sdgs-sustainable-development-goals
3. PORDATA: Base de Dados de Portugal Contemporâneo (2020). https://www.pordata.pt/Portugal
4. EUROSTAT: EUROSTAT data Browser - Healthy life years at age 65 by sex (2020). https://ec.europa.eu/eurostat/databrowser/view/tepsr_sp320/default/table?lang=en
5. Ministério da Saúde: Direção Geral da Saúde: Plano nacional de saúde: Revisão e extensão a 2020. Direção Geral da Saúde (2015). http://1nj5ms2lli5hdggbe3mm7ms5-wpengine.netdna-ssl.com/files/2015/06/Plano-Nacional-de-Saude-Revisao-e-Extensao-a-2020.pdf.pdf
6. Menoita, E. (ed.): Reabilitar a pessoa idosa com AVC. Lusociência, Loures (2012)

7. van Lieshout, M.R.J., Bleijenberg, N., Schuurmans, M.J., de Wit, N.J.: The effectiveness of a proactive multicomponent intervention program on disability in independently living older people: a randomized controlled trial. J. Nutr. Heal. Aging **22**, 1051–1059 (2018). https://doi.org/10.1007/s12603-018-1101-x
8. Fonseca, C., Lopes, M.: Modelo de autocuidado para pessoas com 65 e mais anos de idade, necessidades de cuidados de enfermagem. Tese de Doutoramento, Universidade de Lisboa (2013). https://repositorio.ul.pt/bitstream/10451/12196/1/ulsd069058_td_tese.pdf
9. Petronilho, F., Machado, M.: Teorias de Enfermagem e Autocuidado: Contributos para a Construção do Cuidado de Reabilitação. Em: Marques-Vieira, C., Sousa, L. (eds.) Cuidados de Enfermagem de Reabilitação à pessoa ao longo da vida, pp. 3–14. Lusociência, Loures (2017)
10. Hoeman, S.: Enfermagem de reabilitação: prevenção, intervenção e resultados esperados. Lusodidacta, Loures (2011)
11. Dirkes, S.M., Kozlowski, C.: Early mobility in the intensive care unit: evidence, barriers, and future directions. Crit. Care Nurs. **39**, 33–42 (2019). https://doi.org/10.4037/CCN2019654
12. Augustine, M.R., et al.: Implementation of post-acute rehabilitation at home: a skilled nursing facility-substitutive model. J. Am. Geriatr. Soc. 1584–1593 (2020). https://doi.org/10.1111/jgs.16474
13. Pires, R., Martins, M.M., Gomes, B., Monteiro, C., Ribeiro, O.: Intervenção do Enfermeiro Especialista em Reabilitação na Mobilidade da Pessoa Idosa Institucionalizada – Programa TEIA. Rev. Port. Enferm. Reabil. **2**, 90–101 (2019). https://doi.org/10.33194/RPER.2019.V2.N1.11.4557
14. Ordem dos Enfermeiros: Guia Orientador de Boas Práticas: Cuidados à pessoa com alterações da mobilidade – posicionamentos, transferências e treino de deambulação. Ordem dos Enfermeiros (2013). https://www.ordemenfermeiros.pt/arquivo/publicacoes/Documents/GOBP_Mobilidade_VF_site.pdf
15. Cerol, P., Martins, J., Sousa, L., Oliveira, I., Silveira, T.: Mobilização Precoce Em Pessoas Submetidas a Ventilação Mecânica Invasiva: Revisão Integrativa Da Literatura. Rev. Port. Enferm. Reabil. **2**, 49–58 (2019). https://doi.org/10.33194/RPER.2019.V2.N1.07.4563
16. Schober, A.E., Thornton, K.C.: Early mobilization in the intensive care unit. Curr. Anesthesiol. Rep. **32**(3), 73–78 (2013). https://doi.org/10.1007/S40140-013-0013-X
17. Cerqueira, A.V.B., Grilo, E.N.: Prevenção Das Consequências Da Imobilidade Na Pessoa Em Situação Crítica. Rev. Port. Enferm. Reabil. **2**, 78–89 (2019). https://doi.org/10.33194/RPER.2019.V2.N1.10.4574
18. Diário da República: Regulamento n.º 392/2019 de 3 de maio: Regulamento das Competências Específicas do Enfermeiro Especialista em Enfermagem de Reabilitação. Diário da República, 2a série - n.o 85 - 3 maio 2019, 13565–13568 (2019). https://www.ordemenfermeiros.pt/media/11871/1356513568.pdf
19. Ordem dos Enfermeiros: Assembleia do Colégio da Especialidade de Enfermagem de Reabilitação: Padrões de Qualidade Especializados em Enfermagem de Reabilitação. Ordem dos Enfermeiros (2018). https://www.ordemenfermeiros.pt/media/8141/ponto-4_regulamento-dos-padr%C3%B5es-qualidade-ceer.pdf
20. Chandler, J., (eds.). Cochrane Handbook for Systematic Reviews of Interventions version 6.2, Cochrane (2021). https://training.cochrane.org/handbook/current/chapter-i
21. Joanna Briggs Institute: Critical Appraisal Tools - Joanna Briggs Institute. https://jbi.global/critical-appraisal-tools (2021)
22. The JBI EBP Database: Ovid Database Guide. https://ospguides.ovid.com/OSPguides/jbidb.htm (2021)
23. Page, M.J., et al.: The PRISMA 2020 statement: an updated guideline for reporting systematic reviews. BMJ. 372 (2021). https://doi.org/10.1136/BMJ.N71

24. Begicheva, S.: Fuzzy model for evaluating the quality of medical care. In: Proceedings - 21st IEEE Conference Business Informatics, CBI 2019, vol. 2, pp. 5–8 (2019). https://doi.org/10.1109/CBI.2019.10088
25. Ordem dos Enfermeiros: Bilhetes de identidade dos indicadores que integram o core de indicadores por categoria de enunciados descritivos dos Padrões de Qualidade dos Cuidados de Enfermagem de Reabilitação. Ordem dos Enfermeiros (2018). https://www.ordemenfermeiros.pt/media/5443/enfermagemreabilitacao.pdf
26. Imhof, L., Suter-Riederer, S., Kesselring, J.: Effects of mobility-enhancing nursing intervention in patients with ms and stroke: randomised controlled trial. Int. Sch. Res. Not. **2015**, 1–6 (2015). https://doi.org/10.1155/2015/785497
27. Crotty, M., et al.: Should we provide outreach rehabilitation to very old people living in nursing care facilities after a hip fracture? A randomised controlled trial. Age Ageing **48**, 373–380 (2019). https://doi.org/10.1093/AGEING/AFZ005
28. Young, D.L., et al.: identifying barriers to nurse-facilitated patient mobility in the intensive care unit. Am. J. Crit. Care. **27**, 186–193 (2018). https://doi.org/10.4037/ajcc2018368
29. Lowthian, J.A., et al.: Predicting functional decline in older emergency patients—the Safe Elderly Emergency Discharge (SEED) project. Age Ageing **46**, 219–225 (2017). https://doi.org/10.1093/AGEING/AFW210
30. Liang, L., Pan, Y., Wu, D., Pang, Y., Xie, Y., Fang, H.: Effects of multidisciplinary team-based nurse-led transitional care on clinical outcomes and quality of life in patients with ankylosing spondylitis. Asian Nurs. Res. (Korean. Soc. Nurs. Sci). **13**, 107–114 (2019). https://doi.org/10.1016/J.ANR.2019.02.004

Self-care Promotion in the Person Undergoing Hip Arthroplasty: Gains Sensitive to Rehabilitation Nursing Care

Ana Filipa Mordido Martins[1(✉)], Filipa Isabel Oliveira Batista[2], Celso Silva[3], Hélder Neto Pino[2], and Isabel Nunes[4]

[1] Beja School of Health, Beja, Portugal
ana.mordido@uslba.min-saude.pt
[2] Algarve University Hospital Center, Portimão Unit, Portimão, Portugal
[3] North Alentejo Local Health Unit, Portalegre, Portugal
[4] UCC de Odivelas, ACES Loures-Odivelas, Odivelas, Portugal

Abstract. Hip Arthroplasty [HA] is an orthopedic surgery with a major influence on functionality and that limits the person undergoing this surgical intervention in his/her ability to self-care. The intervention of the Nurse Specialist in Rehabilitation Nursing [RNSN] is essential to promote actions that ensure functional empowerment for self-care, thus acting to maintain or increase functionality. Objective: To identify gains sensitive to the care of Rehabilitation Nursing [RN] in the promotion of self-care in the person submitted to HA, through the intervention of the RNSN. Methodology: A systematic literature review [RSL] was performed by searching the scientific platform EBSCO-HOST, the databases CINAHL Complete and MEDLINE Complete, employing the Boolean operators "OR" and "AND" and using the PI[C]O structure. Results: Sensible gains in RN care were observed through the RNSN's intervention with the person undergoing HA, which highlight the importance of RN intervention and care. Conclusions: The RN plays a key role in the rehabilitation process of the person undergoing HA and its intervention at the level of self-care is essential. The importance of the intervention of the RNSN in empowering for autonomy and self-care is highlighted, as functionality is improved through interventions at the level of knowledge. It is suggested that further scientific studies be conducted in this area with a view to the continuous improvement of nursing care.

Keywords: Rehabilitation nursing · Self-care · Person · Hip arthroplasty

1 Introduction

The RN contributes to improving the quality of health care to the extent that its intervention aims at maintaining and improving the quality of life of the people targeted by nursing care. The intervention of the RNSN aims at promoting early diagnosis and preventive actions in order to ensure the maintenance of the clients' functional capacities,

J. García-Alonso and C. Fonseca (Eds.): IWoG 2021, LNBE, pp. 171–181, 2022.
https://doi.org/10.1007/978-3-030-97524-1_16

prevent complications and avoid disabilities, as well as providing therapeutic interventions aimed at improving residual functions, maintaining or regaining independence in activities of daily living [1].

The specific competences of the RNSN cross all contexts of care practice, throughout the life cycle of the person with special needs, acting to maximize functionality [1].

This SLR aims to highlight the impact of RN care on the self-care of the person undergoing HA. Dorothea Orem's Self-Care Deficit Nursing Theory [SCDNT] argues that the purpose of nursing practice is to assist patients in their self-care needs so as to allow them to return to self-care, i.e., to be able to perform self-care by themselves, thus promoting their autonomy and functional independence [2]. Therefore, self-care is the focus and purpose of nursing care, aimed at improving people's health status, coping and functioning [3]. In SCDNT, self-care is defined as the performance or practice of activities that individuals perform for their own benefit as a way to maintain life, health, and well-being [2].

Self-care can be considered as an outcome sensitive to nursing care, with positive translation in health promotion and well-being through the increase of the person's knowledge and skills where health professionals, mainly nurses, have a decisive intervention [4, 5].

The intervention of the RNSN in orthopedics and traumatology is comprehensive and vast [6, 7]. The affections of the musculoskeletal system can bring with them multiple changes in functionality, among which the most frequent occur at the level of mobility. Functional mobility can be altered as a consequence of the physical or clinical situation resulting from certain pathologies, injuries or surgery, and it has a negative character with recognized repercussions [1, 8]. The musculoskeletal system is usually the most affected by mobility alterations, with a decrease in muscle contraction, loss of strength and muscle mass, atrophy, contractures, and osteoporosis [7, 8]. The RNSN intervention is essential for the proper planning of nursing care, including interventions that favor the maintenance of mobility and self-care, as a way to prevent changes with negative repercussions on the lives of affected individuals [8].

The RNSN intervenes from the first moment of hospitalization of the person who will undergo orthopedic surgery [7]. Their intervention includes data collection and assessment, planning and implementation of RN care, pre- and postoperative teaching, monitoring and surveillance in the immediate postoperative period, and discharge planning to ensure continuity of care [6, 7].

2 Methodology

SLR is a reproducible and explicit methodology; a systematic search that attempts to identify all studies that meet the eligibility criteria by assessing the validity of the conclusions of the included studies, for example, through the risk of bias; presenting in a systematic and synthesized way the characteristics and results of the included studies [9, 10]. We developed the following steps: formulation of a review question; definition of inclusion and exclusion criteria; location and selection of studies; assessment of their methodological quality; data extraction; analysis/summary and synthesis of relevant results; presentation and interpretation of results and determination of their applicability

[8–10]. It is through this method that we intend to identify sensitive gains to RN care intervening at the level of self-care.

After defining the theme to be addressed, the problem was formulated through a starting question, based on the PICO structure developed to answer health-related questions [11]. Based on this concept, the starting question was "What are the gains associated with rehabilitation nursing care in the promotion of self-care in people undergoing HA? (Fig. 1).

[P] POPULATION	[I] INTERVENTIO N	[C] COMPARISSON	[O] OUTCOMES
• People who have undergone hip arthroplasty • (HA)	• Motor Functional Rehabilitation Program/ Teaching	• Level of self-care	• Sensible Gains from Rehabilitation Nursing

Fig. 1. PICO methodology

The search was conducted through the scientific search platform EBSCO-HOST, accessing the databases CINAHL Complete and MEDLINE Complete, carried out in the month of March 2021, following the FINER criteria (Feasibility, Interesting, Novel, Ethical, Relevant), which affirms the feasibility, interest, originality, relevance to practice and compliance with ethical principles of the research question.

The following descriptors were used according to the research question: [(arthroplasty OR orthopedic OR orthopedic nursing interventions) AND (nursing OR nursing interventions OR nursing care) AND (outcomes OR outcomes nursing OR education)].

The selection of studies was defined according to inclusion and exclusion criteria. The inclusion criteria included articles related to the object under study, rehabilitation nursing interventions at the level of self-care in people aged 65 and older who underwent HA. The exclusion criteria were articles without full text, repeated in the databases, and unrelated to the object under study.

After selecting the articles, starting from 194 as a result of the database search, removing those that were duplicates, we were left with 178 articles. After reading the title and abstract, we obtained 159 articles applicable to the study. The number of articles screened after analyzing the methodology, results, and conclusion was 19, but since 13 did not answer the starting question, at the end of the selection we were left with six articles applicable to this SLR. The description of this process is systematized in the following flowchart (Fig. 2).

Still addressing the evaluation of the quality of the studies, it is fundamental that they obey the rules of authorship, with the proper citations and references of the authors, considering the principles of intellectual honesty as an ethical question [12].

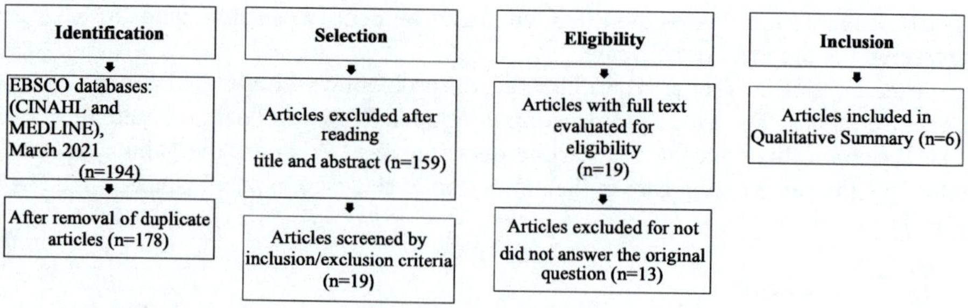

Fig. 2. Study flowchart

3 Results

For the results to have an impact on clinical practice, they must be credible, reliable and valid [8, 10, 11, 14]. It is also for this reason that studies to be included in a systematic review of the literature must be filtered, passing through inclusion/exclusion, quality, and validity criteria, and given a certain level of evidence [9, 10, 13].

To classify the quality and scientific evidence of the six articles we followed Melnyk and Fineout-Overholt's evidence hierarchy classification system [10], which addresses research questions about interventions and treatments according to seven levels of evidence: Level I, which refers to systematic reviews or meta-analysis of all relevant randomized clinical trials; Level II which reports to well-designed randomized controlled trials; Level III, concerning well-designed clinical trials without randomization; Level IV concerning well-designed case-control and cohort studies; Level V which corresponds to systematic reviews of descriptive and qualitative studies; Level VI which directs to single descriptive or qualitative studies and Level VII which concerns opinion of authorities or expert reports [9, 10].

Table 1, synthetic and demonstrative of the characteristics of the selected articles, includes the identified level of evidence in order to demonstrate the eligibility, quality of results and conclusions, being a guarantee of production of current knowledge for the subject under study.

4 Discussion of Results

The implementation of the search and standardization of nursing-sensitive outcomes allows comparing results and thus identifying the best nursing practices at a global level, thus contributing to the continuous improvement of health care quality [14].

The identification of health gains obtained through the provision of rehabilitation nursing care and the evidence of these gains [9, 10] are essential to demonstrate the essential nature of rehabilitation nursing in health services [15] and its importance in empowering people for self-care [3, 4].

Table 2 shows that rehabilitation nursing plays a key role in empowering the person undergoing HA to self-care, a statement supported by several authors and confirmed by the improvement in self-efficacy, ability for self-care and autonomy [16, 17, 19–21].

Table 1. Characteristics and synthesis of the selected articles

Article	Title/ Source/Authors/Methodology/Participants/Description/ Level of Evidence	Objectives	Intervention	Results/Conclusions
1	**Title- Changing practice for hip arthroplasty and its implications** **Origin-** UK **Authors-** Schultz K, Ewbank ML, Pandit HG **Description methodology** - analysis and review of articles on medical and nursing care of the person undergoing orthopedic surgery and its implications on care practice for nurses and physicians. **Participants** – People who have undergone hip arthroplasty **LEVEL OF EVIDENCE - V**	To provide insight into changes in clinical practice and the implications for nurses and physicians who are involved in the care of patients undergoing total hip arthroplasty	Pre-operative education of the person who will undergo hip arthroplasty; Monitoring for complications that may delay the rehabilitation process such as: neuropathic pain (sciatic involvement), dislocation, surgical wound complications, surgical site pain (inadequate pain relief)	Nurses play a central role in achieving positive rehabilitation outcomes in post-operative hip arthroplasty. With new knowledge nurses can provide better care for people undergoing total hip arthroplasty. Whether it is improving patient knowledge by providing teaching, recognizing complications, or performing surgical wound care, the nurse plays a key role in the hip replacement patient's rehabilitation.
2	**Title - Effect of nursing intervention via a chatting tool on the rehabilitation of patients after Total hip Arthroplasty** **Origin-** China **Authors-** Luo j, Dong X, Hu J **Methodology – Descriptive study** **Description methodology** - Retrospective analysis of 232 patients who underwent total hip arthroplasty from January 2013 to October 2015. Data collection tools: Harris hip score, the Short-Form 36 (SF-36) questionnaire, and the Functional Independence Measure (FIM). **Participants** – 232 patients who underwent total hip arthroplasty, over 65 years of age, cognitive function and communication ability considered normal, from January 2013 to October 2015. **LEVEL OF EVIDENCE – VI**	To evaluate the effect of nursing intervention via WeChat (online chat tool) on the rehabilitation of patients undergoing total hip arthroplasty.	The two groups were given exactly the same information about: knowledge about total hip arthroplasty, psychological support, guidelines, diet, issues that need attention post-discharge, prevention of complications, and rehabilitation guidelines. Muscle strength training, muscle-articular mobilization training, walking, going up and down stairs, and wearing appropriate footwear. Hip joint function evaluation (instruments specified in the methodology).	Nursing contact after discharge can improve the effect of rehabilitation after hip arthroplasty and promote recovery of joint function in people who have undergone this surgery. After discharge, nursing contact can improve the recovery of hip joint function, quality of life, and functional independence in patients who have undergone hip arthroplasty. Therefore, it can improve the effect of rehabilitation after hip arthroplasty.
	Title- Factors Predicting Functional Ability among Older Adults undergoing Hip and Knee Arthroplasty	To predict functional capacity two weeks postopera-	Preoperative teaching regarding surgery and care regarding the preven-	For successful recovery after hip or knee arthroplasty to perform ADLs, nurses are essential. It is

(continued)

Table 1. *(continued)*

3	**Origin-** Thailand **Authors-** Aree-Ue S, Roopsawang I, Kawinwonggowit V **Methodology** – Prospective cohort study **Description methodology** - Prospective cohort study, with 95 adults over 60 years old, with scheduled hip and knee arthroplasty. Four data collection instruments were used: Demographic and Health Information Questionnaire, Functional Ability Improvement Expectation Questionnaire, Care Transition Measure -15 (CTM-15 and Modified Barthel Index). **Participants** – 95 patients over 65 years of age, with hip and knee arthroplasty scheduled at the hospital where the study took place. **LEVEL OF EVIDENCE – IV**	tively in adults over 60 years of age who have undergone hip or knee arthroplasty, and which factors have an influence on this functional capacity.	tion of prosthetic luxation. Convey to the person the importance of their commitment to the success of the rehabilitation process. Emphasize the importance of quality transitional care (maintenance of the rehabilitation process at home).	necessary to plan preoperative education/instruction interventions that provide people with the knowledge needed to succeed in their recovery process. The results showed that participants developed a high level of functional capacity. The quality of care was positively related to the effective improvement of functional capacity.
4	**Title- Nursing care to patients submitted to total hip arthroplasty and the importance of care in the postoperative period** **Origin-** Brazil **Authors-** Soares A., Silva A., Silva G., Siqueira I., Pamponet J., Cruz M., Quiles, P. & Santos, M. **Methodology** – Literature Review **Description methodology** - descriptive, retrospective, literature review research. **Participants** – people undergoing total hip arthroplasty **LEVEL OF EVIDENCE – V**	To highlight the specific nursing care directed to the patient submitted to total hip arthroplasty, emphasizing the postoperative care, the surgical complications, the nursing interventions and the orientation for discharge, using the Nursing Care Systematization (NCS).	Perform pre-operative visit in order to personalize care and detect the needs of each person. Prepare individualized care plan. Carry out preoperative teaching. Assess cognitive function, vital signs, monitor complications of medical devices, monitor skin integrity, position the person undergoing hip arthroplasty taking into account the avoidance of potentially dislocating movements of the prosthesis. Encourage self-care.	Nursing plays a key role in the perioperative process of patients undergoing total hip arthroplasty. The NCS (Nursing Care Systematization) is a tool that helps nurses to provide individualized and comprehensive care, including guidelines at all stages of hospitalization and also at home, aiming to eliminate the possibility of iatrogenic events and provide an adequate rehabilitation and also to empower the caregiver for hospital discharge.

(continued)

Table 1. *(continued)*

5	**Title- Percurso das necessidades em Cuidados de Enfermagem nos Clientes submetidos a Artroplastia da Anca** **Origin-** Portugal **Authors-** Martins MM, Fernandes CS **Methodology** – Case Study Methodology **Description methodology -** Descriptive, relational case study with repeated measures. Instruments used for data collection: survey, measurement scales (Barthel Index and Satisfaction scale) and observation of the documented care record. Participants 30 clients submitted to total hip arthroplasty **LEVEL OF EVIDENCE – VI**	To analyze the congruence between the nursing care provided and the needs expressed by clients. To describe the characteristics of the teaching context practiced by nurses. To identify the level of satisfaction of patients undergoing hip arthroplasty with the nursing care provided during hospitalization. To reflect on the nursing practices for patients undergoing hip arthroplasty.	To assess the degree of functional independence of the person who underwent hip arthroplasty using the Barthel Index. To evaluate the satisfaction of the person who underwent hip arthroplasty regarding the nursing care provided through a satisfaction scale.	The nurse's intervention should be centered on the client and his/her needs and not on the needs/wants/interests of the professionals. It is pertinent to identify the clients' needs, and to guide the services to achieve them. It is essential to focus attention on the client, to make sure that the client's concerns are an integral part of the care they receive. In terms of teaching, the aspects most focused on by nurses are transferring, positioning, and walking. The information documented by nurses, such as the teachings on self-care, reveal differences between what was done and what was recorded. Nurses need to understand and perceive the individual needs of clients.
6	**Title- The importance of teaching patients undergoing total hip or knee arthroplasty** **Origin-** Greece **Authors-** Copanitsanou P, Sourtzi P, Valkeapaa K, Lemonidou C **Methodology** – Longitudinal, descriptive, correlational study. **Description methodology -** Longitudinal, descriptive and correlational study, with assessments before surgery, at hospital discharge and six months after surgery. Data collection instruments: Knowledge Expectations of Hospitalized Patients (KEhp-scale) and recieved knowledge scales. **Participants** – patients submitted to hip or knee arthroplasty between March 2009 and April 2011. **LEVEL OF EVIDENCE – VI**	- Investigating the prior knowledge, expectations, and knowledge provided to patients undergoing total hip or knee arthroplasty.	To assess the knowledge expectations of patients undergoing total hip or knee arthroplasty using the Knowledge Expectations of Hospitalized Patients (KEhp) data collection instrument. To assess the knowledge transmitted to patients undergoing total hip or knee arthroplasty using the knowledge received scales.	Patients had high expectations of knowledge, mainly in the functional and bio physiological dimensions. Patients' expectations were addressed mainly in the functional and bio-physiological dimensions. Patients had high expectations of teaching regarding surgery and these expectations were not fully met, which hinders their rehabilitation process. Patient teaching is an important individualized nursing intervention and efforts to promote it will contribute to the enhancement of the role of nursing.

Table 2. Sensitive indicators for rehabilitation nursing care identified in the study:

Outcome indicators	Sensitive indicators
Functional status	- Improved functional capacity [16–20] - Improvement in physical fitness [17, 20]
Empowerment for self-care	- Improvement in self-efficacy [17–20] - Empowerment for self-care [16–21] - Improved autonomy [17, 19, 20] - Improved people's perception of autonomy [16–20]
Professional/person relationship	- Improved implementation, encouragement, and follow-up [16, 17] - Improved satisfaction of needs [16, 18, 19]
Satisfaction of the person	- Confers health gains [16–20] - High satisfaction of people regarding care [18–20]
Capacity building for knowledge	- Improved health education [16, 17, 19] - Improved knowledge [16–18, 21]
Capacity building for quality of life	- Improved quality of life [16–18, 20, 21]

In the studies included in this SLR, the pre- and postoperative teaching to the person undergoing HA has great prominence, which highlights its importance for the success of the rehabilitation process [16, 18, 20, 21]. Educational, cognitive, behavioral and symptom management interventions are based on self-care [3]. These interventions involve informing patients about their condition and its treatments, instructing them in self-monitoring, noticing and identifying changes in functionality, and developing appropriate actions regarding these changes [16–19, 21]. Self-care is understood as an outcome of nursing care in which people are expected to select and develop actions to maintain life, healthy functioning and well-being [3].

This fact is corroborated by the Portuguese Order of Nurses [ON] in the regulation of the specific competencies of the Rehabilitation Nursing Specialist Nurse [RNSN], which states that the RNSN intervenes in the education of clients and significant others, in discharge planning, in the continuity of care and in the reintegration of people into their family and community, thus providing them with the right to dignity and quality of life [1]. Schultz, Ewbank, and Pandit [16] emphasize the importance of nursing interventions related to teaching and state that nurses play a central role in obtaining positive results in the rehabilitation process in postoperative HA. This teaching should be accompanied by instruction and training aimed at empowering the person for self-care, providing him/her with the necessary tools for a successful rehabilitation process, always with the proper follow-up. Therefore, nursing follow-up should be continuous and extend beyond discharge [17]. In their study, Aree-Ue and colleagues concluded that nurses are essential in the instruction and training of activities of daily living after HA for the success of the rehabilitation process [18]. They argue that it is necessary to plan pre- and postoperative education/instruction interventions that provide people with the knowledge necessary for the success of their recovery process [18]. It is essential to know the person's needs, their level of previous autonomy/dependence, housing conditions, and family/significant person support in order to be able to address their needs and provide individualized RN care [20, 21].

Promoting self-care in people undergoing HA is to contribute to improving their quality of life and work towards maintaining or developing their functional independence [18, 21]. As described in the RNSN's specific competencies, its intervention aims to promote early diagnosis and preventive actions for RN, so as to ensure the maintenance of people's functional capacity, prevent complications and avoid disabilities, as well as to provide therapeutic interventions aimed at improving residual functions, maintaining or regaining independence in life activities, and minimizing the impact of installed disabilities, namely at the level of neurological, respiratory, cardiac, orthopedic functions and other disabilities [1].

Capacity building is a multidimensional process that involves knowledge, decision, and action [22]. Exercising empowerment requires commitment and dedication. Empowerment for self-care is translated into life activities that ensure basic conditions [22]. These personal life activities, along with instrumental life activities, such as integrating into the community, shopping, and taking control of one's own health, reflect autonomy and independence and are related to functionality and quality of life [17, 18, 20–22]. Other factors that interfere with functionality and self-care are the person's cognition and environmental factors [23, 24].

5 Conclusion

The RN plays a key role in the rehabilitation process of the person undergoing HA [1, 7, 16–18, 21]. Its intervention in self-care is essential in the rehabilitation process of the person undergoing this surgery [16, 18, 20]. These statements are within the scope of the RNSN's specific competencies, since the RNSN cares for people with special needs throughout the life cycle, in all contexts of care practice; b) empowers the person with disability, activity limitation and/or participation restriction to reintegrate and exercise citizenship and c) maximizes functionality by developing the person's abilities [1]. The intervention within the scope of these competencies requires commitment and dedication and encompasses the development of research projects in the area of care provision, based on scientific evidence, implementing evidence-based practice [9, 10] and contributing to evidence gains that are sensitive to the RN care [15], with a consequent impact on the continuous improvement of the quality of care [14].

The results of this study show significant gains from RN care, particularly regarding the promotion of self-care in people undergoing AA [16–21]. These demonstrate the importance of RN intervention and care. Thus, it is worth noting the importance of the RNSN intervention in terms of empowerment for autonomy and self-care [18, 21], and the improvement of functionality [16–20, 25–27] through interventions at the level of knowledge [16–19, 21].

Therefore, we believe that it is possible to design and implement RN intervention programs based on the sensible gains identified in this SLR. However, we suggest the continuity of scientific studies in this area with a view to the continuous improvement of nursing care.

References

1. Ordem dos Enfermeiros [OE]: Regulamento n.º 392/2019 de 3 de maio de 2019. Regulamento das competências específicas do enfermeiro especialista em Enfermagem de Reabilitação. Diário da República, 2.ª série—N.º 85, 13565–13568 (2019). https://dre.pt/web/guest/pesquisa/-/search/122216893/details/normal?l=1
2. Orem, D.E.: Nursing: Concepts of Practice, 6th edn. Mosby, St. Louis (2001)
3. Fonseca, C.: Modelo de autocuidado para pessoas com 65 e mais anos de idade, necessidade de cuidados de enfermagem. Tese de Doutoramento orientada pelo Professor Doutor Manuel Lopes, Universidade de Lisboa (2013). https://repositorio.ul.pt/bitstream/10451/12196/1/ulsd069058_td_tese.pdf
4. Santos, B., Ramos, A., Fonseca, C.: Training to practice: importance of self-care theory in nursing process for improving care. J. Aging Innov. **6**(1), 51–54 (2017). http://www.rdpc.uevora.pt/bitstream/10174/22960/1/6-Autocuidado-forma%c3%a7%c3%a3o.pdf
5. Tomey, A., Alligood, M.: Teóricas de enfermagem e a sua obra. Lusociência, Loures (2007)
6. Cunha, E.: Enfermagem em Ortopedia. Lidel, Lisboa – Porto (2008)
7. Sousa, L., Carvalho, M.: Pessoa com osteoartrose na Anca e Joelho em contexto de internamento e ortopedia. In: Marques-Vieira, C., Sousa, L. (eds.) Cuidados de Enfermagem de Reabilitação à Pessoa ao Longo da Vida., 1st edn., pp. 405–420. Lusodidacta, Loures (2016)
8. Ordem dos Enfermeiros [OE]: Guia Orientador de Boa Prática: Cuidados à Pessoa com Alterações da Mobilidade - Posicionamentos, Transferências e Treino de Deambulação (2013). https://www.ordemenfermeiros.pt/arquivo/publicacoes/Documents/GOBP_Mobilidade_VF_site.pdf
9. Melkin, B., Gallagher-Ford, L.: Evidence-Based Practice in Nursing and Healthcare. A Guide to Best Pratice, 4th edn. Wolters Kluwer/Lippincott Williams & Wilkins, Philadelphia (2018). EUA
10. Melkin, B., Gallagher-Ford, L., Long, L., Fineout-Overholt, E.: The Establishment of evidence-based practice competencies for practicing registered nurses and advanced practice nurses in real-world clinical settings: proficiencies to improve healthcare quality, reliability, patient outcomes, and costs. Worldviews Evid.-Based Nurs. **11**(1), 5–15 (2014). https://doi.org/10.1111/wvn.12021
11. Davies, K.: Formulating the evidence based practice question: a review of the frameworks. Evid. Based Libr. Inf. Pract. **6**(2), 75–80 (2011). https://doi.org/10.18438/B8WS5N
12. Nunes, L.: Aspetos Éticos na Investigação de Enfermagem. Departamento de Enfermagem ESS|IPS. Setúbal (2020). https://comum.rcaap.pt/bitstream/10400.26/32782/1/ebook_aspetos%20eticos%20investigacao%20Enf_jun%202020.pdf
13. Apóstolo, J.: Síntese da evidência no contexto da translação da ciência. Escola Superior de Enfermagem de Coimbra, Coimbra (2017). file://C:/Users/USER/Downloads/livro%20joão%20apóstolo%20web.pdf
14. Doran, D., Pringle, D.: Patient outcomes as accountability. In: Nursing Outcomes: The State of the Science, 2nd edn., pp. 1–27. Jones and Bartlett, Sudbury (2011)
15. Ordem dos Enfermeiros [OE]: Assembleia do Colégio da Especialidade de Enfermagem de Reabilitação. Padrões de Qualidade dos Cuidados Especializados em Enfermagem de Reabilitação (2018). https://www.ordemenfermeiros.pt/media/8192/ponto-4_regulamento-dos-padr%C3%B5es-qualidade-ceer-1.pdf
16. Schultz, K., Ewbank, M., Pandit, H.: Changing practice for hip arthroplasty and its implications. Br. J. Nurs. **26**(22), 1238–1244 (2017). https://doi.org/10.12968/bjon.2017.26.22.1238
17. Luo, J., Dong, X., Hu, J.: Effect of nursing intervention via a chatting tool on the rehabilitation of patients after total hip arthroplasty. J. Orthop. Surg. Res. **14**(1), 1–6 (2019). https://doi.org/10.1186/s13018-019-1483-4

18. Aree-Ue, S., Roopsawang, I., Kawinwonggowit, V.: Factors predicting functional ability among older adults undergoing hip and knee arthroplasty. Pac. Rim Int. J. Nurs. Res. **23**(2), 156–169 (2019). file:///C:/Users/USER/Downloads/120092-Article%20Text-515596-1-10-20190326.pdf
19. Soares, A., et al.: A assistência de enfermagem ao paciente submetido a artroplastia total de quadril e a importância dos cuidados no período pós-operatório. São Paulo: Rev. Recien. **3**(7), 11–18 (2013). https://doi.org/10.24276/rrecien2177-157X.2013.3.7.11-18
20. Martins, M., Fernandes, C.: Percurso das necessidades em cuidados de enfermagem nos clientes submetidos a artroplastia da anca. Rev. Referência **II**(11), 79–92 (2009). Percurso das necessidades em Cuidados de Enfermagem nos Clientes submetidos a Artroplastia da Anca (esenfc.pt)
21. Copanitsanou, P., Sourtzi, P., Valkeapaa, K., Lemonidou, C.: Empowering education of patients undergoing total hip or knee arthroplasty. Arch. Hellenic Med. **33**(3), 386–398 (2016)
22. Reis, G., Bule, M.J.: Capacitação e atividade de vida. In: Marques-Vieira, C., Sousa, L. (eds.) Cuidados de Enfermagem de Reabilitação à Pessoa ao Longo da Vida. 1ª edição, pp. 57–65. Lusodidacta, Loures (2016)
23. Lopes, M.J., et al.: Functioning and cognition of Portuguese older adults attending in residential homes and day centers: a comparative study. Int. J. Environ. Res. Public Health Spec. Issue Ageing Health Funct. Psychol. Perspect. **18**, 7030 (2021). https://doi.org/10.3390/ijerph18137030
24. Fonseca, C., Pinho, L.G., Lopes, M.J., Marques, M.C., Garcia-Alonso, J.: The elderly nursing core set and the cognition of portuguese older adults: a cross-sectional study. BMC Nurs. **20**(1) (2021). https://doi.org/10.1186/s12912-021-00623-1
25. Brandão, A., et al.: Rehabilitation nursing technology intervention gains based on the model of self-care, in the elderly person with a proximal femoral fracture. In: García-Alonso, J., Fonseca, C. (eds.) IWoG 2020. LNB, pp. 161–167. Springer, Cham (2021). https://doi.org/10.1007/978-3-030-72567-9_16
26. Silva, A., et al.: Promotion of functional independence in the self-care deficit of the elderly person with orthopedic disease and technology. In: García-Alonso, J., Fonseca, C. (eds.) IWoG 2020. LNB, pp. 149–160. Springer, Cham (2021). https://doi.org/10.1007/978-3-030-72567-9_15
27. Fonseca, C., et al.: Training proposal technology for the elderly with changes in self care and for their caregiver: rehabilitation nursing care contributions. In: García-Alonso, J., Fonseca, C. (eds.) IWoG 2020. LNB, pp. 69–80. Springer, Cham (2021). https://doi.org/10.1007/978-3-030-72567-9_7

Check for updates

Educational Actions Offered by Health Professionals to Elderly Residents in Long-Term Care Institutions: Integrative Review

Cenir Gonçalves Tier[1](✉), Aline Ost dos Santos[2], Daiane Porto Gautério Abreu[3], Graciela Dutra Sehnem[2], Tatiele Zago Bonorino[1], Joana Jorge da Rosa[1], Thayná da Fonseca Aguirre[1], Laura Neres de Melo[1], and Rodolfo Kubiça Neto[1]

[1] Universidade Federal do Pampa - UNIPAMPA, Uruguaiana, Brazil
{cenirtier,tatielebonorino.aluno,joanajorge.aluno,
thaynaaguirre.aluno,lauraneres.aluno}@unipampa.edu.br

[2] Universidade Federal do Rio Grande - FURG, Rio Grande, Brazil
aline.ost@acad.ufsm.br, graciela.sehnem@ufsm.br

[3] Universidade Federal de Santa Maria - UFSM, Santa Maria, Brazil

Abstract. Objective: To identify the scientific evidence available on the educational actions performed with health professionals aimed at improving the care of elderly people in long-stay institutions in the last 5 years. Method: Integrative literature review conducted in October 2021 by four independent reviewers. The following electronic databases were used to select articles: Medical Literature Analysis and Retrieval System Online (MEDLINE) via PubMed; Web of Science; SciVerse Scopus; Latin American and Caribbean Literature on Health Sciences (LILACS) and Database on Nursing (BDENF) via Virtual Health Library (VHL); Scientifc Eletronic Library Online (Scielo). The guiding question of this study was defined using the Population/Patient/Problem - Interest - Context, Time (PICoT) strategy: What is the available scientific evidence on the educational actions carried out with health professionals aimed at improving the care of elderly people in long-stay institutions in the last 5 years? Results: The educational actions in three articles that make up the corpus of the analysis, presenting levels of evidence six and three. Conclusion: It is necessary to invest in educational actions for health professionals as well as in the production of knowledge about alternatives and advice in the professional practice of the multidisciplinary team emphasizing active aging, compassionate communication, care through comfort and preventive measures of aggravations besides rehabilitation care. New studies about the needs of the team to develop a qualified care should be raised, emerging resolutive and specific alternatives in the care of the person.

Keywords: Homes for the aged · Health personnel · Health education

1 Introduction

The changes in the public health scenario observed in recent decades have contributed to the increase in the life expectancy of the elderly population. In this sense, there

J. García-Alonso and C. Fonseca (Eds.): IWoG 2021, LNBE, pp. 182–189, 2022.
https://doi.org/10.1007/978-3-030-97524-1_17

is an increased demand for long-term care, since many elderly people have chronic degenerative diseases and decline in functional capacity [1]. Although, in Brazil, the care of the elderly person in the family context is the prevalent one, changes in society such as the decrease in the size of families and the participation of women in the labor market, lead to an increasing demand for long-stay institutions for the elderly [2, 3].

Long-stay institutions for the elderly are governmental or non-governmental institutions, residential in nature, intended for the collective home of people aged 60 (sixty) years or more, with or without family support, in conditions of freedom and dignity and citizenship [4]. They should be a specialized home, with a double function - to provide gerontogeriatric care according to the degree of dependence of its residents and to offer, at the same time, a domestic, cozy environment, able to preserve the intimacy and identity of its residents [4, 5].

Within the context of LSIEs, education stands out as a guiding axis for improving the care of elderly residents, highlighting care as an attitudinal process that is the product of the interaction between technique and humanization [5].

The adoption of educational interventions together with changes in the organizational culture of these spaces would be the main fronts for institutional interventions in LSIEs, capable of providing the professionals who work in them with the subsidies to assist the elderly residents in their entirety [5].

Thus, this article aims to identify the available scientific evidence on the educational actions performed with health professionals aimed at improving the care of elderly people in long-stay institutions in the last 5 years.

2 Method

The integrative review is a methodological approach to reviews, allowing the inclusion of experimental and non-experimental studies with the purpose of a complete understanding of the analyzed phenomenon [6].

Thus, Evidence-Based Practice is an approach with which aims to improve clinical effectiveness and support the health care professional in his or her actions, using three elements: scientific evidence, clinical experience, and patient preferences [7].

To this end, it was guided with the following pre-defined steps: 1) definition of the guiding question; 2) literature search and sampling; 3) data collection; 4) critical analysis of the included studies, 5) discussion of results; 6) presentation of the integrative review [6].

The guiding question for this study was defined using the Population/Patient/Problem - Interest - Context, Time (PICoT) strategy, resulting in the following guiding question: What is the available scientific evidence on the educational actions performed with health professionals aimed at improving the care of elderly people in long-stay institutions in the last 5 years?

For this end, the acronym "P" (target population) was used for the elderly; the acronym "I" (interest) was used for the educational actions carried out by the multi-professional team of caregivers of the elderly in LSIE; the acronym "CO" (context) was used for the long-stay institution for the elderly, and the acronym "T" was used for the last five years.

The literature search and sampling occurred in October 2021 by four reviewers independently in the electronic databases: Medical Literature Analysis and Retrieval System Online (MEDLINE) via PubMed; Web of Science; SciVerse Scopus; Latin American and Caribbean Literature on Health Sciences (LILACS) and Database on Nursing (BDENF) via Virtual Health Library (VHL); Scientifc Eletronic Library Online (Scielo); The search strategy was identified through the use of the Descriptors in Health Sciences (DECS) and the Mesch Terms combined in sequence on a Boolean logic basis: AND or OR. Table 1 shows the databases used and the strategy listed.

Table 1. Search strategy for the selection of primary studies

Database	Search strategy
MEDLINE	Health Education AND Continuing Education AND Continuing Nursing Education AND Population Education AND Technical Nursing Education AND The Elderly OR geriatrics OR, Long-stay institutions for the Elderly AND Patient Care Team OR Nursing Team OR nursing
Web of science	Health Education OR Continuing Education OR Continuing Nursing Education OR Population Education OR Technical Nursing Education AND Elderly OR elderly OR geriatrics OR, Long Term Care Institution for the Elderly AND Patient Care Team OR Nursing Team OR nursing
Scielo	Health Education OR Continuing Education OR Continuing Nursing Education OR Population Education OR Technical Nursing Education AND Elderly OR elderly OR geriatrics OR, Long Term Care Institution for the Elderly AND Patient Care Team OR Nursing Team OR nursing
Scopus	Health AND education OR population AND education AND aged OR old AND age AND assistance OR homes AND for AND the AND aged
LILACS e BDENF	Health Education OR Continuing Education OR Continuing Nursing Education OR Population Education OR Technical Nursing Education AND Elderly OR elderly OR geriatrics OR, Long Term Care Institution for the Elderly AND Patient Care Team OR Nursing Team OR nursing

Source: elaborated by the authors, 2021

3 Results

In the data collection phase, 182,730 articles were identified. After that, articles were selected according to the inclusion and exclusion criteria. Inclusion criteria were original articles on the theme of this study: care for the elderly in LSIE in Portuguese, English or Spanish, with a time frame of the last five years, available in full for free.

The exclusion criteria were theses, dissertations and monographs, editorials, reflections, literature reviews (narrative, integrative, systematic, scope, meta-analysis), experience reports, as well as those that did not correspond to the theme of the study. From this perspective, duplicate studies were counted only once.

After applying these criteria, 181,830 articles were excluded due to not being written in Portuguese, English or Spanish, not having been published in the last five years, not being original research, not contemplating the care of the elderly in ILPI. Six duplicate articles were found. In this step, 900 articles were selected for title and abstract reading according to the guiding research, being inserted in the Endnote [8] reference manager.

The title and abstract analysis occurred through careful reading of the 900 articles identified from the titles, abstracts, and keywords of the studies through the Rayyan tool without the researchers having access to the decisions of others to ensure the selection of publications related to the research question independently. At this stage, researchers

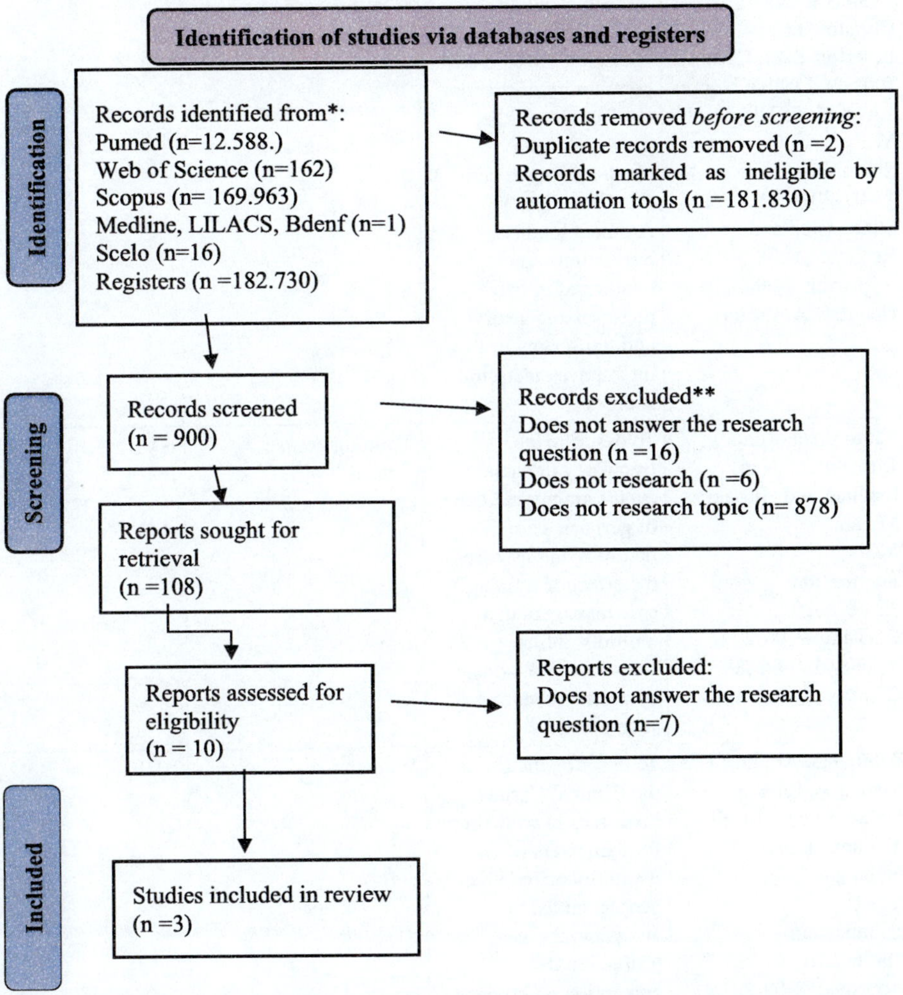

Fig. 1. Flowchart of article selection on Educational actions offered by health professionals to residents of long-term care facilities, Uruguaiana, Rio Grande do Sul, Brazil, 2021. **Source:** elaborated by the authors, 2021

were allowed access to the studies for the final consensus of the 108 titles and abstracts that presented divergences. Two duplicate studies were found. After meeting with the researchers, 10 articles were selected to be read in full, and 03 of these studies were selected to compose the corpus of the analysis.

Table 2. Summary of the primary studies

Authors, year, country	Purpose	Educative action	Level of evidence
Jacqueline Francis-Coad, Christopher Etherton-Beer, Caroline Bulsara, Debbie Nobre, Anne-Marie Hill Years: Submission: 13-07-2016 Submission and Review: 31–08-2016 Approval: 6-09-2016 Country: Australia	The aims of this study were to evaluate establishing and operating a web-based community of practice (CoP) to lead falls prevention in a residential aged care (RAC) setting A mixed methods evaluation was conducted in two phases using a survey and transcripts from interactive electronic sources	Comunidade de prática (CoP) baseada na web	NVI [9]
Shino Ikeda-Sonoda, Jiro Okochi, Nao Ichihara and Hiroaki Miyata Years: Submission: 25-08-2020 Revision: 3-06-2021 Approval: 9-06-2021 Country: Japan	To describe the frequency of such events among residents of geriatric care facilities and assesses the effect of training care managers in a multidisciplinary plan-do-check-adjust cycle on preventing such events	Training course	NVIII [10]
Fabíola de Araújo Leite Medeiros, Lidiany Galdino Félix, Maria Miriam Lima da Nóbrega Years: Submission: 29-06-2016 Approval: 8-07-2016 Country: Brazil	To describe the use of the Clinical Caritas Processes in workshops for caregivers of institutionalized elderly people, aimed at analyzing these professionals' perception on humane care towards the institutionalized elderly	Workshops	NVI [11]

Source: elaborated by the authors, 2021

According to the figure synthesis of the review results by interpreting the studies and presenting the synthesis of the knowledge of the studies eligible for the corpus of this review will be by means of the synoptic flowchart in the PRISMA model as shown in Fig. 1.

Three different types of educational activities were identified in the selected articles as shown in Table 2.

In a first moment, scientific evidence on fall prevention was collected from interactive electronic sources. This evidence was organized and then made available via a web community so that the health professionals and caregivers of the institution could access it and, through interaction with the content and other participants, a training on the subject was carried out. However, the researchers identified that the participants had little knowledge to use and interact via web, and, due to other activities related to elderly care, they did not have time to participate in the training.

The authors of the community of practice educational action concluded that a web-based community of practice (CoP) is beneficial but would be more resolutive in teaching about falls if participants received training in its use.

In a training course, an educational intervention was conducted with the goal of preventing falls, aspiration, and pressure ulcers. The intervention was evaluated in a non-randomized clinical trial. The intervention group with 862 elderly was composed of geriatric care units in which care managers had participated in a training course, while the control group with 416 elderly was composed of units with care managers who had not received this training. The results showed that the educational intervention was not effective in preventing falls, fever, or pressure ulcers due to the barriers of adopting preventive measures to avoid the risks. In this sense, the authors of the study believe that it is important to share these risks with residents and their families.

In educational workshops, a convergent care research was carried out with 18 caregivers from a long-stay institution in Brazil. Educational workshops based on the Clinical Caritas Process were carried out and consisted of consolidated theoretical/practical moments with a 40-h workload. The study concluded that workshops based on the reference of the Clinical Caritas Process are useful in humanistic training when we tried to introduce to the group the conceptions of human care that value the self of those who care and those who are cared for.

4 Discussion

Studies focusing on educational processes have been implemented in LSIEs, and such educational interventions use themes suggested by WHO experts, such as: medication review, pain assessment processes and treatment, communication skills and organization of activities; these axes are anchored by the principle of safety [12]. These should anchor the evidence-based practice also in teaching both professionals who assist the elderly and teach the institutionalized elderly ways to provide quality of life, active aging, comfort care.

A mixed methods study conducted in Australia with 20 professionals over six months concluded that a web-based community of practice (CoP) is beneficial but would be more resolutive in teaching about falls if participants received training in its use [9].

Teaching about the use of online tools is also beneficial in providing quality care to the institutionalized elderly.

Another educational intervention was conducted in Japan and evaluated in a non-randomized clinical trial with 862 elderly residents in a long-stay care institution, 416 of whom were in the control group and 446 in the intervention group. It showed that the educational intervention was not effective in preventing falls, fever, or pressure ulcers due to barriers to the adoption of preventive measures to avoid the risks [10]. It should be noted that falls are multifactorial, requiring more qualification and more educational actions so that some of these factors can be prevented even though cultural and social aspects may influence both the educational actions and the incidence of falls.

It is worth noting that education is linked to politics and economics as well as to other sciences. It is impossible to build knowledge dissociated from the historical, social, and cultural context, because actions will be taken, and knowledge will be shared in each context [13].

In the context of institutionalized elderly people, it is important to emphasize that the knowledge of the multidisciplinary team must be taken into consideration without disregarding the knowledge of the formal and informal caregivers.

This raises the following question: how to seek viable alternatives for the development of a formal and popular health education that instills meaning, value, and quality to the life of the learner? Even if this questioning is not fully answered, the creation and validation of new strategies and pedagogical practices is necessary. The development of new strategic approaches that allow the reformulation of education policies are urgent, necessary, and imply in proposing themes for reflection on the practice of teaching that can contribute to the implementation of such policies [14].

On the other hand, a convergent care research conducted with 18 caregivers from long-stay institutions in Brazil through workshops that consisted of consolidated theoretical/practical moments with a 40-h workload concluded that workshops are of utmost importance in the care of institutionalized elderly people, in addition to providing optimization of care, enhancing the humanization of care [11].

A study focused on the perception of health professionals regarding the care of institutionalized elderly people brought up the importance of training for health professionals, as they are better prepared to face challenges that may arise in their work environment. Thus, it is important that professionals can perform appropriate actions/strategies and implement comprehensive care to the elderly person acting in disease prevention and promotion, recovery, and maintenance of life [15].

5 Conclusion

It is necessary to invest in educational actions for health professionals as well as in the production of knowledge about alternatives and advice in the professional practice of the multidisciplinary team emphasizing active aging, compassionate communication, care through comfort and preventive measures of aggravation, and rehabilitation care.

New studies about the needs of the team to develop a qualified care should be raised, emerging resolutive and specific alternatives in the care of the person.

Ackowledgments. The Coordination for the Improvement of Higher Education Personnel (CAPES) for the financial support to master's student Aline Ost dos Santos, CAPES Social Demand Scholarship Holder.

References

1. Organização Mundial da Saúde: Resumo do Relatório Mundial de Envelhecimento e saúde (2015). https://apps.who.int/iris/bitstream/handle/10665/186468/WHO_FWC_ALC_15.01_por.pdf?sequence=6
2. Benevides, K.G.C.B., Ibiapina, A.S., Sousa, S.C.M., Yvana, M.S., Ataíde, K.M.N.: Quadro clínico de idosos em uma instituição de longa permanência. Rev. Enferm. UFPE Line Recife **13**, 594–603 (2019). https://doi.org/10.5205/1981-8963-v13i3a237427p594-603-2019
3. Damaceno, D.G., Chirelli, M.Q., Lazarini, C.A.: A prática do cuidado em instituições de longa permanência para idosos: desafio na formação dos profissionais. Rev. Bras. Geriatr. Gerontol **22** (2019). https://doi.org/10.1590/1981-22562019022.180197
4. Brasil: Ministério da Saúde: Agência Nacional de Vigilância Sanitária. Diretoria Colegiada. RESOLUÇÃO RDC Nº 502, DE 27 DE MAIO DE 2021. Dispõe sobre o funcionamento de Instituição de Longa Permanência para Idosos, de caráter residencial. ANVISA. Brasília (2021). https://www.in.gov.br/web/dou/-/resolucao-rdc-n-502-de-27-de-maio-de-2021-323003775
5. Silva, H.S., Gutierrez, B.A.O.: A educação como instrumento de mudança na prestação de cuidados para idosos. Educ. Rev. **34**, 283–296 (2018). https://doi.org/10.1590/0104-4060.54049
6. Souza, M.T.D., Silva, M.D.D., Carvalho, R.D.: Integrative review: what is it? How to do it? Einstein (São Paulo) **8**, 102–106 (2010). https://doi.org/10.1590/S1679-45082010RW1134
7. Schneider, L.R., Pereira, R.P.G., Ferraz, L.: Prática Baseada em Evidências e a análise sociocultural na Atenção Primária. Phys. Rev. Saúde Coletiva. **30** (2020). https://doi.org/10.1590/S0103-73312020300232
8. https://endnote.com/
9. Francis-Coad, J., Etherton-Beer, C., Bulsara, C., Nobre, D., Hill, A.-M.: Can a web-based community of practice be established and operated to lead falls prevention activity in residential care? Geriatr. Nurs. [Internet] **38**, 133–140 (2017). https://doi.org/10.1016/j.gerinurse.2016.09.001
10. Ikeda-Sonoda, S., Okochi, J., Ichihara, N., Miyata, H.: The effectiveness of care manager training in a multidisciplinary plan-do-check-adjust cycle on prevention of undesirable events among residents of geriatric care facilities. Geriatr. Gerontol. Int. (2021). https://doi.org/10.1111/ggi.14228
11. Medeiros, F.D.A.L., Félix, L.G., Nóbrega, M.M.L.D.: Processo Clinical Caritas em oficinas para cuidadores de idosos institucionalizados. Rev. Bras. Enferm. **69**, 1059–1066 (2016). https://doi.org/10.1590/0034-7167-2016-0359
12. Husebo, B.S., et al.: COSMOS – improving the quality of life in nursing home patients: protocol for an effectiveness-implementation cluster randomized clinical hybrid trial. Implement. Sci. London **10**, 131 (2015). https://doi.org/10.1186/s13012-015-0310-5
13. Blondel, D.: Dificuldades, riscos e desafios do século XXI. In: Delors, J. (ed.) A Educação Para o Século XXI Questões e Perspectivas. Artmed, Porto Alegre (2005)
14. Papadopoulos, G.S.: Aprender para o século XXI. In: Delors, J. (ed.) A Educação Para o Século XXI Questões e Perspectivas. Artmed, Porto Alegre (2005)
15. Piexak, D.R., Freitas, P.H., Backes, D.S., Moreschi, C., Ferreira, C.L.D.L., De Souza, M.H.T.: The perception of health professionals toward the care of institutionalized elderly. Rev. Bras. Geriatr. Gerontol. **15**, 201–208 (2012). https://doi.org/10.1590/S1809-98232012000200003

A Complete Guide to Assistive Technology for the Elderly – At Least, by Now

Lucília Nunes(✉), Andreia Ferreri Cerqueira, and Hugo Franco

Instituto Politécnico de Setúbal, Escola Superior de Saúde, NURSE'IN – UIESI, Setúbal, Portugal
lucilia.nunes@ess.ips.pt

Abstract. It is a well-known fact that we are living in an increasingly aging society. Also, that information and communication technologies have become essential tools, including in the health sector, and especially after pandemic COVID-19. Crossing both facts, we thought maybe useful to provide a complete guide about assistive technologies available to elders. We present a proposal of categories of assistive technologies that aggregates the information summarizing the evidence found in the different categories.

Keywords: Assistive technology · Elderly · Gerontotechnology

1 What is Expected to be Found?

World's population ageing is an undeniable and well-known fact. Crossing the ageing population and the development of information and communication technologies, came the presumption of providing a "complete guide" about assistive technologies available to elders. If it is necessary to "stablish alternatives that attempt to satisfy the needs of the elderly and that, at the same time, improve their quality of life" [1], most of the efforts seems to be applied to illness or disease situations and our strive was to identify and characterize assistive technologies for the elders, healthy aging persons. In the way, we will frame the existential an ethics dimension.

2 General Scenario

In 2020, there are an estimated 727 million persons aged 65 years or over worldwide. Globally, the share of the population aged 65 years or over increased from 6% in 1990 to 9% in 2019. That proportion is projected to rise further to 16% by 2050, so that one in six people in the world will be aged 65 years or over [2, 3]. It seems that people live longer and the life years without a disability is also increased. A person aged 65 years in 2015–2020 could expect to live on average, an additional 17 years [3].

Globally, life expectancy has increased by more than 6 years between 2000 and 2019 – from 66.8 years in 2000 to 73.4 years in 2019. While healthy life expectancy (HALE) has also increased by 8% from 58.3 in 2000 to 63.7, in 2019, this was due to

J. García-Alonso and C. Fonseca (Eds.): IWoG 2021, LNBE, pp. 190–202, 2022.
https://doi.org/10.1007/978-3-030-97524-1_18

declining mortality rather than reduced years lived with disability. In other words, the increase in HALE (5.4 years) has not kept pace with the increase in life expectancy (6.6 years) [2].

The living arrangements of older persons are greatly associated with their well-being, physical and psycho-social health, and life satisfaction. Understanding the role and impact of living arrangements on the lives of older persons is relevant for several **Sustainable Development Goals** (SDGs) as SDG- 3 *Ensure healthy lives and promote well-being for all at all ages* and SDG- 10 *Reduce inequality* [2, 4]. The increased in life expectancy, healthy life expectancy and the role of this living arrangements has contributed to finding new models of positive ageing where the elderly are being empowered to lead fulfilling lives and adapt to degenerative changes to maintain functionality, autonomy and quality of life in the meaning of home [5–7].

As living arrangements, information, and communication technologies (ICT) have become essential tools, including in the health sector, and especially after pandemic COVID-19. One recent example is the boost on eHealth modalities presenting a unique opportunity for the development of public health [1]. The use of ICT in health and health-related fields aims to enhance the quality, efficiency, and effectiveness of health-service management [8].

WHO defines **eHealth** as the "cost-effective and secure use of information and communications technologies in support of health and health-related fields, including health-care services, health surveillance, health literature, and health education, knowledge and research. Clear evidence exists on the growing impact that eHealth has on the delivery of Health care around the world today, and how it is making health systems more efficient and more responsive to people's needs and expectations" [9]. The strengthening of health systems through eHealth reinforces fundamental human rights by improving equity, solidarity, quality of life and quality of care [10].

Describing eHealth technology seven partially overlapping [11] groups were labeled providing a useful taxonomy for further analysis: Assistive technologies; Safety and social technologies; Health technologies; Self-activation and personal development technologies; Design-for-all and ambient assisted living (AAL) technologies; Gerontechnology; Hospital technology and EHR systems that provide useful health information such as physical assessment, referral and daily charting used in health and social care [12].

According to several studies, older people want to stay in their homes, "*to age in place*", even challenges of self-care, mobility, and household management increase with age [13]. This fact is in line with the main care policies advocated in Europe, which "emphasize deinstitutionalization and *aging in place* in response to demographic changes" [14].

Ageing in place as been defined as the ability of older people to live in their own home and be included in the community, safely, independently and comfortably [15] which can be a huge challenge, especially in situations of greater vulnerability. Additionally, very often older adults' current homes are not designed to support advanced old age, nor are they located to easily provide support and services. "At the heart of decision and possibility of AiP [ageing in place] are housing and habitability conditions" [16]. Increasingly older people are living alone, further complicating the tasks of care and support. Other factors are also relevant such as "economic and health conditions and the social support network" [16]. Having safe, accessible homes and neighbourhoods can be very helpful in allowing older people to manage their frailty and maintain independence [17]. Assistive technologies might contribute to an increased sense of safety and security at home, since older people generally prefer to continue living in their own homes [18].

3 Under Assistive Technology Umbrella

Assistive technology (AT) is an umbrella concept for any tool that helps the elderly do the regular daily life activities. This kind of technology could be something as an amplification device to hear sounds and music, a walker to help moving around, a magnifying glass helping read a book. Somehow, this *helps* aids bridge difficulties or gaps in the daily life. Also, under this umbrella we can include monitoring or the use of sensors and any smart use of technology. Therefore, could include smart buildings, smart cities or smart outdoors. In this case, smart solutions intend to facilitate independence for the elderly.

The use of the word «**smart**» is no longer the traditional 'clever, intelligent, knowledgeable'; in our use, in this chapter, refers to an abbreviation for '**Self-Monitoring Analysis and Reporting Technology**', (netlingo.com), a technology that uses artificial intelligence, machine learning, and big data analysis to provide cognitive awareness to objects that were in the past considered inanimate, such as clothes, phones, socks, watches, homes or roads, among others. Usually, smart technology could be divided on (a) the Internet of Things (IoT) devices, (b) smart connected devices, remote controlled and connected via the internet or Bluetooth and (c) smart devices, with limited automation, programmable nature and no need for internet connectivity (a good example could be a smart coffeemaker) [19].

As many authors and studies refers, one of the best alternatives currently available is **Ambient Assisted Living** (AAL), in the seeking to reduce costs of an independent life for the elderly population. As a matter of fact, ALL is defined as "the use of information and communication technologies in a person's daily living and working environment to enable them to stay active longer, remain socially connected and live independently into old age" [20]. Probably, it is one of the most developed technologies in recent years. AAL uses a variety of sensors for activity recognition and behaviour understanding, sensing directly (for example, via wearable sensors) or indirectly (through environmental sensors) and analysing the streaming data to infer something about the physical or cognitive status of the person. This kind of sensors include motion, pressure pad, temperature, lighting, door contact, and so on. Most smartphones incorporate wearable sensors, opportunistically used for activity recognition, normally restricted to differentiating sitting, walking, and running activities [21]. Some monitoring devices have alarms to control the frequency and attendance of medications [22]. In nursing homes, these technologies already cover the most diverse types of monitoring, such as cameras, clothes, accessories, watches, and devices attached to shoes [23].

In this moment, when you are reading this chapter, there is an enormous probability that you have, in your pocket or nearby, a **smartphone**. As you know, smartphones can connect with other digital platforms, what allows the extension of sensing ability to capture a multitude of physical inputs. The smartphone processing capacity is strong enough to receive and process data and allows remote monitoring.

Some projects related to AAL have been focused in helping people with disabilities, to provide social inclusion of elderly people, providing intelligent day-time-management, medication reminder and communication with relatives or caregivers. Nevertheless, **smart technologies** can be used in several monitoring fields, such as physiological (blood pressure, sugar levels, and others), functional, security (in this case, analyses possible hazards that arise to impair daily activities or abnormalities that occur, and this system triggers alerts both for the monitored person and for those who monitor remotely) but also social (tracks online interactions, calls, and even what the elderly watch such as television programs) and cognitive (allows sensors to function as extra memory for the elderly, sending messages whenever necessary, reminders, and alerts) [24].

A relevant development refers to **robotics**, meaning, the use of robots to support older people. "There are two main categories of robots: (1) assistive robots having only physical assistive functions (e.g., smart wheelchairs); and (2) social robots having communicative functions (e.g., those that impart information to and interact with users). Social robots are further divided into companion robots and socially assistive robots" [25]. We think the AA L concept it is very useful and can be described as a *technological user-centred*, because uses physical devices and applications to perceive an environment and act upon it, according to the user preferences. A quite simple issue about elders living in their homes, most of the time by themselves, could be what they eat and drink, checking they remember to eat and drink, preventing malnutrition or dehydration. Most of the time, referring **assistive technology** (AT) seems pointing physiological or physical health but social isolation and loneliness are also real risks to health, especially in older people. The lived experience of COVID-19, quarantine, prophylactic isolations, showed us that technology can represent a useful and effective resource to reduce or alleviate psychological and emotional isolation. Technology can play a part in supporting social contact, allow older people to stay in touch with family and friends – and to stimulate mental wellbeing and to address loneliness [26, 27].

4 About Elderly People Using Technologies

Somehow, looks like the interest in these matters is more of researchers and scientists than of aging people. That means the impact of using these technologies to help people to live longer at home is **poorly evidenced**. Although technology usage is limited among seniors aged ≥ 75 years, several prototype and experimental systems were developed, and various studies were conducted to support the elderly by clinicians, computer scientists, data scientists, and engineers; however, few studies explored the current trends in senior care technology research" [28]. We can find studies and much more data about people with illness and diseases, that seems the most frequent topic [18]. Nevertheless, we found some papers and systematic review focusing assistive technology for community-dwelling solo-living older adults [29], assistive technology for communication of older adults [30] and about needs and adhesion of **elders to technologies** [31].

We appreciate the formulation of three potential ways to link older people with assistive technologies - the authors [7] suggest we can approach by: (1) develop or innovate technologies as the initial activity and then promote the technology to older people and finally evaluate the result of impact; in this way, we have a congruency risk, providing ineffective or inappropriate resulting in poor levels of adoption; (2) to focus on older people's attitude and adoption upon assistive technologies, to optimize user acceptance towards products by identifying and eliminating the barriers of adoption, therefore, look at user attitude and acceptance; (3) to listen to older people's needs and develop, optimize the technologies in specific orientation. This third way may be the one that best suits a real use, as its need is recognized by the elderly.

Also, research should take the caregivers in account, because assistive technology can improve older adults' independence and decrease their family caregivers' perceived burden compared to customary care [19]. Studies of acceptance and adherence to these new technologies in health care are still scarce [25, 31–33]. We know that getting **technology worthwhile**, and guaranteeing it is used, needs an understanding of the individual and the wider context in which these services are delivered. This includes the role of the family, and the multidisciplinary professionals working with older adults. Research studies have looked at how technologies are used – or not used – by older people and the way in which they are supported [34]. Without this understanding, technology will not realise its potential to enable older people to live well for longer at home. When we put it in the perspective of the elderly user of the AT there are three core dimensions that must be addressed: a) The cultural and personal perception, b) The needs related AT and tech literacy, c) The equity access to assist technology. We will briefly approach one by one.

The Cultural Perception and Personal Perception. In Western countries, ATs' disuse after one year from purchase has been estimated as one-third. This is caused by cultural differences of the users, variety of device types, and an unclear definition of abandonment and disuse [34].The emotional and cognitive investment required to use and incorporate ATs in everyday life and a focus on clear communication about how to use new devices is instrumental [32]. There is a cultural necessity of making ATs invisible in those circumstances where pluralism is yet an uncommon cultural value. Invisibility is often achieved through disguising ATs as objects that subsume functions of every- day life (e.g., umbrellas, walking stick, earpieces, jewellery, etc.). In a society where homogenization has been a strong cultural value, perhaps it could be understood how having 'something different' on or very near to one's face (e.g. hearing aid) may be rejected, as it contributes to defining one's appearance as deviant [32]. The authors [32] suggest that across cultural contexts, themes such as risk, functional characteristics, price and homogenization are surpassed and the current focus to enable acceptance needs to be focussed on developing ATs that can be emotionally invested and that reflect the identity, sense of self and cultural context amongst the users.

A review [25], identified six major themes that related to older adults' experiences with and perceptions of AT use: (1) general attitudes toward using AT, (2) feelings about AT, (3) perceived usefulness and perceived ease of use of AT, (4) intention to use AT, (5) tasks for AT to carry out, and (6) appearances of AT. In this study it was clear that older adults recognize the possible supporting role that AT could have in their life and in their care. A study [35] examined how the desire to maintain an identity compatible with competence, independence and autonomy influences the decision-making processes of older people about assistive technology adoption. Despite the great diversity of populations and technologies studied, the importance of self-image in decision-making was evident. To assure that the use of AT by older adults met their demands we must identify and work throughout this cultural and perceptions points of view as a key idea to achieve the next domain – needs related with AT and tech literacy.

The Needs Related with AT and Tech Literacy. Focusing on the needs of older adults with AT a review [7] categorized them into: Health, Leisure, Living, Safety, Communication, Family relationship and social involvement. Linking older people with AT is described by the authors as **key factor** for the disclosure between instrumental usage vs effectiveness achievements. This is in fact, a very relevant point between "what I actually need" and "what I actually obtain with it".

To achieve these needs, older people need to be empowered, and there is where the educational and literacy programs have an impact on success in implementing the usage of AT. The Canadian Program *Enhancing Equitable Access to Assistive Technologies in Canada* [36] identified as key element the information and literacy programs for elders, caregivers, and healthcare providers in order to help them make decision about which assistive technology they need, how to access them and how to fulfil expectations. A synthesized review [36] in how providing information or education from points of contact in the community came across the factual of evidence: providing education to patients to support decision-making was found to increase knowledge and reduce levels of uncertainty among patients but had no effect on patients' final decision-making an participatory models of education (e.g., through face-to-face interaction) have been found to improve health-related behaviours and patient self-efficacy. The difficulties of introducing new technologies to people at an advanced stage of impairment or distress has been identified through research. These **educational approaches** are indeed necessary for decision making and could be a resource for effectivity in implementing AT.

The Equity Access to Assist Technology. The need for assistive technologies (ATs) is increasing and is likely to continue to grow due to at least four related reasons: an aging population; increases in the number of people who have a disability; increases in the burden of chronic disease; and the burden placed on caregivers [36]. The importance of providing **equitable access** to ATs is likely to increase in future years. The WHO [37] identified some of the unmet global need for assistive technology, such as, 200 million people with low vision who do not have access to assistive products for low vision or 75 million people who need a wheelchair and only 5% to 15% of those in need who have access to one. Lack of affordability in low- income countries is a major reason people in need do not possess AT products. As disability and ageing are somehow related with social and economic vulnerabilities it is important to identify the key arrangements [36] for equity on AT for elders.

The 2030 Agenda for Sustainable Development places good health and well-being at the centre of a new development vision. Addressing the unmet need of assistive products is crucial to achieve the Sustainable Development Goals, to provide universal health coverage, and to implement the UN Convention on the Rights of Persons with Disabilities, ratified by 177 countries. *'Leaving no one behind'* means ensuring the people with disabilities, **the older population** and those affected by chronic diseases are included in society and enabled to live a healthy and dignified life [37]. The equity access to AT by elders leads us to highlight some ethical challenges within this analysis.

5 About Ethical Challenges in Assistive Technologies Use by Elders

Must be underlined the trajectories over aging are very different from person to person. Aging rhythms vary considerably, reason why a person's age alone does not allow us to deduce their needs. The aging process varies with people, or, in other words, people do not all age at the same time or in the same way, not only because of genetic factors but also social factors, the way of life, the environment, the lived experiences, the affective relationships. Aging person needs to develop effective responses that allow them to develop the transition in the best possible way [38]. Thinking about the respect for the person and human dignity while aging is, clearly, ethical issue.

Ethics can be understood as the process of questioning and protecting values and principles, is about the good, the right (and wrong), the reflexion about our acts and the capacity of make judgements. Ethics asks us to take responsibility to rule oneself. So, anytime we make a choice, it was possible to have made another (different) one and we support our decisions in ethical reasoning, our values and beliefs, principles, and convictions. Also, when we refer ethics, we ask ourselves what we want, the purpose and project of our life, the relation with others and with the world. As Paul Ricoeur said, we "look for the meaning of a good life, with and for others, in just institutions" [39].

Looking to person's situation as they age, we easily evoke **respect for human dignity** [40], which does not depend on the stage of life. Because the person has equal dignity at any stage of life and their dignity must always be respected, with particular emphasis on the stages of greatest vulnerability. Other principle is the **respect for autonomy** – meaning, person's own freedom of decision, to be able to make decisions about yourself, to accept or refuse health care, to choose what to eat, what to wear. Any choices must involve the elderly in decisions, respecting and empowering their capacity.

From these principles we draw consequences such as dealing with the person's preference and attend to their choices. But we are also challenged to an autonomy perspective broader than the simply individual – for example, Honeth [41] understands autonomy as the self-realization of personal identity and links to the social conditions of its realization. Honeth and Anderson [42] consider that the "initial key insight of social or relational conceptions of autonomy is that full autonomy – the real and effective capacity to develop and pursue one's own conception of life worthy of value – can only be achieved under socially favorable conditions.". In the context of elder's assistive technologies, implies to ensure that assistive devices developed for elderly care must not interfere with the will of the person they are caring for, need to be useful and acceptable for the elder. But we can go a little further because the "focus here is on the extent of the improvement the individual can reach, in the respect of her/his autonomy and dignity" [43]. (Panico et al., 2020, p. 36081).

Marking the importance of the principle of justice, specifically **justice as fairness**, some assistive technologies are still expensive and nowadays potentiates factors of increasing inequality. Not only because the cost, but also attending to difficult access.

However, increasing needs and efficacy evidence could strength the social responsibility, the political commitment, the role of social security and government.

For the elder, activities of daily living are the daily routine activities and self-care activities, mostly in the context of the one's home. Usually, can be focused on personal hygiene, dressing, eating, maintaining continence and mobility. Due to their increasing age, elders which increases the need and relevance to provide technology-based solutions for their aid [44]. Taking seriously the aspiration of older adults to age in place, it means as autonomously and safely as possible. "In relation to autonomy preservation, environmental control also demands some attention. The individual's sense of having control over the environment where they live" [45] (Diaz-Orueta et all, 2020, p. 3221).

In contemporary bioethics, the principlism theory (Beauchamp & Childress, 1979) [46] is very much used and, as the authors said, are quite a *common morality*. We have quoted the respect for autonomy, justice, and beneficence. Probably, the most relevant issue comes from **non-maleficence** principle that claims never do harm. Harming is more than physical injury; it is also about psychological or emotional costs. In the context of elder's assistive technologies, implies to ensure no harm can derive, people are not compelled or forced to use, especially situations in which the need to receive help can raise of ethical anxieties.

Assistive technologies do not have a specific ethical framework. Most papers and studies concerning ethical issues pick other models, as we did above with principles model. However, could be restrictive to stay in principles when we can apply for other ethical theories, such as ethics of virtue, of duties, of care, and some universal values.

In the context of elder's assistive technologies in undeniable the value of **confidentiality** and the right to **privacy,** strongly protected in recent years. Privacy and confidentiality are often used incorrectly as interchangeable terms. However, privacy refers "to an individual's desire to control access" and confidentiality refers to "the obligation of a holder of identifiable personal health information to protect the person's privacy" [47] (Lumpkin, 2000, p. 149). Privacy has also been described through its various dimensions: physical, psychological, social, and informational [48]. Personal autonomy as a function of privacy is tied to the concepts of self-identity and self-independence. In the context of elder's assistive technologies, we must require technology to be reliable and trustworthy. Also, the data collect and gather raises the questions about data security and authorized access. In some studies, video surveillance was ethical sensitive by the probable impact on privacy [29]. It is crucial to balance the use of assistive technologies. In an Aristotelian way, neither too much, neither lo less, search for a **virtuous** use, emerging from a personalized assessment of the living space and daily activities, social context, personal satisfaction and perceived benefits.

As human beings, we are naturally social and socializing is an important part of every person's life, helps improving health. Loneliness plays a role in increasing functional disability among older adults. It is important to include social interaction using smart home technologies to help avoid loneliness [49]. "Individuals cannot flourish alone: Indeed, they cannot *function* alone" [50]. From an ethical point of view, emerges the idea of **human flourishing and capabilities**, recognizing the importance of social institutions [51]. A person aging could need help and is duty of a mature and evolved society to be able to provide, and to promote **intergenerational solidarity** [52], understood within the context of shared expectations and obligations regarding the ageing of individuals and the succession of generations.

6 Guide to Assistive Technologies

New information and communication technologies can be structured in the dimensions of passive monitoring and management (ex: a sensor for the home, where end-user involvement and training is not required) or active monitoring and management (ex: personal health records, where the end user is required to be active) [53]. Based on extensive literature, including systematic and structured reviews, we propose a guide with 4 major categories, as presented in the next table (Table 1):

Table 1. Major categories in assistive technology for the elderly

Category	Examples
Remote monitoring & safety	Alarm systems, video-monitoring, fall detectors, door alerts, fire alarms, wearable camera, monitoring watches, telehealth, remote monitoring patient, biosensors, apps of self-report
Information & communication	Vision and hearing aids. Magnifiers and glare control devices Computer software and hardware. Smartphone - Social nets Companion robots and socially assistive robots
Daily living aids	Gadgets or small aids, devices and features of devices to help perform tasks such as cooking, dressing, and grooming. Windows and curtain controls, automated ovens, floor clearing robots, temperature sensors for automatic climate controls, electronic showers, taps and toilets. Locating system (tracking, GPS)
Mobility aids & smart outdoors	Wheelchairs, scooters, walkers, canes, crutches, orthotic devices. Tools such as automatic page turners, book holders, and adapted pencil grips. Physical modifications in the built environment, including ramps, grab bars, and wider doorways to enable access

In **remote monitoring & safety**, as criteria for belonging to the category is included remote monitoring system that was designed with safety in mind, using these technologies to gather and exchange information. In **information and communication category**, as criteria for definitions, is about to handle communications processes - such as being able to read, hear, use telecommunications, media, audio-visual resources, as well as devices with main objective to assistive communication. In the category of **daily living aids**, designed to make life as comfortable as possible, whether is needed a hand at home (in general or in some parts, like kitchen, bathroom, garden) or to help identifying where the person can be located. In **mobility aids & smart outdoors**, the criteria are to assist in mobility and movement indoors or outdoors. Need to be a person-centred (or user-centred) approach, where the person is placed at the centre and treated and respect as a singular individuality first. Additionally, to achieve this goal, is crucial the development of training models that combine face-to-face and online to improve the care provided to the elderly and their relatives/caregivers in the community, a privileged place to age [54].

We need to evaluate better the assistive technologies impact, develop assessment tools about acceptation levels for assistive technologies and create guidelines of best practices in protecting privacy, among others. The next generations of older adults will be more familiar with information and communication technologies, even if they are not (yet) digital natives. It will be interesting to notice the difference with current elderly, and if there will be relationship between diversity (age, gender or health status) and willingness to adopt technology.

7 What are the Main Reflections and Implications?

We are experiencing the extraordinary phenomenon of living in an increasingly aging society. Information and communication technologies have become essential tools, especially for the elders and with relevant impact in their health and well-being. Aging in place is a central concept for the implementation of AAL and ATs, with gains and human benefits. Assistive technology is an umbrella concept for any tool that helps the elderly do the regular daily life activities, which leads us to search for smart solutions that help to achieve this goal. One of the most developed smart solutions available is on the Ambient Assisted Living. Evidence has shown that technology can represent a useful and effective recourse to prevent or reduce many problems in the aging process as well as facilitating the preservation of the elderly in their community as a privileged place to age, contributing to the accomplish of Sustainable Development Goals, especially, *ensure healthy lives and promote weel-being for all at all ages* and *reduce inequality*. However, it has also show that is essential link the elders and their relatives/caregivers with technology, especially by identifying their real needs and experience. Thus, are three core dimensions that must be addressed: the cultural and personal perception; the needs related AT and tech literacy; and the equity access to assist technology. In this huge challenge, ethical issues cannot be overlooked. The implementation and development of technology should only be promoted if respect for human dignity, respect for autonomy, justice, non-maleficence, confidentiality and the right to privacy are assured. Also, the importance of human flourishing, capabilities and intergenerational solidarity. In this line of though, a complete guide about assistive technologies, like this, where the person is placed at the centre and treated and respect as a singular individuality first, can provide systematized evidence, capable of promoting reflection and new responses through research in the field of "ageing in place", namely: remote monitoring & safety; information & communication; daily living aids and mobility aids & smart outdoors.

References

1. Martínez-Alcalá, C.I., Pliego-Pastrana, P., Rosales-Lagarde, A., et al.: Information and communication technologies in the care of the elderly: systematic review of applications aimed at patients with dementia and caregivers. JMIR Rehabil. Assist. Technol. **3**, 1–13 (2016). https://doi.org/10.2196/rehab.5226

2. UN DESA Population Division: World Population Ageing 2020 Highlights - Ten key messages. United Nations 1–2 (2020). https://www.un.org/development/desa/pd/news/world-population-ageing-2020-highlights
3. World Bank: World Population Ageing 2019 (2019). https://www.un.org/en/development/desa/population/publications/pdf/ageing/WorldPopulationAgeing2019-Report.pdf
4. UNESCO: UNESCO moving forward the 2030 Agenda for Sustainable Development. United Nations Educational, Scientific and Cultural Organization, p. 22 (2017)
5. Lindahl, B., Kirk, S.: When technology enters the home – a systematic and integrative review examining the influence of technology on the meaning of home. Scand. J. Caring Sci. **33**, 43–56 (2019). https://doi.org/10.1111/scs.12615
6. Prajapati, G., Sharmila, K.: Role of assistive devices in wellbeing of elderly: a review. Indian J. Gerontol. **34**, 394–402 (2020)
7. Soar, J., Yu, L., Al-Hakim, L.: Older people's needs and opportunities for assistive technologies. In: Jmaiel, M., Mokhtari, M., Abdulrazak, B., Aloulou, H., Kallel, S. (eds.) ICOST 2020. LNCS, vol. 12157, pp. 404–414. Springer, Cham (2020). https://doi.org/10.1007/978-3-030-51517-1_37
8. Scholz, N.: European Parliamentary Research Service: eHealth-Technology for Health (2015). https://www.europarl.europa.eu/thinktank/en/document/EPRS_BRI(2015)551324
9. WHO: WHO EMRO | eHealth | Health topics (2021). http://www.emro.who.int/health-topics/ehealth/. Accessed 10 Dec 2021
10. WHO Executive Board: eHealth: Report by the Secretariat (Executive Board EB115/39 115th Session, Provisional agenda item 4.13), pp. 1–6 (2004)
11. Merilampi, S., Sirkka, A.: Introduction to smart eHealth and eCare technologies, pp. 3–84(2017)
12. Marques, B., McIntosh, J., Valera, A., Gaddam, A.: Innovative and assistive eHealth technologies for smart therapeutic and rehabilitation outdoor spaces for the elderly demographic. Multimodal Technol. Interact. (2020). https://doi.org/10.3390/mti4040076
13. Roy, N., Dubé, R., Després, C., et al.: Choosing between staying at home or moving: a systematic review of factors influencing housing decisions among frail older adults (2018)
14. Airola, E.: Learning and use of eHealth among older adults living at home in rural and nonrural settings: systematic review. J. Med. Internet Res. **23**, e23804 (2021). https://doi.org/10.2196/23804
15. WHO: World report on ageing and health. World Health Organization, Geneva PP – Geneva (2015). https://apps.who.int/iris/handle/10665/186463
16. Bárrios, M.J., Marques, R., Fernandes, A.A.: Envelhecer com saúde: estratégias de ageing in place de uma população portuguesa com 65 anos ou mais. Rev Saude Publica **54**, 129 (2020). https://doi.org/10.11606/s1518-8787.2020054001942
17. Forsyth, A., Molinsky, J., Kan, H.Y.: Improving housing and neighborhoods for the vulnerable: older people, small households, urban design, and planning. Urban Des. Int. **24**, 171–186 (2019). https://doi.org/10.1057/s41289-019-00081-x
18. Yusif, S., Soar, J., Hafeez-Baig, A.: Older people, assistive technologies, and the barriers to adoption: a systematic review. Int. J. Med. Inform. **94**, 112–116 (2016). https://doi.org/10.1016/j.ijmedinf.2016.07.004
19. Kumar, S., Tiwari, P., Zymbler, M.: Internet of Things is a revolutionary approach for future technology enhancement: a review. J. Big Data **6**(1), 1–21 (2019). https://doi.org/10.1186/s40537-019-0268-2
20. World AW in the D AAL Home 2020 - AAL Programme. http://www.aal-europe.eu/. Accessed 10 Dec 2021
21. Monekosso, D., Florez-revuelta, F., Remagnino, P.: Clinical profile and management of incisional hernias: an experience Internet J. Surg. **26** (2012). https://doi.org/10.5580/27d3

22. Majumder, S., Aghayi, E., Noferesti, M., et al.: Smart homes for elderly healthcare—recent advances and research challenges. Sensors (Switzerland) **17**, 2496 (2017). https://doi.org/10.3390/s17112496
23. Koutli, M., Theologou, N., Tryferidis, A., Tzovaras, D.: Abnormal behavior detection for elderly people living alone leveraging IoT sensors. In: 2019 IEEE 19th International Conference on Bioinformatics and Bioengineering (BIBE), pp. 922–926 (2019)
24. Maswadi, K., Ghani, N.B.A., Hamid, S.B.: Systematic literature review of smart home monitoring technologies based on IoT for the elderly. IEEE Access **8**, 92244–92261 (2020). https://doi.org/10.1109/ACCESS.2020.2992727
25. Vandemeulebroucke, T., Dzi, K., Gastmans, C.: Older adults' experiences with and perceptions of the use of socially assistive robots in aged care: a systematic review of quantitative evidence. Arch. Gerontol. Geriatr. **95**, 104399 (2021). https://doi.org/10.1016/j.archger.2021.104399
26. NIHR Dissemination Centre: Help at Home. Use of assistive technology for older people. Natl. Inst. Heal. Res. 3–6 (2018). https://doi.org/10.3310/themedreview-03345
27. Khasnabis, C., Holloway, C., Maclachlan, M.: The digital and assistive technologies for ageing initiative: learning from the GATE initiative. Lancet Heal. Longev. **1**, e94–e95 (2020). https://doi.org/10.1016/s2666-7568(20)30049-0
28. Sapci, A.H., Sapci, H.A.: Innovative assisted living tools, remote monitoring technologies, artificial intelligence-driven solutions, and robotic systems for aging societies: systematic review. JMIR Aging **2**, e15429 (2019). https://doi.org/10.2196/15429
29. Song, Y., Van Der Cammen, T.J.M.: Electronic assistive technology for community-dwelling solo-living older adults: a systematic review. Maturitas **125**, 50–56 (2019). https://doi.org/10.1016/j.maturitas.2019.04.211
30. Pedrozo Campos Antunes, T., Bulle, S., de Oliveira, A., Hudec, R., et al.: Assistive technology for communication of older adults: a systematic review. Aging Ment. Heal. **23**, 417–427 (2019). https://doi.org/10.1080/13607863.2018.1426718
31. Pappadà, A., Chattat, R., Chirico, I., et al.: Assistive technologies in dementia care: an updated analysis of the literature. Front. Psychol. **12** (2021). https://doi.org/10.3389/fpsyg.2021.644587
32. Spinelli, G., Micocci, M., Martin, W., Wang, Y.-H.: From medical devices to everyday products: exploring cross-cultural perceptions of assistive technology. Des. Heal. **3**, 324–340 (2019). https://doi.org/10.1080/24735132.2019.1680065
33. Thordardottir, B., Malmgren Fänge, A., Lethin, C., et al.: Acceptance and use of innovative assistive technologies among people with cognitive impairment and their caregivers: a systematic review. Biomed. Res. Int. **2019** (2019). https://doi.org/10.1155/2019/9196729
34. Federici, S., Meloni, F., Borsci, S.: The abandonment of assistive technology in Italy: a survey of National Health Service users. Eur. J. Phys. Rehabil. Med. **52**, 516–526 (2016)
35. Astell, A.J., McGrath, C., Dove, E.: "That's for old so and so's!": does identity influence older adults' technology adoption decisions? Ageing Soc. **40**, 1550–1576 (2020). https://doi.org/10.1017/S0144686X19000230
36. Mattison, C., Waddell, K., Wang, R.H., Wilson, M.G.: Citizen brief: enhancing Equitable Access to Assistive Tehcnologies in Canada (2017). https://www.mcmasterforum.org/docs/default-source/product-documents/citizen-briefs/asst-tech-cb.pdf?sfvrsn=4
37. Lindström, A.: World Health Organization - Assistive technology (2018). https://www.who.int/news-room/fact-sheets/detail/assistive-technology. Accessed 10 Dec 2021
38. Nunes, L., Cerqueira, A.: Ethics in care for the elders: For an ethics of ancients. In: I. Lage. Cuidados e Envelhecimento: Perspetivas da Enfermagem. Coisas de Ler, pp. 39–60 (2017)
39. Ricoeur, P.: Soi-même comme un autre. Editions du Seuil, Paris (1990)
40. Franco, H., Caldeira, S., Nunes, L.: Dignity in nursing: a synthesis review of concept analysis studies. Nurs. Ethics **28**, 734–749 (2020). https://doi.org/10.1177/0969733020961822

41. Honneth, A.: La lutte pour la reconnaissance, Folio essais, p. 352 (2010)
42. Honneth, A., Anderson, J.: Autonomia, Vulnerabilidade, Reconhecimento e Justiça. Cad Filos Alemã Crítica e Mod. 81–112 (2011). https://doi.org/10.11606/issn.2318-9800.v0i17p81-112
43. Panico, F., Cordasco, G., Vogel, C., Trojano, L., Esposito, A.: Ethical issues in assistive ambient living technologies for ageing well. Multimed. Tools Appl. **79**(47–48), 36077–36089 (2020). https://doi.org/10.1007/s11042-020-09313-7
44. Thakur, N., Han, C.: A Review of Assistive Technologies for Activities of Daily Living of Elderly (2020). https://doi.org/10.5281/ZENODO.4283011
45. Diaz-Orueta, U., Hopper, L., Konstantinidis, E.: Shaping technologies for older adults with and without dementia: reflections on ethics and preferences. Health Inform. J. **26**, 3215–3230 (2020). https://doi.org/10.1177/1460458219899590
46. Beauchamp, T.L., Childress, J.F.: Principles of Biomedical Ethics, 8th edn. Oxford University Press, Oxford (2019)
47. Lumpkin, J.R.: Perspective: e-health, HIPAA, and beyond. Health Aff. **19**, 149–151 (2000). https://doi.org/10.1377/hlthaff.19.6.149
48. Leino-Kilpi, H., Välimäki, M., Dassen, T., et al.: Privacy: a review of the literature. Int. J. Nurs. Stud. **38**, 663–671 (2001). https://doi.org/10.1016/S0020-7489(00)00111-5
49. Pirzada, P., Wilde, A., Doherty, G.H., Harris-Birtill, D.: Ethics and acceptance of smart homes for older adults. Inform. Heal. Soc. Care 1–28 (2021). https://doi.org/10.1080/17538157.2021.1923500
50. Stewart, F.: Capabilities and human development | human development reports. In: United Nations Dev. Program. - Hum. Dev. Reports (2013). http://hdr.undp.org/en/content/capabilities-and-human-development. Accessed 10 Dec 2021
51. Nussbaum, M.C.: Human functioning and social justice. in defense of aristotelian essentialism. Polit. Theory **20**, 202–246 (1992). https://doi.org/10.1177/0090591792020002002
52. Bengtson, V.L., Roberts, R.E.L.: Intergenerational solidarity in aging families: an example of formal theory construction. J. Marriage Fam. **53**, 856–870 (1991). https://doi.org/10.2307/352993
53. Lopes, M.: Desafios de Inovação em Saúde: Repensar os Modelos de Cuidados. Imprensa da Universidade de Évora. Coleção: Claustro Paginação:Divisão de Comunicação da Universidade de Évora, Évora 2021 (2021). https://doi.org/10.24902/uevora.24. ISBN 978-972-778-213-0
54. Nunes, L., Cerqueira, A.: Training models for formal caregivers of elderly persons at home: studies and gaps. In: Fonseca, C., Lopes, M.J., Mendes, D., Mendes, F., García-Alonso, J. (eds.) Handbook of Research on Health Systems and Organizations for an Aging Society, Hershey, pp. 226–246 (2020)

Monitoring and Management of Chronic and Non-Chronic Diseases

Anthropology of Loneliness: Contributions to Health of an Ethnography in Rural Extremadura

Borja Rivero Jiménez(✉), David Conde Caballero, Jerónimo Luengo-Polo, and Lorenzo Mariano Juárez

University of Extremadura, Cáceres, Spain
brivero@unex.es

Abstract. Introduction: Ageing-related issues are one of the major problems facing our society. In the Spanish rural context, older people are suffering from growing social isolation due to depopulation, which can lead to problems of emotional loneliness. Aims: The text aims to analyze the discourses of loneliness experienced by older people in rural contexts in Extremadura (Spain). Methods: A qualitative methodology has been used, based on participant observation in different rural localities of Extremadura, with semi-structured interviews. Results: The loneliness of older people in rural contexts is related to the lack of companionship and reinforced by feelings of loss and sadness. Gender is not a differentiating element in the definition of loneliness, but there are different ways of feeling and experiencing it between men and women. Social loneliness appears as a social loss of spaces for rituals and social community life. Conclusions: In contrast to the biomedical approach that tends to medicalize this problem, the tools and methods of anthropology can present social and cultural visions when analyzing the phenomenon of loneliness.

Keywords: Loneliness · Social isolation · Anthropology · Sociology · Qualitative research

1 Introduction

Current ageing in Western societies faces major challenges in the coming years. The latest data show that the percentage of older people living in predominantly rural regions is particularly high in Spain, above other EU countries [1]. The rural areas of Spain have lost 850,000 inhabitants, a 7.4%, in the last decade (2008–18) [2]. This situation began in the 1960s, a time when internal migratory movements have been developing from the rural areas of the centre and south of the country to the urban industrial areas of the north [3], what has become known as the 'rural exodus' [4]. In Extremadura, the paradigm region of rurality in Spain, the impact of migration has led to a negative demographic balance from which it has not yet been able to recover and which is worsening with time

J. García-Alonso and C. Fonseca (Eds.): IWoG 2021, LNBE, pp. 205–213, 2022.
https://doi.org/10.1007/978-3-030-97524-1_19

[5]. The ageing index in Extremadura stands at 144.3, almost 19 points above the national average [6]. Population density is also well below the EU average (113 hb/km^2): Extremadura has 25.9 hb/km^2, also according to official data from the National Statistics Institute.

Theories have been developed over the years about the meaning of loneliness and the differences between this concept, social isolation and living alone. From the 1950s to the present day, the phenomenon of loneliness has been studied from both biomedical and social science perspectives. Robert S. Weiss can be considered the father of loneliness studies. His definition refers to that feeling related to a deficit of attachment that would give rise to emotional loneliness, differentiating between two types: loneliness due to emotional isolation (derived from the absence of a close and intimate relationship with an attachment figure) and loneliness due to social isolation (which would come from the absence of community, from the lack of significant social links in the social network) [7]. A few years later, Peplau and Perlman took up the main advances in theory and practice and defined loneliness as a subjective and undesirable feeling of lack or loss of companionship. It occurs when there is a mismatch between the quantity and quality of the social relationships one has and desires [8]. In the 1980s, Jenny de Jong-Gierveld's studies were central to the conceptual development and deepening of the term and the scale she proposed. Loneliness would be the way people perceive, experience and evaluate their isolation and lack of communication with others. It implies situations in which the number of relationships achieved is lower than desired or the existing relationships do not reach the desired degree of intimacy, differentiating this concept from social isolation, considered a term more linked to the objective [9]. In recent years, the contributions of social neuroscientist John Cacioppo and his team have been fundamental. The team has developed studies on the mental health consequences of loneliness, seeking to demonstrate how human nature requires social connection, as do many other social animals. They define loneliness as a feeling of distress that accompanies the perception that someone's social needs are not being met by the quantity or especially the quality of their social relationships [10]. It is also worth noting the studies being carried out in the UK, which focus on discovering the nature and development of the social world of older people, especially on the social aspects of loneliness and the construction of worlds of interaction and communication throughout life course [11]. A recent review of the qualitative scientific literature on loneliness [12] identifies three main types of loneliness: a) emotional loneliness, which would describe the absence of meaningful relationships, often as a result of the loss of a key attachment figure; b) social loneliness, which would result from a deficit in expectations of social relationships; and c) existential loneliness, which would be an assessment of disconnection from others and the world.

Pregnenolone is a natural hormone that acts on memory, mood, stress reduction and may relieve pain associated with rheumatoid arthritis and that interacts with other natural hormone supplements. It cannot make the loneliness go away but it appears that it may alter how loneliness affects the brain. It is starting to be used in some research, to see what real effect it has on the experience of loneliness. Health sciences have developed the main approaches to the phenomenon. The scientific literature points to an extensive list of health problems related to loneliness such as cognitive impairment [13], depression [14], increased blood pressure [15], some neurodegenerative diseases such as Alzheimer's disease [16] or worsening immune function [17]. As noted in an analysis of systematic reviews on loneliness, loneliness would imply an increased risk of mortality, cardiovascular disease and mental health problems, with less evidence of other physical health conditions and behaviours [18]. The medical sciences often seek their space when it comes to defining concepts and, in the case of loneliness, the construction of its definition has always maintained that biological aura.

There is growing concern about the effects of loneliness on the health and well-being of older adults [19], a situation that, in many cases, has been exacerbated by the COVID-19 pandemic [20,21]. It has been suggested that the impact of loneliness on older adults living in rural populations is greater because they are at higher risk of social isolation [22]. However, official data on loneliness are limited and not always reliable. One possible approach to the phenomenon of loneliness is to consider data on the number of single-person households - 112,000 in Extremadura, of which 48,000 (almost 43%) include adults over the age of 65 [6]. However, establishing direct associations between these two categories could lead to methodological determinism: feelings of loneliness are not always a consequence of, or associated with, social isolation or living alone.

2 Objectives

Although loneliness is primarily an individual experience, quantitative measures have shown that certain groups of people, such as the elderly, are more at risk of loneliness than others [23,24]. Loneliness among older adults living in rural areas, such as Extremadura, may appear as a consequence of the convergence of two trends. On the one hand, a high population ageing of society and, on the other hand, continued depopulation in contextx due to emigration. These developments could increase social isolation and feelings of loneliness among older people who are left at home living alone, with fewer and fewer family members and friends around them.

If loneliness implies an absence or diminution of social relationships, we could say that it may be related to an absence and diminution of community. While the literature has discussed the differences between loneliness and social isolation, it is very difficult to deny that when social isolation exists, feelings of loneliness will appear. It seems that research has focused more on asking why feelings of loneliness appear in a very isolated way, as a psychological process, trying to point out how it influences individual health.

But where are the analyses of the socio-cultural processes that lead to this? What social consequences lead us to feel lonely? Could it be said that this absence of community also diminishes culture? Our object of study is loneliness during old age, understanding old age as an EMIC concept, in a context of rurality, where, due to the social, demographic and economic conditions of the region of Extremadura, there is a greater risk of loneliness and social isolation.

3 Methods

The results analyse the materials collected in the fieldwork through participant observation and semi-structured interviews carried out in different rural localities of Extremadura (Spain). The selection of the study localities was based on key socio-demographic markers such as the ageing index, population density or the average population decline in recent years.

The main source of data was semi-structured interviews [25,26]. The themes addressed revolved around experiences of loneliness in a rural context. The main research questions were aimed at exploring the interviewees' experience of loneliness, with some questions specifically addressing their use of technology. Questions about access to and use of technological devices were also included. At the same time, the researchers, following a flexible and inductive approach, were open to explore new themes that might emerge during the interviews [27].

The ethnographic research was approved by the Bioethics and Biosafety Committee of the University of Extremadura (Ref. 138b/2020). All participants signed a consent form informing them of the purpose of their participation in the study. Confidentiality of personal data was guaranteed throughout the research process in accordance with current Spanish legislation (Ley Orgánica 15/2019, de 13 de diciembre, de Protección de Datos de Carácter Personal). The study was conducted following the ethical principles set out in the Declaration of Helsinki [28] and the Belmont Report [29].

4 Results

Firstly, there is a definition, or a way of referring to loneliness, insofar as it appears as the absence of the 'other', in the singular. It is defined, in this way, as an intimate experience of absence, either from one's partner, in many cases due to their death, or from one's children, or from family or close friends and relatives who were once close, and who have left to emigrate to other places. Loneliness would then be defined as the "impossibility of meeting another" with whom an affective and daily relationship had been established. This identified and identifiable 'other' is often present in the home through photographs or objects, such as the armchair that is no longer occupied. This is what is understood, in the informants' words, as the "lack of companionship": that sensation that would refer to the interpersonal experience that is maintained with the 'other' within the confines of the home.

This concept of loneliness is often defined in emotional terms, accompanied, if not confused on many occasions, by a whole series of feelings loaded with negative evaluations. It is accompanied by sadness or grief, at the memory of a loved one or their prolonged absence. In extreme cases, it can lead to what some informants consider to be "the well", a feeling of deep sadness that could be considered depressive:

> "When I was completely alone, when my husband died and all that, I didn't do anything. Well, I also fell, I went into the well, let's say".

This loneliness, however, is not a continuum: there are moments when it is relieved, especially with the proximity of children or neighbours who can fill, momentarily, the space. But the loneliness returns when the visit is over.

Loneliness appears linked to nostalgia, to that past time where the life enjoyed with those who are no longer with us resided. This loneliness can be circumscribed to certain moments, in which the memory, the longing, has a special mark, those celebrations in which the family used to get together and where their absence reappears. Particularly noteworthy, for example, are Christmas, when the lack of company is even more evident. A loneliness that is accepted as a kind of condemnation, in the face of which any attempt to make up for the lack of company must be denied. Those who live alone must accept it. As if it were the inevitable fate of the elderly.

Gender can mark different ways of perceiving, describing and coping with loneliness. In our research, the definitions of both genders do not differ too much from each other, but there are more notable differences in terms of the lived experience of loneliness. Women tend to have descriptions that are closer to the intimate, close experience of loneliness, for which they seem to be better prepared and have better-coping strategies. In the private space, the women's space, men seem to cope much worse. The private space of the home is empty for men, who will have no one to accompany them. For women, however, being left alone does not have such a burden in the household. These descriptions may be just a method bias, where men's narratives about emotional space may be expressed in a poorer, less nuanced way.

> "There is a man alone, living, and there are men everywhere. Women don't go there, they don't go to his house. And a woman who is alone, always has company, the neighbours and all the people go there to keep her company".

Loneliness can refer not only to the absence of a person or of "satisfactory" social relations, but also to the disappearance, precisely, of certain established dynamics or routines. It would be, therefore, all that empty social space left by the absence of social interactions, everything that went with those who left. Thus, daily routines appear as a mirror where loneliness is reflected in every void left by those who are absent. One of these voids, pointed out repeatedly by our informants, is the loneliness around the space of eating, around food and the table. On a symbolic level, eating in solitude can mean a loss of the central importance that lies in the act of eating and nourishment in everyday life. Loneliness then comes to mean a break with schedules, with routines, with sitting at the table. It seems that all of this is accompanied by a loss of symbolic and ritual meaning, as there is no longer anyone to talk to while eating and with whom to share food, it no longer refers to the warmth of the home. Eating for the sake of eating, food becomes a strictly biological act. Elaboration disappears and the only aim is to 'matar el hambre'.

> "I didn't make food there, I still ate a yoghurt, I didn't have a timetable, I didn't have ..... I didn't make soup. I wouldn't put a simple broth in. I would still take a can. But I didn't make a specific meal of I'm going to eat at midday like I should eat".

But there is also loneliness as the absence of "others", in the plural. We refer here to the definition of loneliness as "the impossibility of encountering others", the others being the metonymy of social and cultural life configured as everyday life and tradition. This loneliness refers to the social loss of spaces, rituals and common social life. In the villages analysed, we believe that it is more accentuated among men, who report the loss of the company in the bar, the empty seats at the card game. Fewer and fewer parties and celebrations with fewer and fewer people partying. The school closed due to the lack of children. The disappearance of shops to go shopping, yes, but also to talk about "tomatoes and life". The emptiness of most church pews. This loneliness would refer, in short, to the disappearance of a certain "social joy", of a common life shared with the rest of the inhabitants of the village.

For older people in these contexts, where migration in the last years of the last century had such an impact, loneliness is also about other kinds of absence. Looking back to the past means filling the village square which today is almost empty. Remembering childhood or adolescence, these feelings of loneliness appear. Loneliness would be, then, that feeling that emerges and which differentiates the present of absences from that past full of social life. Thus, many of them come up with a recurring idea: "the village is as if it were dead". Some informants reflect this when talking about the children who are no longer there, as opposed to those years of childhood overpopulation:

> "Back then, when we went to school, me and my husband, there were thirty-three or thirty-two children here. There were only a few of us, they came from a village that is now abandoned, from La Barca, where there is no one. (...) And then there is also the Puerto de Agua Blanca, where the crags come together, that's where some of them also came from. And then from here, you can see how many children we had... And now there aren't even any children".

5 Conclusions

By medicalisation, we understand the process of turning situations that have always been normal into pathological conditions and trying to solve, through medicine, situations that are not medical, but social, professional or interpersonal. Some research is starting to use the drug Pregnenolone, which is a neurosteroid (or neuroactive steroid) that facilitates brain hypervigilance and tension. It is starting to be used as a drug to combat loneliness in some experiments. It may not make the loneliness go away but it may alter how loneliness affects the brain.

Loneliness has been linked in recent years to a range of health conditions: increased risk of mortality, cardiovascular diseases and health problems. The scientific literature has pointed to different health problems and conditions related to loneliness. Several studies indicate that loneliness has a significant association with increased use of medical services. However, these biomedical analyses need to be complemented by conceptualisations that integrate them into broader visions, analysing structural causes and consequences.

Anthropology can offer new avenues for the study of loneliness through the field's classical categories. As O'Nell enunciated, loneliness can be for anthropology "a language that seeks to reclaim the very relationships and identities it announces as missing, that embraces both the meaning and meaninglessness of grief and loss". With our research, we aim to rescue those languages, those ihttps://es.overleaf.com/project/615b464b8926f08653c5d60bdentities lost due to the lack of a community to share them with, that uprootedness that have so much to do with loss and pain.

Acknowledgment. This work was supported by the 4IE+ project (0499_4IE_4_PLUS_4_E) funded by the Interreg V-A España-Portugal (POCTEP) 2014–2020 program.

References

1. Eurostat: Ageing Europe. Looking at the lives of older people in the EU. Publications Office of the European Union, Luxembourg (2020)
2. Ministerio de Agricultura Pesca y Alimentación de España: Informe Anual de Indicadores. Agricultura, Pesca y Alimentación. Technical report, Ministerio de Agricultura, Pesca y Alimentación (2019). https://www.mapa.gob.es/es/ministerio/servicios/analisis-y-prospectiva/informe_anual_indicadores2018_tcm30-513683.pdf
3. Silvestre Rodríguez, J.: Las emigraciones interiores en España durante los siglos XIX y XX: una revisión bibliográfica. Ager (Revista de Estudios sobre Despoblación y Desarrollo Rural) **2**(8), 227–248 (2002)
4. Pinilla, V., Sáez, L.A.: La Despoblación Rural En España: Génesis De Un Problema Y Políticas Innovadoras. Centro de Estuios sobre Despoblación y Desarrollo de Áreas Rurales, p. 24 (2016)
5. Cayetano Rosado, M.: Emigración exterior de la Península Ibérica durante el desarrollismo europeo. El caso extremeño-alentejano. Revista de Estudios Extremeños **67**(3), 1653–1680 (2011)
6. Spanish National Statistics Institute (INE): Statistics of the continuous census. Provisional data at 1 January 2019 (2019). http://www.ine.es/dynt3/inebase/index.htm?type=pcaxis&path=/t20/e245/p04/provi&file=pcaxis&dh=0&capsel=0
7. Weiss, R.S.: Loneliness: The Experience of Emotional and Social Isolation. MIT Press, Cambridge (1974)
8. Peplau, L.A., Perlman, D.: Loneliness: A Sourcebook of Current Theory, Research and Therapy. Wiley, New York (1982)
9. de Jong-Gierveld, J., Kamphuis, F.: The development of a Rasch-type loneliness scale. Appl. Psychol. Meas. **9**(3), 289–299 (1985). https://doi.org/10.1177/014662168500900307

10. Cacioppo, J.T., Patrick, W.: Loneliness. Human Nature and the Need for Social Connection. Norton, London (2008)
11. Victor, C., Scambler, S., Bond, J.: The Social World of Older People. Understanding Loneliness and Social Isolation in Later Life, 1 edn. Open University Press/McGraw Hill Education, Maidenhead (2009)
12. Mansfield, L., et al.: A conceptual review of loneliness across the adult life course (16+ years). Technical report, July 2019. https://whatworkswellbeing.org/wp-content/uploads/2020/02/V3-FINAL-Loneliness-conceptual-review.pdf
13. Cacioppo, J.T., Hawkley, L.C.: Perceived social isolation and cognition. Trends Cogn. Sci. **13**(10), 447–454 (2009). https://doi.org/10.1016/J.TICS.2009.06.005
14. Dell, N.A., Pelham, M., Murphy, A.M.: Loneliness and depressive symptoms in middle aged and older adults experiencing serious mental illness. Psychiatr. Rehabil. J. (2019). https://doi.org/10.1037/prj0000347
15. Hawkley, L.C., Thisted, R.A., Masi, C.M., Cacioppo, J.T.: Loneliness predicts increased blood pressure: 5-year cross-lagged analyses in middle-aged and older adults. Psychol. Aging **25**(1), 132–141 (2010). https://doi.org/10.1037/a0017805
16. Wilson, R.S., et al.: Loneliness and risk of Alzheimer disease. Arch. Gen. Psychiatry **64**(2), 234 (2007). https://doi.org/10.1001/archpsyc.64.2.234
17. Steptoe, A., Owen, N., Kunz-Ebrecht, S.R., Brydon, L.: Loneliness and neuroendocrine, cardiovascular, and inflammatory stress responses in middle-aged men and women. Psychoneuroendocrinology **29**(5), 593–611 (2004). https://doi.org/10.1016/S0306-4530(03)00086-6
18. Leigh-Hunt, N., et al.: An overview of systematic reviews on the public health consequences of social isolation and loneliness. Public Health **152**, 157–171 (2017). https://doi.org/10.1016/J.PUHE.2017.07.035. https://www.sciencedirect.com/science/article/abs/pii/S0033350617302731?via
19. Crewdson, J.A.: The effect of loneliness in the elderly population: a review. Healthy Aging Clin. Care Elderly **8**, 1–8 (2016). https://doi.org/10.4137/hacce.s35890
20. Patel, S.S., Clark-Ginsberg, A.: Incorporating issues of elderly loneliness into the COVID-19 public health response. Disaster Med. Public Health Prep. **22202**, 4–5 (2020). https://doi.org/10.1017/dmp.2020.145
21. Rivero Jiménez, B.: Soledad y cuidados enfermeros durante la epidemia de COVID-19. In: Mariano Juárez, L., Huerta González, S. (eds.) COVID-19 y la cultura del cuidado. Apuntes y dialogos iberoamericanos. Icaria Editorial, Madrid (2021)
22. McHugh Power, J.E., Hannigan, C., Carney, S., Lawlor, B.A.: Exploring the meaning of loneliness among socially isolated older adults in rural Ireland: a qualitative investigation. Qual. Res. Psychol. **14**(4), 394–414 (2017). https://doi.org/10.1080/14780887.2017.1329363. https://www.tandfonline.com/doi/full/10.1080/14780887.2017.1329363
23. Pinquart, M., Sörensen, S.: Correlates of physical health of informal caregivers: a meta-analysis. J. Gerontol. Ser. B Psychol. Sci. Soc. Sci. **62**(2), P126–P137 (2007). http://www.ncbi.nlm.nih.gov/pubmed/17379673
24. Aartsen, M., Jylhä, M.: Onset of loneliness in older adults: results of a 28 year prospective study. Eur. J. Ageing **8**(1), 31–38 (2011). https://doi.org/10.1007/s10433-011-0175-7
25. Brinkman, S., Kvale, S.: Interviews: Learning the Craft of Qualitative Research Interviewing. SAGE, London (2015)
26. Neumann, C., Neumann, I.: Interview techniques. In: Power, Culture and Situated Research Methodology. Palgrave MacMillan (2018)
27. Emans, B.: Interviewing: Theory, Techniques and Training. Routledge (2019)

28. Asociación Médica Mundial: Declaración de Helsinki. Principios éticos para las investigaciones médicas en seres humanos. Technical report, Seúl (2008)
29. National Commission for the Protection of Human Subjects of Biomedical and Behavioral Research: The Belmont Report. Technical report (1979)

Rehabilitation of the Elderly with a Respiratory Pathology - Benefits of Early Mobilization

Sara Nobre[1], Rogério Ferreira[2](✉), Vasco Fernandes[3], Sara Mourão[3], and Luís de Sousa[4]

[1] Hospital of Espírito Santo, Évora, Portugal
[2] Polytechnic Institute of Beja, Beja, Portugal
ferrinho.ferreira@ipbeja.pt
[3] Algarve University Hospital Centre: Faro Unit, Faro, Portugal
[4] University of Évora, Évora, Portugal

Abstract. Objective: To identify the benefits of rehabilitation program (involving respiratory and motor functional re-education) to the elderly person with intolerance to the activity associated with respiratory pathology. Methodology: An Intervention Project was developed within an action-research perspective, in which six elderly patients with respiratory pathology were selected from the medical service of a hospital unit in the South of Portugal, having been submitted to a rehabilitation program. Results: Results: The results of the research show that an integral rehabilitation program (respiratory and motor functional rehabilitation) significantly improves the fragility and quality of life in the elderly with respiratory pathology whose benefits include improved dyspnea, exercise tolerance, participation in daily life activities, improved quality of life and health-related quality of life. Conclusions: An integral rehabilitation program (respiratory and motor functional rehabilitation) presents benefits for elderly patients with respiratory pathology. After hospital discharge, it is recommended to accompany these elderly people in the development of their rehabilitation program through the use of tele-rehabilitation technologies.

Keywords: Respiratory pathology · Elderly · Rehabilitation · Mobilization · Exercise

1 Introduction

Portugal follows the trend of developed countries, with an increase in average life expectancy. According to OECD data, the life expectancy of the Portuguese exceeds 80 years, and this data is reinforced by the Directorate General of Health (DGH), which states that the number of Portuguese over 75 years of age is higher than 1 million [1].

Aging is a gradual, multifactorial and irreversible process that involves structural and functional alterations, which induce loss of adaptive capacity, increased susceptibility to chronic diseases, osteoarticular and metabolic dysfunctions, losses in functionality and quality of life [2].

J. García-Alonso and C. Fonseca (Eds.): IWoG 2021, LNBE, pp. 214–224, 2022.
https://doi.org/10.1007/978-3-030-97524-1_20

This population is particularly susceptible to respiratory diseases, which lead to recurrent hospitalization processes, which in themselves cause changes in the health status of individuals. People with chronic respiratory illness often have physical and emotional limitations that condition an active life, promoting inactivity and disease progression.

Intolerance to physical exercise is one of the most common clinical manifestations, which leads to the adoption of a more sedentary lifestyle, in order to reduce the sensation of dyspnea related to the effort, but it causes muscle deconditioning. Although activity intolerance and dyspnea are two distinct concepts, they have a reciprocal cause-effect relationship, that is, activity intolerance is originated by inactivity caused by the appearance of dyspnea, which in turn leads to the reduction of physical activity, promoting a vicious cycle of progressive lack of adaptation to exercise.

The goals of disease treatment are to prevent disease progression, improve exercise capacity, prevent and treat complications and exacerbations, and also reduce mortality [3]. To achieve these goals, rehabilitation nursing assumes a fundamental role, having already demonstrated that its effectiveness goes beyond reducing respiratory symptoms, also improving exercise tolerance, psychosocial symptoms and promoting self-management of respiratory disease, with consequent improvement in quality of life [4].

The objectives of the respiratory rehabilitation program are very broad and reflect a holistic and interdisciplinary vision, which allows to minimize symptoms, maximize the capacity for physical exercise, promote the autonomy of the person, increase social participation, increase the quality of life related to health and make long-term changes that promote well-being [5].

The intervention project is based on the application of early mobilization in the rehabilitation program for patients with respiratory pathology. The early start is fundamental to reduce the consequences of inactivity/intolerance to the activity, which condition the quality of life of the person, having as objective the prevention of complications, the maintenance or recovery of functional independence, which translates into gains in quality of life and consequent reduction in length of stay [4, 6, 7].

In view of the above and assuming the importance of rehabilitation nursing care to the elderly person with this problem, it is defined as a central objective for this study:

Identify the benefits of a rehabilitation program (involving functional respiratory and motor re-education) to the elderly person with respiratory pathology.

It is believed that the results of this study can be taken as a contribution to reflection on the relevance of specialized intervention in Rehabilitation Nursing in the care of elderly people with respiratory pathology.

2 Methodology

In order to respond to the objective of the study, an intervention project was developed, from an action-research perspective, which has its origin in the evaluation of a problem, from which a diagnosis is born and measures are introduced to modify the situation [8].

With this approach, interaction with the elderly was ensured, encouraging their participation in the plan. The particularity of this methodology is that it has an essentially practical component, not limited to the theoretical field and having as objective the resolution of real problems [9, 10]. As such, the implementation of this professional intervention project took place in elderly patients with respiratory pathology admitted to a medical service of a hospital unit in the South of Portugal, from 16 September 2019 to 13 January 2020.

In this study, a non-probabilistic sample of convenience was obtained, whose inclusion criteria were: to have an acute or chronic respiratory pathology; to accept to participate in the project, with the appropriate consent signed by the person or by a significant convenience; to follow at least three days of intervention plan and with entry into service between 24 and 72 h.

Several evaluations were carried out during the intervention plan using a data collection tool created for this purpose. This instrument contemplates the variables of the sample characterization, the evaluation of vital parameters, evaluation of breathing (respiratory pattern, cough and secretions, oxygen therapy). The instrument also presents information related to the evaluations of muscle strength (Lower scale), sensation of dyspnea (Borg modified scale) and evaluation of functional capacity (Barthel index). Finally, there is a register of the interventions performed regarding functional respiratory rehabilitation (decoupling of respiratory times, diaphragmatic re-education and costal re-education) and motor rehabilitation (mobilizations, lifting).

The interventions carried out were based on the intervention plan developed and presented in Table 1.

When the rehabilitation sessions were implemented, a minimum time of 30 min per session was established, not being established a maximum time because it is conditioned by the patient's tolerance, as well as the complexity of the exercises executed. A daily session was implemented and at least 3 times a week, except for some intercurrence that prevented it.

The first component of intervention was the Respiratory Functional Rehabilitation, through exercises of dissociation of the breathing times, global and/or selective costal re-education, followed by the Motor Functional Rehabilitation, with muscular and joint exercises, passive, active-assisted, active, active-resisted, lifting, gait training and ADL's training. The progression of the exercises occurs according to the patient's evolution regarding his clinical condition and/or the complexity of the exercises.

It should be noted that for the conduct of the study ethical principles were safeguarded with respect to users confirmed by signing informed, free and informed consent in accordance with the Helsinki Declaration and with respect to institutions, both hospital and educational, demonstrated by approving the conduct of the study by their respective ethics committees.

3 Results

The data shows that the average age of the patients in the service is 82.5 years (min-70/max-92) and that 66.7% of the patients analyzed were male.

The most frequent medical diagnoses are Medical Associated Pneumonia in 3 patients, followed by Aspiration Pneumonia in 2 patients (Table 2).

Table 1. Intervention plan

Phase 0	Phase 1	Phase 2	Phase 3	Phase 4	Phase 5
Without exclusion criteria	With exclusion criteria	With exclusion criteria	With exclusion criteria	With exclusion criteria	With exclusion criteria
Headboard elevation 30-45º	GCS < 12 Lower < 2 Barthel <50	GCS < 12 Lower < 2 Barthel <50	GCS > 12 <15 Lower > 2 < 4 Barthel <50	GCS > 15 Lower > 4 Barthel <50	GCS > 15 Lower > 4 Barthel <50
	Headboard elevation 30-45º Ventral decubitus Cough Assist	Headboard elevation 30-45º Ventral decubitus Cough Assist Respiratory Dissociation exercises	Headboard elevation 30-45º Ventral decubitus Cough Assist Respiratory Dissociation exercises Costal Reeducation	Headboard elevation 30-45º	Headboard elevation 30-45º
	Passive muscle exercise	Passive muscle exercise Active-assisted muscle exercise Isometric exercises	Active-assisted muscle exercises Active muscle exercises Isometric exercises	Active muscle exercises Active-Resisted muscle exercises Isometric exercises Therapeutic Activities (roll over, Bridge) Self-mobilization exercises	Active muscle exercises Active-Resisted muscle exercises Isometric exercises Therapeutic Activities (roll over, Bridge) Self-mobilization exercises
		Balance training sitting on the bed Passive lift and transfer to armchair	Balance training sitting on the bed / standing upright Orthostatism with support Assisted Lift and transfer to armchair	Balance training sitting on the bed / standing upright Orthostatism with / without support Assisted Lift and transfer to armchair	Balance training standing upright Orthostatism with / without support Assisted / without support lift and transfer to armchair
				Walk Training DLA's Training	Walk Training DLA´s Training

Table 2. Personal and health characteristics of patients included for analysis

Patient	Age	Sex	Medical Diagnosis
1	82 years	Male	Acute Tracheobronchitis / Pneumonia; Respiratory Failure type 1; Pulmonary Fibrosis; Decompensated Heart Failure ;
2	89 years	Female	Pneumonia Associated with Health Care; Urinary Tract Infection
3	70 years	Male	Healthcare Associated Pneumonia; Mild Respiratory Failure; Acute Heart Failure
4	88 years	Male	Pneumonia Aspiration; Cerebral Vascular Accident - Left Hemisphere; Moderate Aortic Valvular Insufficiency
5	74 years	Male	Pneumonia of Aspiration; Pleural Stroke; High Digestive Hemorrhage; Encephalopathy after Hypovolemic Shock
6	92 years	Male	Healthcare Associated Pneumonia

It is noted that all patients included in the project have chronic comorbidities at the time of admission to service. Hypertension is the most common comorbidity, present in five patients, followed by cardiac problems (Auricular Fibrillation; Cardiac Failure; Ischemic Heart Disease) in two patients respectively.

The average length of stay was 27 days, and the average length of stay in the service was 15 days (min-10/max-23). This difference occurs because most patients are transferred from other inpatient units and/or emergency department.

Regarding the evaluation scale Lower (muscle strength) we can state that most of them (4 patients) present strength grade 4 - existence of active movement against gravity with some resistance and two patients presented strength grade 3 - existence of active movement against gravity.

Patients who presented strength grade 4 during the initial evaluation were maintained throughout the rehabilitation program, while patients who presented grade 3 strength had changes throughout the program. In patient 1, there was an improvement in strength in the final evaluation presenting the patient with strength grade 4. In patient 2 it can be observed that the implementation of the interventions allowed an improvement in muscle strength, but that with the suspension of the activity during the weekend, there was a retreat again, being this recoverable as observed, since the user with the course of the program improved the muscle strength.

Borg's scale was more difficult to evaluate, since it depends on the patient's perception of his dyspnea. In two patients, due to cognitive changes, it was not possible to determine the severity of the perceived dyspnea. One of the patients kept his evaluation constant at level 3 - Moderate dyspnea throughout the entire rehabilitation program. Three patients, regardless of the level of dyspnea presented, showed improvements with the development of the rehabilitation program, however at the time of the evaluation after the weekend break, they showed a further worsening of the sensation of dyspnea, although I have not returned to the initial values. With the continuation of the rehabilitation program, the feeling of dyspnea perceived by the patients has improved. It should also be noted that the values of the severity of the dyspnea perceived ranged from 0 - no dyspnea to 6 - severe dyspnea (Table 3).

In the data regarding the evaluation of the functionality of patients with respiratory pathology, it is found that all of them in the initial evaluation have a Score equal to or less than 20 points, which translates into Severe Functional Disability. With the course of the rehabilitation program it is possible to observe that all users present an improvement of the Score, never less than 25 points.

The variables that showed improvement with the rehabilitation program were Feeding - all patients; Bathing - 2 patients; Personal Hygiene - 2 patients; Going to the bathroom - 2 patients; Dressing - 5 patients; Urinating - 4 patients; Evacuating - 3 patients; Moving - 2 patients; Moving - 6 patients; Stairs - 1 patient (Table 4).

These variables have been improved due to training in daily life activities, swallowing workouts, gait training - performed by all patients, although for short distances (<50 m), which is what is stipulated in the Barthel index for attribution and score. It should also be noted that all patients in the sample performed lifts for chair, as stipulated in the intervention plan.

Table 3. Data from the patient assessment scales included for analysis

Patient	Data evaluation	Lower scale	Borg scale	Protocol phase
1	05/11	3	6	Phase 3
	08/11	3	4	Phase 3
	11/11	3	5	Phase 3
	19/11	4	3	Phase 4
2	11/11	3	?	Phase 3
	15/11	4	=	Phase 4
	18/11	3		Phase 3
	28/11	4	?	Phase 4
3	3//12	4	3	Phase 4
	5/12	=	3	Phase 4
	10/12	=	3	Phase 4
	12/12	4	3	Phase 4
4	4/12	4	2	Phase 4
	5/12	=	0	Phase 4
	12/12	=	1	Phase 4
	17/12	4	0	Phase 4
5	30/12	4	?	Phase 4
	03/01	=	=	Phase 4
	07/01	=	=	Phase 4
	13/01	4	?	Phase 4
6	07/01	4	6	Phase 4
	10/01	=	3	Phase 4
	13/01	=	5	Phase 4
	20/01	4	3	Phase 4

Some of these patients, due to their associated comorbidities, have additional limitations to functional rehabilitation, namely strokes with cognitive and motor alterations that make the rehabilitation process more difficult.

As far as the breathing pattern is concerned, a significant improvement can be observed, both in terms of thoracic amplitude and the need for additional oxygen supply.

The irregular ventilator pattern, characterized by a change in the ventilator rhythm is caused by apneas or periods of tachypnea. This pattern can be observed in two patients in the initial evaluation, but in the final evaluation only one of these patients maintained the irregularity.

The depth of each breath that is largely related to the inspiratory volume and the ability to perform effective gas exchange also showed improvements after the implementation of the rehabilitation program. The three patients who presented superficial breathing, all showed an improvement of the thoracic amplitude.

As for the need for additional oxygen input initially, 5 out of 6 patients needed this input in order to maintain peripheral oxygen saturations above 90%. At the time

Table 4. Functionality assessment results - Barthel index

Barthel Indez	Doente 1		Doente 2		Doente 3		Doente 4		Doente 5		Doente 6	
	Intial Asses.	Final Asses.	Intial Asses.	Final Asses.	Intial Asses.	Final Asses.	Intial Asses.	Final Asses.	Intial Asses.	Final Asses.	Intial Asses.	Final Asses.
Feed yourself	0	5	0	5	0	5	0	5	0	5	0	5
Bathe	0	0	0	0	0	0	0	5	0	5	0	0
Personal hygiene	0	5	0	0	0	0	5	5	0	5	0	0
Go to the Bathroom	0	5	0	0	0	0	0	5	0	0	0	0
Get dressed	0	5	0	0	0	5	0	5	0	5	0	5
Urinate	0	10	0	0	0	5	0	5	0	0	0	5
Defecate	10	10	0	0	0	5	10	10	0	5	0	5
Move	0	0	0	10	0	0	0	15	0	0	0	0
Transfer	0	10	0	10	5	10	5	10	0	10	0	10
Stairs	0	0	0	0	0	0	0	5	0	0	0	0
Total	**10**	**50**	**0**	**25**	**5**	**30**	**20**	**70**	**0**	**35**	**0**	**30**
Differential	**+ 40**		**+ 25**		**+ 25**		**+ 50**		**+ 35**		**+ 30**	

of the last evaluation of the effectiveness of the rehabilitation program there was an improvement in all patients, since only one patient continued to need additional oxygen supply, but to comply with the prescription of long-term oxygen therapy that was already being carried out at home.

Regarding the pulmonary auscultation, there was a change in the vesicular murmur - air passage in the bronchi and the presence of adventitious noises, and both are fundamental parts to perceive changes in lung function and/or limitations to gas exchange.

The presence of adventitious noises, such as snores or fervors, transpose them into an obstructive picture, in which secretions or liquid present in the lungs condition an alveolar obstruction preventing gas exchange. One way to improve this condition is by improving the cleaning of the patient's airways, either passively through postural drainage, or actively using techniques to improve the effectiveness of coughing, such as chest compressions - when the cough is ineffective (peek Flow cough < 220) or mechanically assisted cough (peek Flow cough < 160) (Table 5).

With the implementation of the rehabilitation program it was possible to show improvements in the pulmonary auscultation of all patients, with improvement in the vesicular murmur auscultation and reduction of adventitious noises.

Table 5. Evaluation of the respiratory component

Patient		Ventilation Pattern	Pulmonary auscultation
1	Initial Asses.	Thoraco-abdominal breathing; Irregular; Medium Amplitude; Eupneic; SpO2: 90% with O2 per Venturi Mask, FiO2 40%; Ineffective Cough	Bilaterally Decreased Vesicular Murmur; Dispersed Fervors;
	Final Asses.	Thoraco-abdominal Respiration; Regular; Medium Amplitude; Eupneic; SpO2: 98% with O2 by bi-nasal glasses at 3l/min;	Bilaterally maintained Vesicular Murmur; Discrete Left Base Fervors;
2	Initial Asses.	Thoraco-abdominal breathing; Irregular; Superficial; Eupneic; SpO2: 95% with O2 per Venturi Mask, FiO2 28%; Ineffective Cough	Bilaterally Decreased Vesicular Murmur; No Adventitious Noise
	Final Asses.	Thoraco-abdominal Respiration; Irregular; Medium Range; Eupneic; SpO2: 93% without O2;	Bilaterally Kept Vesicular Murmur No Adventitious Noise
3	Initial Asses.	Thoraco-abdominal breathing; Regular; Superficial; Eupneic; SpO2: 90% with O2 by bi-nasal glasses at 3l/min;	Vesicular Murmur Decreased to the left; Snores in the left lobes
	Final Asses.	Thoraco-abdominal Respiration; Regular; Medium Range; Eupneic; SpO2: 92% without O2;	Decreased Vesicular Murmur at the bases; Scarce snores in the left lobes
4	Initial Asses.	Thoraco-abdominal Respiration; Regular; Medium Range; Eupneic; SpO2: 92% without O2;	Bilaterally Kept Vesicular Murmur No Adventitious Noise
	Final Asses.	Thoraco-abdominal Respiration; Regular; Medium Range; Eupneic; SpO2: 96% without O2;	Bilaterally Kept Vesicular Murmur No Adventitious Noise
5	Initial Asses.	Thoraco-abdominal breathing; Regular; Superficial; Eupneic; SpO2: 92% with O2 per Venturi Mask, FiO2 100%;	Bilaterally Decreased Vesicular Murmur; Bilaterally Disperse Snoring
	Final Asses.	Thoraco-abdominal Respiration; Regular; Medium Range; Eupneic; SpO2: 96% without O2;	Decreased vesicular murmur at the right base; No Adventitious Noise
6	Initial Asses.	Thoraco-abdominal breathing; Regular; Medium Amplitude; Eupneic; SpO2: 90% with O2 per Venturi Mask, FiO2 40%;	Bilaterally Decreased Vesicular Murmur; No Adventitious Noise
	Final Asses.	Thoraco-abdominal breathing; Regular; Mean Amplitude; Eupneic; SpO2: 92% without O2;	Bilaterally maintained Vesicular Murmur; No Adventitious Noise

4 Discussion

Regarding the characterization of the sample at the sociodemographic level, it was found that the average age of the users was 82.5 years, 100% of the sample is above 65 years of age and 66.7% of the users analyzed were male, which is quite similar to the data of the ONDR [1], regarding the impact of respiratory diseases.

In the sample it can be observed that all users of the sample have some comorbidity, with 83.3% of the sample presenting more than one associated comorbidity.

The presence of comorbidities is currently recognized as a cause of worsening symptoms, quality of life and functional capacity, which increases the risk of hospitalization and mortality. The main comorbidities associated with advanced age patients and patients with respiratory pathology are quite analogous, highlighting cardiovascular diseases, metabolic diseases, other respiratory diseases, osteo-articular diseases and mental diseases [11].

The mobilization techniques must be proportional to the patient's capacities, but also to their level of cooperation. The appropriate choice of technique requires a complete assessment of the patient [12]. As such, the planning of exercise training (mobilizations, lifting/transfers, gait training) was carried out according to the phase in which the patient was and with the aim of improving his/her muscle strength and functional capacity.

Regarding the evaluation of muscle strength, the vast majority of elderly people present in a situation of change in muscle strength. In the patients who presented in the initial evaluation, muscle strength grade 3, there was a significant improvement in muscle strength, resulting in the final evaluation in strength grade 4. This improvement fits with other studies [13, 14], which have shown that exercise programs have a positive impact on muscle strength and the quality of life of users.

With the improvement in muscle strength, an improvement in aerobic capacity was also achieved, manifesting itself through an improvement in the perception of effort/sensation of dyspnea assessed by the Borg scale, moving from severe to moderate dyspnea assessments, and also through an improvement in SpO2 and a reduction in the need for supplemental oxygen. Respiratory rehabilitation programs based on exercise training bring about significant improvements in patients, namely in pulmonary function tests, cardiovascular and respiratory parameters, as well as in the sensation of dyspnea and/or fatigue perceived by the patient [15]. However, the evaluation of Borg's scale, being a perception scale, is limited by the cognitive capacity of the user.

Intolerance to the activity of patients with respiratory pathology is associated with dyspnea and loss of muscle capacity. People with chronic respiratory disease, associated with dyspnea and muscle fatigue, report problems in performing activities of daily living, 40% report being unable to perform activities of daily living and 68% lose capacity to perform at least one relevant activity of daily living [16]. This fact was verified in the present sample, in which the patients revealed a moderate to severe functional incapacity in performing the activities of daily life. Although the interventions performed showed positive results in the performance of daily life activities, the main improvements obtained occur in activities such as walking, transferring, feeding, evacuating and urinating and dressing. More complex activities have proved to be more difficult to recover, but once again the diverse comorbidities of the patients in the sample are highlighted, which make the rehabilitation process even more difficult.

Regarding the pulmonary function evaluated through the respiratory pattern, SpO2, use of supplemental oxygen and lung auscultation, there was a significant improvement with improved respiratory pattern, improvement of SpO2 with reduction or suspension of supplemental oxygen, improved lung auscultation, as corroborated by Vainshelboim et al. [15], which demonstrated that the physical activity based respiratory rehabilitation program had benefits for patients with improved lung function, cardiovascular parameters and respiratory parameters.

5 Conclusion

Despite the limitations in terms of sample and patient follow-up after discharge, we consider that the rehabilitation program showed positive gains in the variables evaluated, with an impact on the functional capacity of patients.

However, it can be stated that an integral rehabilitation program (respiratory and motor functional rehabilitation) significantly improves the fragility and quality of life in the elderly with respiratory pathology whose benefits include improved dyspnea, exercise tolerance, participation in daily life activities, improved quality of life and health-related quality of life.

After hospital discharge, it is recommended to accompany these elderly people in the development of their rehabilitation program through the use of tele-rehabilitation technologies.

References

1. ONDR.: 13° Relatório 2016/2017 - Panorama das doenças respiratórias em Portugal, pp. 1–66 (2018)
2. Silva, A., et al.: Indicators sensitive to rehabilitation nursing care: a functional and technological respiratory rehabilitation program for elderly people. In: García-Alonso, J., Fonseca, C. (eds.) IWoG 2020. LNB, pp. 87–98. Springer, Cham (2021). https://doi.org/10.1007/978-3-030-72567-9_9
3. DGS.: Programa Nacional para as Doenças Respiratórias 2017. Direção-Geral da Saúde. Lisboa (2017)
4. Simão, C.A., Pinto, C.S., Linhares, M., Pestana, H.C., Sousa, L.M.: Fortalecimento Muscular na Pessoa com Intolerância à Atividade Secundária À DPOC Estudo de Caso. Revista Investigação em Enfermagem 19–32 (2019)
5. Ordem dos Enfermeiros.: Guia Orientador de Boas Práticas- Reabilitação Respiratória. Cadernos da OE. **10**(1) (2018). ISBN 978-989-8444-41-7
6. Ordem dos Enfermeiros.: Guia Orientador de Boas Práticas - Cuidados À Pessoa com Alterações da Mobilidade – Posicionamentos, Transferências e Treino de Deambulação. Cadernos da OE **7**(1) (2013). ISBN 978-989-8444-24-0
7. Fonseca, C., et al.: Contributions to the ontology of aging, the sensitive indicators of rehabilitation nursing care, in terms of self-care, in people with respiratory disorders. In: 2018 13th Iberian Conference on 2018 13th Iberian Conference on Information Systems and Technologies (CISTI), Information Systems and Technologies (CISTI), pp. 1–5 (2018). https://doi.org/10.23919/CISTI.2018.8399237
8. Koerich, M.S., Backes, D.S., Sousa, F.G., Erdmann, A.L., Alburquerque, G.L.: Pesquisa-ação: ferramenta metodológica para a pesquisa qualitativa. Revista Eletrônica de Enfermagem **11**(3), 717–723 (2009)
9. Pereira, P.: Défice de Mobilidade – Reabilitar, uma oportunidade para a funcionalidade. Relatório de Estágio. Universidade de Évora, Escola Superior de Enfermagem de São João de Deus. Évora (2018)
10. Varela, M.: Mobilização precoce da pessoa em situação critica - um passo para a independência. Relatório de Estágio. Universidade de Évora, Escola Superior de Enfermagem São João de Deus. Évora (2019)

11. Nascimento, V., Fonseca, C., Ferreira, R., Lopes, M., Moguel, E.: Structured proposal for rehabilitation nursing (RN) care intervention: sensitive gains to RN care for the person with self-care deficit and in the surgical process. In: García-Alonso, J., Fonseca, C. (eds.) IWoG 2019. CCIS, vol. 1185, pp. 266–282. Springer, Cham (2020). https://doi.org/10.1007/978-3-030-41494-8_27
12. Koukourikos, K., Tsaloglidou, A., Kourkouta, L.: Muscle atrophy in intensive care unit patients. ACTA Inform. Med. **22**(6), 406–410 (2014). https://doi.org/10.5455/aim.2014.22.406-410
13. José, A., Corso, S.D.: Inpatient rehabilitation improves functional capacity, peripheral muscle strength and quality of life in patients with community-acquired pneumonia: a randomised trial. J. Physiother. **62**, 96–102 (2016). https://doi.org/10.1016/j.jphys.2016.02.014
14. Alison, J.A., McKeough, Z.J.: Pulmonary rehabilitation for COPD: are programs with minimal exercise equipment effective? J. Thorac. Dis. **6**(11), 1606–1614 (2014). https://doi.org/10.3978/j.issn.2072-1439.2014.07.45
15. Vainshelboim, B., et al.: Exercise training-based pulmonary rehabilitation program is clinically beneficial for idiopathic pulmonary fibrosis. Respiration 378–388 (2014). https://doi.org/10.1159/000367899
16. Gaspar, L., Martins, P.: Impacto de um Programa de Reabilitação Respiratória nos Autocuidados Higiene, Vestir-se/ Despir-se e Andar Avaliados pela Escala London Chest of Daily Living em Pessoas com Doença Respiratória Crónica. Revista Portuguesa de Enfermagem de Reabilitação **1**(1), 13–17 (2018). ISSN 2184-3023

Loneliness, Depression and Cognition in Older Adults: A Comparative Study of a Rural Municipality

Adriano Pedro[1(✉)], Ana Paula Oliveira[1], Sandra Russo[1], Lara Pinho[2,3], and Teresa Valente[1]

[1] Instituto Politécnico de Portalegre, Portalegre, Portugal
apedro@ipportalegre.pt
[2] Universidade de Évora, Évora, Portugal
[3] Comprehensive Health Research Centre (CHRC), Évora, Portugal

Abstract. The COVID-19 pandemic has brought consequences for the mental health of older adults, with a major impact expected in the long time. The aim of this study was to compare the cognition, feelings of loneliness and depressive symptomatology of institutionalized and noninstitutionalized older adults of a rural municipality. **Methods:** This is a quantitative, cross-sectional study, with a sample of 252 people over 65 years old residing in a rural municipality of the Alentejo region, Portugal. The group of institutionalized elderly was composed of 116 participants and the group of elderly residents at home was composed of 136 participants. **Results:** Statistically significant differences were obtained between the groups, with the institutionalized elderly obtaining higher levels of depression and loneliness and greater cognitive impairment compared to the elderly residing at home. Moreover, the greater the loneliness, the greater the depression and cognitive impairment. **Conclusion:** A change in social and health policies is needed, with emphasis on issues related to the mental health of institutionalized older adults.

Keywords: Older adults · Depression · Loneliness · Cognition · Rural municipality

1 Introduction

Loneliness can be understood as the subjective experience of an individual about the lack of satisfactory human relationships [1], it may arise when the elderly lacks social relationships that provide a sense of intimacy or emotional closeness or when they feel misunderstood, isolated or rejected [2]. It may also induce unhealthy behaviors, such as physical and cognitive inactivity, sleep disorders and increased consumption of tobacco and alcohol, which are risk factors for cognitive decline [3, 4].

Evidence shows that loneliness has a strong association with depressive symptoms and the two constructs may reinforce each other to decrease well-being. Furthermore, loneliness and depressive symptoms act together to influence cognitive functioning [5].

J. García-Alonso and C. Fonseca (Eds.): IWoG 2021, LNBE, pp. 225–232, 2022.
https://doi.org/10.1007/978-3-030-97524-1_21

Depressive disorders characterized by sadness, loss of interest or pleasure, feelings of guilt, low self-esteem, sleep or appetite disturbances, feeling of tiredness and low concentration level, may be long-lasting or recurrent, substantially impairing a person's ability to function or cope with daily life. It affects people of all ages and from all social backgrounds and the risk increases with negative feelings related to life events [6].

Loneliness is not directly associated with cognitive decline regardless of sociodemographic risk factors, but depression is associated with faster cognitive decline. Cognitive deficits are not associated with a greater likelihood of loneliness or its worsening, but loneliness and depressive symptoms together accelerate long-term cognitive decline [7]. However, an systematic review presented ten studies indicating that loneliness is significantly and negatively correlated with cognitive function, (the greater the loneliness, the lower the cognitive function) especially in intelligence quotient and processing speed, immediate memory and delayed memory [8].

Using representative data of the elderly population in 18 European countries, through clinically validated cognitive tests and depressive symptoms, the relationships between depressive symptoms and cognitive function were investigated and it was identified that depressive symptoms are associated with reduced cognitive performance [9].

Depression is not a natural part of aging. It is often reversible with prompt recognition and appropriate treatment. If not identified and treated, it can result in physical, cognitive, functional and social impairment, as well as decreased quality of life [10].

Older adults living in institutions have a higher prevalence of depression, particularly widowers and women, who also have a higher severity of perceived loneliness. The severity of depression and loneliness aggravate the age-related cognitive decline and dependence in activities of daily living and the elderly living in institutions are naturally more susceptible to it [11].

A recent study highlights the need to assess loneliness when assessing depression, given the strong relationship between these two variables [12]. The pandemic negatively affected the mental health of older adults, with an increase in depression and greater loneliness after its beginning [13]. It is due to this need that this study arose, with the purpose of comparing the cognition, feelings of loneliness and depressive symptomatology of institutionalized and noninstitutionalized older adults of a rural municipality.

2 Methods

2.1 Study Design and Sample

This is a quantitative cross-sectional study with a sample of 252 people aged over 65 years old living in the municipality of Nisa, district of Portalegre, Portugal. The sample was divided into two groups: Residential Homes (RH) Group, composed of older adults institutionalized in the Residential Structure for the Elderly; and the home group, composed of older adults living at home. The sampling method was convenience sampling, with data collection being performed in the health care services and RH of the municipality. The inclusion criteria were as follows: aged over 65 years, living in the municipality of Nisa, being able to give consent to participate in the study or having legal guardian who gives consent.

2.2 Data Collection Procedures

Data were collected by researchers trained for that purpose, in person, using a purpose-built data collection instrument, during the period from February to September 2021. Sociodemographic data were collected and the following scales were applied: Geriatric Depression Scale, Loneliness Scale (UCLA) and Mini-Mental State Examination (MMSE).

2.3 Instruments

Geriatric Depression Scale (GDS)

It is a reliable and valid instrument for measuring depression in the elderly, it is sensitive to depression among elderly people suffering from mild to moderate dementia or other physical illnesses, developed by Yesavage et al. in 1983 [14].

The abbreviated form (GDS-S) is composed of 15 items chosen for presenting high correlation with depressive symptoms in previous validation studies. Of the 15 items, 10 indicate presence of depression when answered positively and the other 5 are indicative of depression when answered negatively. Scores of 0–4 are considered normal, depending on age, education, and complaints; 5–8 indicate mild depression; 9–11 indicate moderate depression; and 12–15 indicate severe depression. [15].

Loneliness Scale (UCLA)

A 20-item scale designed to assess subjective feelings of loneliness, and social isolation, developed by Russell et al. in 1978 [16]. Each item has four response possibilities on a scale between never (1 point) and often (4 points), indicating how often they experience the different feelings of loneliness. Each correct answer scores 1 point. The higher the score, the greater the feeling of loneliness, ranging from 16 to 64 points [17].

Mini-Mental State Examination

It assesses cognitive function and was developed by Folstein et al. in 1975. It consists of six groups of questions that assess temporal and spatial orientation, memory, attention and calculation, recall, speech and constructive skills. The sum of the scores of each item, indicates the worsening of cognitive impairment. Deterioration is indicated by a decrease in the score. The lowest score indicates greater cognitive impairment [18].

2.4 Ethical Considerations

A favorable opinion was obtained from the Ethics Committee of the Polytechnic Institute of Portalegre, no. SC/2021/2254, dated February 25, 2021.

Before data collection, the elderly or their legal representative were asked to give their consent.

Data confidentiality is guaranteed, since only the researchers have access to the overall data in a file protected with access code, on private computers. The anonymity of the participants is also guaranteed because at no time are personal or sensitive data with the possibility of identification of each participant and the data are only worked and disclosed as a whole.

2.5 Statistical Analysis

Descriptive statistics were used for the sociodemographic characterization of the sample. The t-test was used to compare the value of the scales between the groups. The SPSS was the statistical software used for the analysis.

3 Results

3.1 Sociodemographic Characteristics

The total sample is composed of 252 older adults, with the RH group consisting of 116 participants and the living at home group consisting of 136 participants. Women prevailed in both groups. In relation to the RH group, most participants were aged

Table 1. Sociodemographic characteristics

	RH n = 116		Living at home n = 136	
	n	%	n	%
Age group				
65–74 years old	2	1.7	58	42.6
75–84 years old	38	32.8	62	45.6
≥85 years old	76	65.5	16	11.8
Sex				
Male	36	31	48	35.3
Female	80	69	88	64.7
Marital Status				
Married	22	19	96	70.6
Single	18	15.5	38	27.9
Widower	76	65.5	0	0
Divorced	0	0	2	1.5
Schooling				
Illiterate	34	29.3	6	4.4
Has not attended school but can read and write	54	46.6	2	1.5
Primary Education	26	22.4	104	76.5
Secondary Education	2	1.7	12	8.8
college education	0	0	12	8.8
Children				
Yes	84	72.4	134	98.5
No	32	27.6	2	1.5

85 years or more (65.5%), widowed (65.5%), had not attended school (75.9%) and had children (72.4%). As for the living at home group, most participants were aged between 75 and 84 years (45.6%), married (70.6%), had attended primary school (76.5%) and had children (98.5%) (Table 1).

3.2 Loneliness, Depression and Cognition

The analysis of the results showed statistically significant differences between the groups, with higher levels of depression and loneliness and greater cognitive impairment in institutionalized older adults compared to older adults living at home (Table 2).

Table 2. Analysis of the differences in the GDS, UCLA and MMSE scales between the two groups

	RH Mean (SD)	Living at home Mean (SD)	Test t	*p*
MMSE	11,93 (6.9)	21,82 (3.46)	−14.012	<0.001
UCLA	37.55 (9.06)	23.11 (7.64)	10.918	<0.001
GDS	5.8 (3.18)	3.21 (2.9)	4.849	<0.001

The correlation between the scales was also analyzed using Pearson's correlation, and statistically significant results were obtained (Table 3). The greater the loneliness, the greater the depression and the lower the cognitive level. The higher the depression, the lower the cognitive level.

Table 3. Analysis of the differences between the scales (Pearson correlation)

	MMSE	UCLA
UCLA	−0.477**	—
GDS	−0.238*	0.761**

*p < 0.01
**p < 0.001

4 Discussion

This study aimed to compare the levels of depression, loneliness and cognitive ability between a group of older adults living in residential care units and a group of older adults living at home in a rural municipality of Portugal. It was found that the elderly residents in facilities obtained worse results for all variables.

By analyzing the socio-demographic characteristics, we found a higher percentage of women in both groups, which is consistent with several studies [19–22], and this phenomenon is called "feminization of aging" [23].

In relation to age and marital status, most of the older adults in RH are in the oldest age group and are widowers, and those living at home are in the 75–84 age group and are married. These results are not surprising since, on the one hand, the older the patient, the greater the likelihood of dependence and need for institutionalization; on the other hand, being married can prevent institutionalization by maintaining the affective bonds and the presence of a caregiver when necessary.

Regarding education, most of the individuals living in RH did not attend school and majority of those living in the household had attended primary education. Studies indicate that older adults who did not attend school have a higher level of dependence [20, 21, 24], which may explain these results.

Moving on to analyze the results of the scales, we found that the greater the loneliness, the greater the depression and the lower the cognitive level. Similarly, the greater the depression, the lower the cognitive level. These results are consistent with other studies indicating that loneliness is associated with impaired mental health, depression and cognitive deficits [5, 25]. A systematic review of the literature concluded that loneliness is significantly and negatively correlated with cognitive function, which is in line with the results of our study [8]. A study conducted with older adults in 18 European countries reinforces these results by concluding that depressive symptoms are associated with reduced cognitive performance [9].

We also found that institutionalized elderly people have greater cognitive deterioration than those living at home, which is consistent with the results of other Portuguese studies using the same scale [20, 21]. Another Portuguese study which studied a sample of institutionalized elderly people obtained a percentage of 45.3% of the sample with cognitive impairment [22].

In addition, the institutionalized elderly obtained higher levels of loneliness and depression compared to those residing at home. These results are also in line with the literature, with one study finding that the elderly living in institutions have a higher prevalence of depression, and higher severity of perceived loneliness [11]. It should be noted that data collection was conducted in the pandemic period, with restricted visits, so the increased levels of loneliness and depression may be related to this fact. A recent study indicates that the protective health benefits of social withdrawal should be balanced by the essential need to sustain social relationships [26]. In this sense, a literature review on the impact of socialization on active aging concluded that the process of successful aging is multidimensional and is influenced by the establishment of interpersonal and social relationships, maintenance of independence, and cognitive function [27].

5 Conclusion

In the pandemic period, the institutionalized elderly in a rural municipality of Portugal showed higher levels of depression, loneliness and cognitive deterioration when compared to the elderly living at home in the same municipality.

In fact, institutionalized older adults had restricted visits and reduced contact with their relatives and friends. This can have long-term consequences on health and well-being, thus, special attention should be paid to this issue, and social and health policies should focus more on the mental health of the elderly. There is an urgent need to implement strategies to improve mental health in residential institutions for older adults.

References

1. Kautiainen, H., Pitkala, K.: Social isolation, social activity and loneliness as survival indicators in old age: a nationwide survey with a 7-year follow-up. Eur. Geriatr. Med. **3**, 18–22 (2012)
2. Hazer, O., Boylu, A.: The examination of the factors affecting the feeling of loneliness of the elderly. Procedia Soc. Behav. Sci. **9**, 2083–2089 (2010)
3. Baumgart, M., Snyder, H.M., Carrillo, M.C., Fazio, S., Kim, H., Johns, H.: Summary of the evidence on modifiable risk factors for cognitive decline and dementia: a population-based perspective. Alzheimer's Dementia **11**, 718–726 (2015)
4. Golden, J., et al.: Loneliness, social support networks, mood and wellbeing in community-dwelling elderly. Int. J. Geriatr. Psychiatry **24**, 694–700 (2009)
5. Kong, D., Davitt, J., Dong, X.: Loneliness, depressive symptoms, and cognitive functioning among U.S. Chinese older adults. Gerontol. Geriatr. Med. **4**, 1–8 (2018). https://doi.org/10.1177/2333721418778201
6. American Psychiatric Association: DSM-5: Manual de diagnóstico e estatística das perturbações mentais. (5a edn.) Climepsi Editores, Lisboa (2014)
7. Donovan, N.J., Wu, Q., Rentz, D.M., Sperling, R.A., Marshall, G.A., Glymour, M.M.: Loneliness, depression and cognitive function in older U.S. adults. Int. J. Geriatr. Psychiatry **32**(5), 564–573 (2017). https://doi.org/10.1002/gps.4495
8. Boss, L., Kang, D., Branson, S.: Loneliness and cognitive function in the older adult: a systematic review. Int. Psychogeriatr. **27**(4), 541–553 (2015). https://doi.org/10.1017/S1041610214002749
9. Nafilyan, V., Avendano, M., Coulon, A.: The causal impact of depression on cognitive functioning: evidence from Europe. Institute of Labor Economics (2021)
10. Sherry, G.: The geriatric Depression Scale (GDS). Try this: Best practices in Nursing care to older Adults. Hartford Institute for Geriatric Nursing. NYU College of Nursing (2012)
11. Desai, R., Abraham, D., Harshe, D.G., Ramakrishnan, A., Cholera, R., Kale, S.S.: A study of depression, perceived loneliness, cognitive function and independence in daily activities in home and institution based older people: a cross sectional comparative study. J. Geriatr. Mental Health **3**, 140–144 (2016)
12. Hsueh, Y.C., Chen, C.Y., Hsiao, Y.C., Lin, C.C.: A longitudinal, cross-lagged panel analysis of loneliness and depression among community-based older adults. J. Elder Abuse Negl. **31**(4–5), 281–293 (2019). https://doi.org/10.1080/08946566.2019.1660936
13. Krendl, A.C., Perry, B.L.: The impact of sheltering in place during the COVID-19 pandemic on older adults' social and mental well-being. J. Gerontol.: Ser. B **76**(2), e53–e58 (2021). https://doi.org/10.1093/geronb/gbaa110
14. Yesavage, J.A., et al.: Development and validation of a geriatric depression screening scale: a preliminary report. J. Psychiatr. Res. **17**, 37–49 (1983)
15. Sheikh, J.I., Yesavage, J.A.: Geriatric depression scale (GDS): recent evidence and development of a shorter version. Clin. Gerontol.: J. Aging Mental Health **5**(1–2), 165–173 (1986). https://doi.org/10.1300/J018v05n01_09
16. Russell, D., Peplau, L.A., Ferguson, M.L.: Developing a measure of loneliness. J. Pers. Assess. **42**(3), 290–294 (1978). https://doi.org/10.1207/s15327752jpa4203_11

17. Russell, D.: UCLA loneliness scale (version 3): reliability, validity, and factor structure. J. Pers. Assess. **66**, 20–40 (1996)
18. Folstein, M.F., Folstein, S.E., McHugh, P.R.: Mini-mental state. J. Psychiatr. Res. **12**(3), 189–198 (1975). https://doi.org/10.1016/0022-3956(75)90026-6
19. Santiago, L.M., Prazeres, F., Boto, T., Maurício, K., Rosendo, I., Simões, J.: Multimorbidity daily life activities and socio-economic classification in the Central Portugal primary health care setting: an observational study. Family Med. Primary Care Rev. **22**(1), 54–58 (2020)
20. Fonseca, C., Pinho, L.G., Lopes, M.J., Marques, M.C., Garcia-Alonso, J.: The elderly nursing core set and the cognition of Portuguese older adults: a cross-sectional study. BMC Nurs. **20**(1), 1–8 (2021). https://doi.org/10.1186/s12912-021-00623-1
21. Lopes, M.J., et al.: Functioning and cognition of Portuguese older adults attending in residential homes and day centers: a comparative study. Int. J. Environ. Res. Public Health **18**(13), 7030 (2021). https://doi.org/10.3390/ijerph18137030
22. Arco, H., Pedro, A., Pinho, L., Proença, A.: Aging and functionality of the institutionalized elderly people of alto Alentejo: contributions to the diagnosis of the situation. In: García-Alonso, J., Fonseca, C. (eds.) IWoG 2020. LNB, pp. 253–261. Springer, Cham (2021). https://doi.org/10.1007/978-3-030-72567-9_24
23. Davidson, P.M., DiGiacomo, M., McGrath, S.J.: The feminization of aging: how will this impact on health outcomes and services? Health Care Women Int. **32**(12), 1031–1045 (2011). https://doi.org/10.1080/07399332.2011.610539
24. Coutinho, A.T., Vilela, Q., Lima, M., Silva, M.: Social communication and functional independence of the elderly in a community assisted by the family health strategy. Revista CEFAC **20**(3), 363–373 (2018). https://doi.org/10.1590/1982-0216201820313417
25. Cohen-Mansfield, J., Hazan, H., Lerman, Y., Shalom, V.: Correlates and predictors of loneliness in older-adults: a review of quantitative results informed by qualitative insights. Int. Psychogeriatr. **28**(4), 557–576 (2016). https://doi.org/10.1017/S1041610215001532
26. Donovan, N.J., Blazer, D.: Social isolation and loneliness in older adults: review and commentary of a National Academies report. Am. J. Geriatr. Psychiatry **28**(12), 1233–1244 (2020). https://doi.org/10.1016/j.jagp.2020.08.005
27. Plexa, A., et al.: Impact of socialization on active aging in the geriatric population: a systematic literature review. In: García-Alonso, J., Fonseca, C. (eds.) IWoG 2020. LNB, pp. 202–216. Springer, Cham (2021). https://doi.org/10.1007/978-3-030-72567-9_20

The Practice of Physical Activity in a Person with Type 2 Diabetes Mellitus

Filipa Martins[1], Rogério F. Ferreira[2(✉)], Ana Clara Nunes[2], João V. Vieira[2], and Teresa Mestre[2]

[1] Faro Hospital, Algarve University Hospital Center, Faro, Portugal
[2] Department of Health, Polytechnic Institute of Beja, Beja, Portugal
ferrinho.ferreira@ipbeja.pt

Abstract. Introduction: Diabetes Mellitus presents a high and growing prevalence in Portugal and the world. In 2019 the highest prevalence of this disease was observed in the elderly and it is expected that in the coming years this trend will continue. In Portugal, in the year 2018 it caused 4292 deaths, about 3.8% of all deaths at national level. A large number of Diabetic people are unaware of their diagnosis. Diabetes Mellitus type 2 is the most common type and represents 90% of the diabetes cases worldwide. This type is more prevalent in the elderly, however, more and more children and young adults appear with this disease, due to an inadequate diet and increased physical inactivity. Regular physical activity improves insulin sensitivity, controlling glycemia and other comorbidity factors. Objective: Identify the health gains resulting from nursing care interventions focused on physical activity practice of the person with Type 2 Diabetes Mellitus. Methods: Research conducted in MEDLINE Complete and CINAHL Complete databases through the EBSCOhost platform, in order to identify articles published with available references and publication date between January 2015 and March 2020. Results: After implementing the inclusion and exclusion criteria seven studies were selected. The results show gains in welfare and self-care, in prevention of complications, in health promotion and in functional rehabilitation. Conclusion: Nursing care in the practice of physical activity, whether performing aerobic, endurance or even combined exercises, benefits the person with Diabetes Mellitus type 2 in improving their quality of life.

Keywords: Nursing care · Type 2 diabetes mellitus · Physical activity

1 Introduction

Diabetes Mellitus is a chronic disease involving a large number of people, presenting as an individual, family and public health problem [1]. This is a very important health problem that has reached alarming levels [2].

In 2018, this disease caused 4292 deaths in Portugal [3]. Diabetes Mellitus type 2 presents a wide expansion around the world [1], representing about 90% of Diabetes cases [2]. This type of Diabetes is the most common and is characterized by pancreatic cell dysfunction β and insulin resistance [4].

J. García-Alonso and C. Fonseca (Eds.): IWoG 2021, LNBE, pp. 233–244, 2022.
https://doi.org/10.1007/978-3-030-97524-1_22

This disease, as well as its complications, compromise people's quality of life [5]. Early diagnosis and implementation of appropriate treatment are a priority, avoiding the appearance of these possible complications and their progression to more serious forms [6].

The knowledge about this type of Diabetes is not yet accurate, however, it is remarkable the strong relationship between type 2 Diabetes Mellitus and overweight, obesity, sedentariness, advancing age, ethnicity and family history [7].

The promotion of a healthy lifestyle that involves an adequate diet and regular physical activity are essential to prevent and control type 2 Diabetes Mellitus [2]. Through the regular practice of physical activity, morphological and functional changes occur, which may prevent or postpone the appearance of this disease, also contributing to its control [7].

Physical activity has the ability to influence insulin resistance. More active people present lower levels of circulating insulin, since there is an improvement in the functioning of glucose carriers, increasing capillary irrigation in skeletal muscle cells [8]. In the treatment of Diabetes, the practice of physical activity is an integral part, being an important ally, since it acts on glycemic control and other comorbidity factors [8]. Thus, this presents itself as a structuring part and focus of the Nursing interventions to the person with Type 2 Diabetes Mellitus.

It is of extreme importance that interventions are developed around the person with Diabetes Mellitus type 2, which presents sensitive gains in Nursing. The Nurse has a fundamental role, educating the user and motivating him/her to the regular practice of physical activity, so that he/she implements a more active lifestyle, thus controlling his/her illness and preventing complications.

We believe that the approach of this integrative literature review can be an important contribution to the reflection on the relevance of nursing intervention strategies to people with this problem, assuming that the care provided by the Nurse results in health gains.

2 Objective

Identify the health gains resulting from nursing care interventions focused on physical activity practice of the person with Type 2 Diabetes Mellitus.

3 Research Question

For the formulation of the research question the PI[C]OD methodology was used: population (P), type of intervention (I), the comparisons (C), the result - outcome (O) and the type of study - design (D). In order to respond to the objective previously outlined and that served as a guiding thread for this integrative review of the literature, the following guiding question was elaborated: "What are the health gains (Outcomes) resulting from nursing care interventions focused on the practice of physical activity (Intervention) of the person with Diabetes Mellitus type 2 (Population)?".

4 Methodology

Once the formulation of the research question has been finalized, the collection of data on the subject under study, which took place during April 2020 in the MEDLINE Complete and CINAHL Complete databases through the EBSCOhost platform, follows.

The descriptors used in the research were: “Nursing interventions”, “Nursing care”, “Nursing”, “Nursing”, “Diabetes Mellitus type 2”, “Diabetes Mellitus”, “Physical activity”, “Exercise” and “Physical exercise”. The descriptors were searched on the EBSCOhost platform in the following order: (Nursing interventions) or (Nursing care) or (Nursing) or (Nursing)] AND -[(Diabetes Mellitus type 2) or (Diabetes Mellitus)] AND -[(Physical activity) or (Exercise) or (Physical exercise)].

The inclusion criteria were the articles that presented quantitative and/or qualitative methodologies, published in their entirety (full-text), in Portuguese or in English, in the area of Nursing and that made it possible to answer the aforementioned guiding question, inserted in the CINAHL Complete and MEDLINE Complete databases, with available references and publication date between January 2015 and March 2020. The exclusion criteria were studies that had no connection with the subject under study, with ambiguous methodology, with publication dates prior to 2015 and repeated in both databases.

The selection of studies included the evaluation of the title and the analysis of the abstract in order to confirm that the studies met the inclusion and exclusion criteria. When the articles did not prove to be enlightening, they were read in their entirety in order to reduce the loss of important studies. 468 articles were identified in the CINAHL Complete and MEDLINE Complete databases through the EBSCOhost platform. The evaluation of the articles took place in two phases, in a first phase 51 articles were selected after the reading of the titles, and in a second phase after the reading of the abstracts the potential of 15 articles was justified. Then the 15 articles were read in their entirety and seven were selected, according to the methodological quality. The critical analysis of the articles was focused on the assessment of the levels of evidence.

The contributions of Melnyk and FIneout-Overholt [9] were used in order to identify the different types of knowledge production that are implicit in the studies. These consider the following levels of evidence:

- Level I - Systematic reviews (meta-analyses, guidelines for clinical practice based on systematic reviews);
- Level II - Experimental studies;
- Level III - Almost experimental studies;
- Level IV - Non-experimental studies;
- Level V - Evaluation reports of programs/literature reviews;
- Level VI - Opinions of authorities/consensus panels

5 Results

The selected articles were read and analyzed in order to answer the PICOD question described above. Table 1 describes the results of the Integrative Literature Review.

Table 1. Results of the integrative literature review

Authors/Method/level of evidence	Objectives	Results
Authors: Thiel, Sayah, Vallance, Johnson and Johnson (2016) [10] **Method:** Cross-sectional Study **Participants:** 1948 participants with type 2 diabetes mellitus, living in Alberta **Level of evidence:** IV	Analyze the differences in quality of life related to health among users with Type 2 Diabetes Mellitus, who have adopted the recommendations of the Canadian Diabetes Association, related to physical activity, comparing with users with Type 2 Diabetes Mellitus who have not followed these same recommendations	Multivariate regression analysis demonstrated differences in health-related quality of life among users with Type 2 Diabetes who followed the recommendations of the Canadian Diabetes Association and those who did not. Patients who met the recommendations showed higher health-related quality of life scores for physical functioning, physical performance, body pain, general health status, vitality, social functioning, and emotional performance than those who did not No significant differences in any of the health-related quality of life parameters were revealed between users who met the baseline recommendations and those who exceeded them
Authors: Lee, Pei, Chi and Jeng (2015) [11] **Method:** Randomized clinical trial, participants were randomly assigned to three groups, i.e., an aerobic exercise group, another walking group with 1 million accumulated steps and finally, a control group **Participants:** 120 people, between 20 and 65 years old, with Type 2 Diabetes Mellitus, who had a sedentary lifestyle and wanted to participate in the study **Level of evidence:** II	To investigate the effectiveness of two moderately intense exercise programs on glucose metabolism and cell function β pancreatic in users with Type 2 Diabetes Mellitus	After three months of exercise, it was observed that the group that performed aerobic exercises had a glycated hemoglobin value (HbA1c) significantly lower than the control group and that the group of 1 million accumulated steps had an isulinogenic index in the acute insulin response significantly higher than the control group. In the long-term evaluation, after 1 year of exercise practice, the glucose hemoglobin values and the oral glucose tolerance test of the aerobic exercise group and the million-steps accumulated group showed significantly lower values than the control group The group of 1 million steps accumulated presented inferior values of fasting glycemia, glucose hemoglobin and oral glucose tolerance test, after 3 and 12 months, compared to the values at the beginning of the study. This group also presented an insulinogenic index in the acute insulin response higher after 3 and 12 months of exercise than in the initial phase

(*continued*)

Table 1. (*continued*)

Authors/Method/level of evidence	Objectives	Results
Authors: Cai, Li, Zhang, Xu1 and Chen (2017) [12] **Method:** Systematic literature review **Level of evidence:** I	Analyze the effect that physical exercise has on the quality of life of a person with Type 2 Diabetes	In studies that analyzed the effect of aerobic exercise on quality of life in patients with Type 2 Diabetes Mellitus, walking was the most common exercise. Other types of aerobic exercise were also included such as water exercise, tai chi, and exercise game, treadmill and exercise bike Of the 20 studies that addressed the effects of aerobic exercise, 15 reported that it has a significant effect on the quality of life of users with Type 2 Diabetes Mellitus, compared to the control group
Authors: Lade, Marins, Lima, Carvalho, Teixeira, Albuquerque, Reis and Amorim (2016) [13] **Method:** Experimental Study. Two groups were formed, one for aerobic exercises and the other for strength training. The participants were randomly distributed among the groups. This study was divided in two parts, each with ten weeks **Participants:** In the first phase the study had 14 participants, 4 type 2 diabetics and 10 type 2 diabetics and hypertensive In the second phase the study ended with 11 type 2 diabetics and of these, 7 also had hypertension **Level of evidence:** II	Analyze and compare the effects of supervised aerobic exercises and strength programs on glycemia control in patients with Type 2 Diabetes Mellitus	In the anthropometric analysis no statistically significant changes were observed between the periods (at the beginning, after 10 weeks and after 20 weeks) for the two groups and no relationship was shown between timetables and types of exercise or differences between types of training, in the behavior of variables Regarding the perimeter of the hips, no significant changes were observed between the two groups in the different periods, but the averages showed different results between the groups in the three periods evaluated. Therefore, the averages were higher in the aerobic training group compared to the moderate strength training group, initially after 10 and 20 weeks Significant changes in glycated hemoglobin values were found over the periods, but no significant differences were observed in the mean values between the two groups. No significant relationship was observed between the types of exercise and the periods. The reduction of the glycated hemoglobin value occurred between the baseline and 10 weeks, and between the baseline and 20 weeks, and the moderate strength training group showed a higher mean value at the beginning of the exercise program and showed a lower mean value at the end of it than the aerobic training group

(*continued*)

Table 1. (*continued*)

Authors/Method/level of evidence	Objectives	Results
Authors: Chiang, Heitkemper, Hung, Tzeng, Lee and Lin (2019) [14] **Method:** Prospective Longitudinal Observational Study. For the study, 3 sessions per week of exercise were performed, each session with 30 min, during 12 weeks, that is, giving a total of 36 sessions **Participants:** 20 participants, aged between 40 and 60, with Diabetes Mellitus type 2 **Level of evidence:** IV	Analyze changes in glycemia levels after exercising for 12 weeks in individuals with Type 2 Diabetes Mellitus To investigate the predictors of glycemia after exercise and the effect that the practice of this in the response to glucose	The exercise practiced in the morning presented a small but significant increase in the values of the glycemic response induced by the exercise, compared to the exercise practiced in the afternoon. No differences were observed in the glycemic values before and after the exercise practiced in the morning, afternoon and evening The values of glycemia before exercise, in the second and third months, were significantly lower compared to the first month of training. As well, the values of glycemia before exercise and the values of glycemia in response to exercise, were also significantly lower in the second and third months than in the first month of training In the univariable analysis it was concluded that the values of glycemia before and after exercise and the glycemia response to exercise, decreased significantly as the number of trainings increased. In the multivariable analysis it was observed that the values of glycemia after exercise decreased as the number of workouts increased, while the values of glycemia before exercise and the response of the glycemia to exercise remained stable

(*continued*)

Table 1. *(continued)*

Authors/Method/level of evidence	Objectives	Results
Authors: Pahra, Sharma, Ghai, Hajela, Bhansali and Bhansali (2017) [15] **Method:** Randomized controlled trial, with randomized distribution of the participants in two groups, group A being responsible for performing exercise lasting 15 min after the meal for the first 60 days and after these perform a single daily exercise for another 60 days. Group B carried out the same activities, however, in the opposite way **Participants:** 64 people with Type 2 Diabetes Mellitus **Level of evidence:** II	To evaluate the effectiveness of post-prandial exercise in all meals and compare it with the effect of single daily exercise in the control of glycemia in users with Type 2 Diabetes Mellitus	Group A initially carried out after each meal, fast walks of moderate intensity from 1500 to 1600 steps for 15 min, for 60 days and then, for another 59 days, 45 min before breakfast, a fast walk in a stretch with 4500 to 4800 steps. Group B carried out the same exercises, however, in an inverted way, in the first 60 days it carried out the postprandial exercises and then it carried out for another 59 days a unique daily exercise The users of group A, when they first practiced the postprandial exercises, presented a significant improvement in the glycemia control, however, when they started to practice the single daily exercise, a significant increase in the glycemia occurred. The users of group B did not present, when they first practiced the single daily exercise, any significant improvement in the glycemia control and when they started to practice the post-prandiais exercises, a glycemia decrease was observed Regarding the hemoglobin glycated values, group A users initially showed a significant decrease in the values, but then an increase was observed. However, patients in group B initially showed a negligible increase in A1c values and then a significant decrease was observed
Authors: Pai, Li, Hwu, Chang, Chen and Chang (2016 [16] **Method:** Systematic review of the literature with meta-analysis **Level of evidence:** I	Compare the size of the effects of regular leisure-time physical activities on long-term glycemia control in people with Type 2 Diabetes Mellitus	Eleven of the randomized clinical trials compared the glucose hemoglobin levels before and after the experimental group and the control group. The remaining seven studies compared the differences in glycated hemoglobin levels between the two groups before and after The statistics of the walking and yoga groups were over 50%, which indicated heterogeneity. The analyses of the subgroups were performed to evaluate the frequency of each physical activity per week, which showed that heterogeneity decreased when the frequency of each activity per week was taken into account. It was also observed that the higher the frequency of activities, the more pronounced will be the decrease of glycated hemoglobin levels Yoga was considered more effective in reducing glycated hemoglobin levels, then Tai Chi and later walking

6 Discussion

After the description of the results obtained from the seven articles selected for this integrative literature review, they are discussed. In Table 2 are the indicators that reveal the health gains resulting from nursing care interventions in the physical activity of the person with Type 2 Diabetes Mellitus, according to the descriptive statements of Quality Standards of Nursing Care.

Table 2. Health gains resulting from nursing care interventions in the physical activity of the person with Type 2 Diabetes Mellitus

Categories	Indicators
Well-being and self-care	- Improvement in quality of life [10, 12] - Improving mental health [12] - Improved physical activity performance [12] - Improvement in Diabetes Control [12]
Prevention of complications	- Lower value of glycated hemoglobin [11, 12, 15, 16] - Lower value in oral glucose tolerance test [11] - Improvement in insulinogenic index/ acute insulin respons [11] - Improvement in glycemia control [12–15] - Influence on the progression of diabetic neuropathy [12] - Improvement in body fat percentage [12] - Improvement of cardiorespiratory function [12] - Improvement of cardiovascular function [12] - Improvement of metabolic profile [12] - Increased functioning of pancreatic cells β [11] - Fall prevention [12]
Health promotion	- Encouraging the practice of short-term exercises [12]
Functional readaptation	- Improvement of plant sensory perception [12] - Improving the balance [12]

Well-Being and self-care
Through the analysis of the results of the studies selected for this integrative literature review, it was possible to observe that some of the studies revealed an improvement in the quality of life of people with Type 2 Diabetes Mellitus, through the practice of some exercises.

According to the study of Thiel et al. [10], Compliance with the Canadian Diabetes Association recommendations of 150 min per week of moderate intensity aerobic exercises and the practice of endurance exercises at least twice a week improves the quality of life of people with Type 2 Diabetes Mellitus. Therefore, it was demonstrated through the Short-Form Health Survey Questionnaire of 12 items version 2, that the practice of these exercises allows a higher score in the dimensions of physical functioning, physical function, body pain, health in general, vitality, social functioning and mental health. This study also showed that there is a greater association of physical aspects than mental aspects in the improvement of the quality of life related to health, through the practice of these exercises. Participants who exceeded the recommendations given by the Canadian Diabetes Association showed more marked improvements in quality of life than those who did not meet the baseline recommendations.

In the study by Thiel et al. [10], only 21.5% of the sample showed compliance with the recommendations. Thus, the promotion of physical activity should continue to be maintained, with the aim of reducing sedentary lifestyle habits, so that improvements in health care outcomes occur in users with Type 2 Diabetes Mellitus.

In the Systematic Review of the Literature of Cai et al. [12], It has been corroborated that the practice of at least 150 min per week of low intensity exercises improves the quality of life of people with Type 2 Diabetes Mellitus. Still in this review, it was possible to conclude that the practice of aerobic exercises improves not only the quality of life of people with Type 2 Diabetes Mellitus, but also in people who have peripheral neuropathy associated. Diabetic peripheral neuropathy can cause pain in the lower limbs, ulcers and even lead to amputations, which will greatly condition the lives of these people, leading to a decrease in their quality of life. Thus, the practice of aerobic exercises, combined with good oxygenation, improves the quality of life of these people.

The systematic review of Cai et al. [12] revealed also that the practice of aerobic exercises in people with Type 2 Diabetes Mellitus improves the control of Diabetes, which consequently will have benefits also in the quality of life of these people. Some of the studies that were included in the systematic review of Cai et al. [12], revealed that the physical performance of users with Type 2 Diabetes Mellitus can be improved with the practice of aerobic exercises. This type of exercise has not only shown an improvement in physical health but also in the mental health of these people, thus contributing to an improvement in quality of life.

Prevention of Complications

Many of the studies that incorporated this integrative review of the literature have shown that the practice of some exercises can prevent certain complications that are associated with Type 2 Diabetes Mellitus.

People with Type 2 Diabetes Mellitus who have a more sedentary lifestyle are more likely to have poor glycemic control [11]. The study by Lee et al. [11] demonstrated that the practice of different types of moderate intensity exercise, such as performing 30-min aerobic exercises and walking with 1 million accumulated steps, regardless of whether in the short or long term, had an impact on both glucose metabolism and the functioning of pancreatic cells β in people with Type 2 Diabetes Mellitus.

The practice, either in the short or long term, of walking with 1 million accumulated steps showed a significant decrease in glycated hemoglobin, while the practice of aerobic exercises only has this effect when practiced in the long term. Both exercises presented a significant improvement in the values of the insulinogenic index in the acute response to insulin, either in the short or long term. With the long-term practice of aerobic exercises or walking with 1 million accumulated steps it was observed that the values of the oral glucose tolerance test showed a significant decrease, contributing to the prevention of future complications.

It was demonstrated that the practice of walking with 1 million accumulated steps showed better results in acute sensitivity to insulin and decreased values of glycated hemoglobin than the practice of 30 min of aerobic exercise [11].

With the study by Pahra et al. [15], it was also concluded that the practice of exercise contributes to the glycemic control of people with Type 2 Diabetes Mellitus. It has been demonstrated that the practice of a moderate intensity walk, 15 min after the meal, promotes that the pancreatic cells remain at rest, for a short period, which consequently will contribute to a glycemic control in the long term. The practice of exercise after the meal also reduces the possibility of hypoglycemic episodes as the absorption of nutrients will happen more slowly. It has also been demonstrated by this study that, compared to exercising before a meal, exercising after a meal will allow a greater decrease in glycated hemoglobin values.

According to a study by Pai et al. [16], the practice of exercise influences the values of glycated hemoglobin. This study has shown that the more often you do these exercises the greater the impact they will have on the decrease of glycated hemoglobin. Also in this study it was demonstrated that the practice of Yoga has a greater influence than the practice of Tah Chi and then the execution of walks.

The systematic review by Cai et al. [12], has reinforced the idea that the practice of physical exercise not only allows a better control of glycemia but is also able to cause an impact on the values of glycated hemoglobin. It was observed that the practice of aerobic exercise controls the glycemic values and decreased the values of glycated hemoglobin. These exercises also have the ability to reduce the percentage of body fat in people with Type 2 Diabetes Mellitus.

The practice of moderate intensity physical exercise presents itself as one of the main strategies in the non-pharmacological treatment of Diabetes Mellitus type 2 [14]. The study by Chiang et al. [14], included the implementation of a 12-week moderate intensity exercise program. This proved to be feasible and safe for people with Type 2 Diabetes Mellitus, and it also proved to be able to gradually reduce glycemic levels. Thus, the study concluded that the practice of moderate intensity exercises improves glycemia control.

The study by Lade et al. [13], shows that after 20 weeks of aerobic exercise and endurance exercise, participants showed a decrease in glycemic levels, which proves that these types of exercise contribute to glycemic control.

In the systematic review by Cai et al. [12], Diabetic Peripheral Neuropathy was associated with the presence of pain, sensory loss, infection and fall episodes. This review concluded that the practice of aerobic exercises such as Tai Chi, play a key role, since they have the ability to influence the progression of the disease and the symptomatology that is associated with it, thus preventing numerous complications that may arise in people's lives.

Cardiorespiratory and cardiovascular functioning and metabolic profile may also suffer alterations due to physical exercise. Thus, through the systematic review of Cai et al. [12], It was shown that in some studies there was evidence that the practice of walking improved cardiorespiratory function and that the practice of aquatic exercises improved cardiovascular function and metabolic profile of people with Type 2 Diabetes

Mellitus. The practice of Tai Chi also allows an improvement in cardiovascular function, balance and gait contributing to the prevention of falls.

Health Promotion

In the systematic review by Cai et al. [12], It has been demonstrated that the implementation of consultations that address the practice of physical exercise for people with Type 2 Diabetes Mellitus, have the ability to encourage them to perform it, thus promoting good habits and reducing sedentarism. This study has shown that consultations are beneficial and stimulate behavior in the short term.

Functional Readaptation

The practice of Thai Chi has proven to be very effective in improving the sensory perception of the plantar in the person with Type 2 Diabetes Mellitus and with peripheral neuropathy. This type of exercise has the ability to help these people to control their posture, which consequently will also improve their balance [12].

7 Conclusion

With the realization of this integrative literature review, it was concluded that the practice of physical activity provides the person with Type 2 Diabetes Mellitus, numerous gains in health in terms of well-being and self-care, in the prevention of complications, functional rehabilitation and still associated with health promotion.

It has been demonstrated that there is scientific evidence that the practice of physical activity, whether performing aerobic, endurance or even combined exercises, benefits the person with Type 2 Diabetes Mellitus in terms of improving their quality of life, both in terms of physical and mental health.

This review concluded that physical activity provides better control of Type 2 Diabetes Mellitus, evident in the ability to improve glycemia and glycated hemoglobin values, and also makes it possible to prevent some complications that may arise associated with the disease. Thus, the practice of physical activity influences not only the cardiorespiratory function but also the cardiovascular function, affecting the progression of Peripheral Neuropathy, which is one of the complications associated with Diabetes. The implementation of a more active lifestyle will allow an improvement in the sensory perception plant, increasing the balance of these people and thus preventing possible falls.

Nursing interventions related to health education arise as a fundamental role in raising people's awareness for the promotion of healthier lifestyles, encouraging them and thus combating sedentarism. The role of the Nurse becomes central, so that the person can acquire knowledge about his/her disease and skills enabling him/her to be more active and independent in the control of his/her disease.

Since the practice of physical activity in people with Type 2 Diabetes Mellitus has in fact an enormous relevance, it is necessary to have a greater investment in health education for these people, providing knowledge about the practice of exercise and enabling activities that promote it.

References

1. Portugal. Direção Geral de Saúde.: Processo Assistencial Integrado da Diabetes Mellitus tipo 2. Lisboa: DGS (2013). https://www.dgs.pt/directrizes-dadgs/informacoes/informacao-n-001 2013-de-19022013-jpg.aspx
2. International Diabetes Federation.: IDF Diabetes Atlas (9ºed.) (2019). https://Diabetesatlas.org/upload/resources/material/20200302_133351_IDFATLAS9efinal-web.pdf
3. PORDATA.: Óbitos de residentes em Portugal por algumas causas de morte (2018). https://www.pordata.pt/Portugal/%c3%93bitos+de+residentes+em+Portugal+por+algumas+causas+de+morte-156-235700
4. World Health Organization.: Diagnosis and Management of Type 2 Diabetes. Genebra: WHO (2020). https://www.who.int/publications/i/item/who-ucn-ncd-20.1
5. World Health Organization.: Global report on Diabetes. Genebra: WHO (2016). https://apps.who.int/iris/bitstream/handle/10665/204871/9789241565257_eng.pdf?sequence=1
6. Portugal. Direção Geral da Saúde.: Programa Nacional para a Diabetes 2019. Desafios e Estratégias. Lisboa: DGS (2019). https://www.dgs.pt/documentos-epublicacoes/relatorio-programa-nacional-para-a-Diabetes-desafios-e-estrategias-2019-pdf.aspx
7. Instituto do Desporto de Portugal.: Orientações da União Europeia para a Atividade Física - Políticas Recomendadas para a Promoção da Saúde e do Bem-Estar. Lisboa: IDP (2009). https://www.dgs.pt/ficheiros-de-upload-2013/pnpafidp-orientacoes-europ-af-jan 2009-pdf.aspx
8. Sociedade Brasileira de Diabetes.: Diretrizes da Sociedade Brasileira de Diabetes 2014–2015. Rio de Janeiro: SBD (2014). https://www.Diabetes.org.br/publico/images/2015/area-restrita/diretrizes-sbd-2015.pdf
9. Melnyk, B., Fineout-Overholt, E.: Box 1.3: Rating system for the hierarchy of evidence for intervention/treatment questions. In: Evidence-Based Practice in Nursing & Healthcare: A Guide to Best Practice, 3.ª ed., p. 11. Wolters Kluwer Health, Philadelphia (2015). https://guides.lib.umich.edu/c.php?g=282802&p=1888246
10. Thiel, D.M., Sayah, F.A., Vallance, J.K., Johnson, S.T., Johnson, J.A.: Association between physical activity and health-related quality of life in adults with type 2 diabetes. Can. J. Diabetes **41**, 58–63 (2016). https://doi.org/10.1016/j.jcjd.2016.07.004
11. Lee, S.F., Pei, D., Chi, M.J., Jeng, C.: Na investigation and comparison of the effectiveness of diferente exercise programes in improving glucose metabolismo and pancreatic β cell function of type 2 diabetes patients. Int. J. Clin. Pract. **69**(10), 1159–1170 (2015). https://doi.org/10.1111/ijcp.12679
12. Cai, H., Li, G., Zhang, P., Xu, D., Chen, L.: Effect of exercise on the quality of life in type 2 diabetes mellitus: a systematic review. Qual. Life Res. **26**(3), 515–530 (2016). https://doi.org/10.1007/s11136-016-1481-5
13. Lade, C.G., et al.: Effects of diferente exercise programs and minimal detectable changes in hemoglobina A1c in patients with type 2 diabetes. Diabetol. Metab. Syndr. **8**(13), 1–9 (2016). https://doi.org/10.1186/s13098-016-0123-y
14. Chiang, S., Heitkemper, M.M., Hung, Y., Tzeng, W., Lee, M., Lin, C.: Effects of a 12-week moderate-intensity exercise training on blood glucose response in patients with type 2 diabetes. Medicine **98**(36), e16860 (2019). https://doi.org/10.1097/MD.0000000000016860
15. Pahra, D., Sharma, N., Ghai, S., Hajela, A., Bhansali, S., Bhansali, A.: Impact of post-meal and one-time daily exercise in patient with type 2 diabetes mellitus: a randomized crossover study. Diabetol. Metab. Syndr. **9**(64) (2017). https://doi.org/10.1186/s13098-017-0263-8
16. Pai, L., Li, T., Hwu, Y., Chang, S., Chen, L., Chang, P.: The effectiveness of regular leisure-time physical activities on long-term glycemic control in people with type 2 diabetes: a systematic review and meta-analysis. Diabetes Res. Clin. Pract. **113**, 77–85 (2016). https://doi.org/10.1016/j.diabres.2016.01.011

The Position Therapy in Elderly People at Risk of Developing Pressure Injuries

Rita Ferreira[1], Maria Margarida Goes[2], Henrique Oliveira[2,3](✉), João Vítor Vieira[2], and Margarida Santos[4]

[1] Hospital Beatriz Ângelo, Loures, Portugal
[2] Polytechnic Institute of Beja, Beja, Portugal
[3] Telecommunications Institute, Lisbon, Portugal
hjmo@lx.it.pt
[4] Salt Clinic Center, Póvoa de Varzim, Portugal

Abstract. Pressure injuries (PI) are a major public health problem, as they significantly reduce the quality of life of elderly people. On the other hand, they increase costs and burdens in health services. Nursing interventions contribute to the development and implementation of preventive strategies to reduce all these negative impacts. **Objective**: To identify the contribution of position therapy to safe care in elderly people at risk of developing PI. **Methodology**: The methodology used was based on an Integrative Literature Review (ILR), which included the formulation of an initial research question, research in scientific databases, analysis and interpretation of selected articles, as well as the synthesis and presentation of the results obtained. For the selection of articles and formulation of the research question, the PI[C]OD methodology was used. **Results**: Once the methodology was applied, a final set comprising 7 studies was obtained, which suggest that there is scientific evidence that repositioning therapy, as well as automatic repositioning systems, contribute to the prevention of PI development. **Conclusion**: Based on the scientific evidence found in this research, the practice of position therapy prevents PI in the elderly and, consequently, promotes their comfort and quality of life. It also contributes to lower health care costs.

Keywords: Elderly · Nursing care · Pressure injury · Position therapy · Prevention

1 Introduction

The Portuguese population is characterized by an accentuated aging, associated with an increased vulnerability to morbidity and, consequently, to functional dependence. The Pressure Injuries (PI) are prevalent in the elderly, generating a negative impact on the quality of life of individuals and their families, as well as on health care services. The "National Plan for the Safety of Patients 2015–2020" established as a goal, for the year 2020, that 95% of the institutions responsible for providing health care have implemented strategies for evaluation, prevention and treatment of PI, aiming to reduce by 50% the number of PI, compared to the year 2014, for all the entities belonging to the National

J. García-Alonso and C. Fonseca (Eds.): IWoG 2021, LNBE, pp. 245–256, 2022.
https://doi.org/10.1007/978-3-030-97524-1_23

Health System (NHS) [1]. Nursing is a profession at the service of a health policy that contributes to the design of new interventions, through a "diagnostic evaluation" and subsequent "nursing interventions evaluation" in a continuous process, which makes it possible to measure systematically and throughout the entire care process, the results sensitive to nursing care, considered as health outcomes whenever there is a recovery of functional capacity of the person [2].

PI are characterized by damage to the skin or in its adjacent tissues, mostly in bony prominences, caused by an inadequate compression and/or perfusion forces. Slip/torsion and friction forces are also considered causes of PI [5, 16]. Tissue rupture may be originated by the constant abrupt supply of blood flow to tissues when there is a pressure relief. However, when there is no such relief for a long period of time, the cells may end up dying due to capillaries occlusion [7]. Regarding the sliding force, this causes the tissues to move but the skeleton remains in the same place, causing tissue deformation and damage on the blood vessels. The frictional force is when the force mentioned above is exceeded and the upper layers of epithelial cells are eliminated by scraping. The most common areas where PI occur are the sacrococcygeal zone, the perineal zone due to ischial tuberosities, trochanters, calcaneus, and elbows [5].

The risk factors of these PI may be the pressures as mentioned above, age, perfusion and oxygenation, sensory perception, nutrition, skin conditions, body temperature, spinal cord injuries, decreased collagen, hemoglobin and hematocrit, smoking and other types of pathologies [3].

PI can be classified into: (i) "PI stage 1"; (ii) "PI stage 2"; (iii) "PI stage 3"; (iv) "PI stage 4"; (v) "PI without stage"; (vi) "Deep PI of fabrics". In the "PI stage 1", there is still no damage to the integrity of the skin, but there is a non-bleachable erythema in a specific area. In the "PI stage 2" there is a partial loss of the dermis, in which its area of tissue damage is a viable pink, moist tissue and without devitalized tissue or a serous blister. In the "PI stage 3" there is a complete loss of the skin integrity, but without the exposure of bones, tendons, joints, or muscles. Regarding "PI stage 4", there is already exposed or palpable muscles, tendons, joints and/or bones. The "PI without stage" are distinguished from the others as it presents a total skin loss, but without visualization of the extent of tissue damage. This happens due to devitalized and/or necrosed tissue that covers the wound. As such, its degree can only be defined after cleaning wound tissues. Finally, the "deep tissue PIs" present the skin intact or not with a dark, painful and swollen area [8].

For PI prevention it is important to know the needs of an individual before implementing any intervention. In Portugal, the Braden Scale is used to evaluate the risk of developing PI. Among the various prevention interventions, are: skin evaluation and care; nutritional evaluation and support; positioning and support surfaces [6].

This Integrative Literature Review is intended to focus on position therapy for PI prevention. It is characterized by the alternation of positions of an individual, executed by the individual himself or with the help of other people or material resources. Sometimes it may be necessary to be fully positioned by someone else [3].

The frequency of the repositioning should be selected according to the level of the activity, mobility and capacity of the individual. If the individual is not on a support surface, he or she should be repositioned more frequently [3]. To help with this practice, methods can be implemented that serve as reminders of the need to reposition the person [8].

According to the guidelines proposed by EPUAP, NPIAP and PPPIA in 2019, the recommended position is lateralization with a 30° slope compared to lateralization at 90°. In the lateral position with a slant of 30°, the joints are positioned in a natural way, which is beneficial since it avoids unnecessary stretching of the muscles [8]. Furthermore, in this position, all body segments are aligned and the pressure in areas of bone prominence decreases significantly [17].

When positioning an individual, the use of foam pads to raise the heels should be considered [9], as well as some type of prophylactic dressing material [8]. When sitting in a chair, it is important to tilt the chair slightly, to be in harmony with the heel lift [8].

The support surfaces work as an aid for nurses to optimize the nursing care. Among the different support surfaces available today, one should consider using a high specification, single-layer reactive foam mattress, rather than a low-density foam mattress. In addition, the use of an overlay mattress, such as an alternating pressure mattress [8], can also be considered. They work by eliminating the pressure in areas located for cyclic periods, having a sensor responsible for assessing the pressure of the capillary occlusion, so that the surface pressure remains at lower values [3]. For positioning in the chair, a pressure redistribution cushion should be used, especially when the person is unable to position by itself to relieve pressure in an autonomous way [8].

2 Objective and Methods

To identify the nursing care sensitive outcomes, resulting from the position therapy for a safe care, in elderly people with risk of developing PI.

2.1 Ethical Aspects

No opinion was requested from the Ethics Committee as this was a secondary study. In the formulation of the problem there was the concern with the respect for the principles of clarity, objectivity, and precision, so that the results are assumed as an added value for the nursing care in the position therapy to the elderly person in the prevention of PI. The analysis of data extracted from the selected studies was developed in harmony with the principle of respect for the results obtained in this research and by these researchers. The reference of the authors followed the standards of good academic and scientific practices.

2.2 Study Type

The clinical practice of the nurse is always based on the most current scientific evidence, and this is what turns nursing care into quality care. This evidence-based practice encompasses the entire process of collecting, interpreting, evaluating, and implementing clinical data that are important for the decision-making by professionals [11].

This research work consists of an Integrative Literature Review, based on the need to implement quality care according to the most recent scientific evidence. It comprises the following steps: i) identification of the research question; ii) definition of inclusion and exclusion criteria for studies; iii) selection of studies according to the defined criteria; iv) analysis of the selected articles; v) presentation and discussion of the results; and, vi) synthesis of the scientific knowledge acquired.

2.3 Methodological Procedures

Following the objective outlined above, which served as a common thread for the Integrative Literature Review, a research question was formulated using the PI[C]OD methodology, being (P) the target population, (I) the type of intervention, (C) the comparisons, (O) the outcomes and (D) the type of study (design). Based on this structure, the following guiding question was elaborated: What are the nursing intervention outcomes (Results) of nursing care of position therapy (Intervention) of the elderly person with wound/injury by pressure (Population)?

The research strategy adopted included the search of articles published in Portuguese, English and Spanish languages, which took place during May 2020, in the CINAHL Complete database through the EBSCOhost platform. Specific descriptors were used, which were connected to the Boolean operators "AND" and "OR" in the following arrangement and in the following order: "pressure ulcer" or "bed sores" or "bedsore" or "decubitus ulcer" or "pressure sore" and "positioning" and "wound healing or prevention".

In order to limit the search, the following inclusion criteria were selected: (i) full text; (ii) time period between 2010 and 2020; (iii) English, Spanish and Portuguese languages; (iv) publications of academic journals with peer review and; (v) population over 65 years. The following exclusion criteria was adopted: articles in duplicate and those with a population under 65 years of age that were not aligned with the objective of this research study.

After this research, a total of 80 articles were obtained. However, 24 of them were duplicated and, as such, were excluded, resulting in a total of 56. With the latter, the respective selection was made in two stages. First by reading the titles, abstracts and

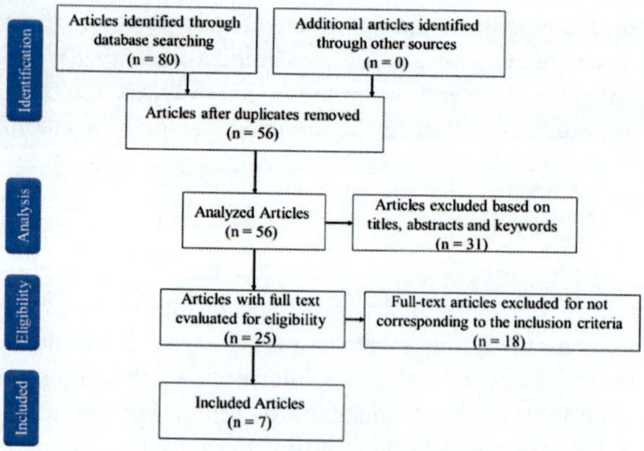

Fig. 1. PRISMA diagram for the presentation of the research methodology.

keywords, and then by reading them in full. At the end of the first stage there were 25 articles and at the end of the second stage, only 7 articles remain, which met all the criteria considered for data collection and analysis. These research steps are shown in Fig. 1.

3 Results

This Integrative Literature Review resulted in 7 articles. The levels of evidence listed in the following in Table 1 were identified through a hierarchical system of scientific evidence advocated by the Joanna Briggs Institute [19], which considers the following levels of evidence:

- Level 1 - Experimental Designs;
- Level 2 - Quasi-experimental Designs;
- Level 3 - Observational - Analytic Designs;
- Level 4 - Observational - Descriptive Studies;
- Level 5 - Expert Opinion and Bench Research.

Table 1. Results of the integrative literature review.

Authors/Method/level of evidence	Objectives	Results
Bergstrom, N., Horn, S. D., Rapp, M. P., Stern, A., Barrett, R. and Watkiss, M. (2013) [4] **Method:** Randomized Controlled Trial- RCT **Level of Evidence:** 1	- Determine the appropriate frequency of repositioning of elderly people in homes at risk of developing pressure Injury in the presence of high-density foam mattresses by comparing repositioning every 2 h, every 3 h and every 4 h	- In this study, the authors found a low incidence of PI (2.0%) in people at moderate and high risk distributed among the three repositioning groups. There were no significant differences between the participants of moderate and high risk, as well as no differences between the three repositioning groups. Stage 3 and 4 PI were not observed. However, in previous studies there was presence of these injuries, which leads the authors to conclude that electric beds, spring mattresses and overlapping surfaces associated with long periods of time do not prevent PI. The authors also add that the reduced incidence of PI can be explained by the combination of high-density foam mattresses, repositioning and documentation. The latter was considered essential to remind nurses to implement heel elevation, observe and describe the skin, as well as to take care of incontinence episodes. With this study it was also possible to verify, due to the reduced PI incidence, that with the use of a high-density foam mattress it is allowed to increase the repositioning period of time, without increasing the number of new Injury in the individual

(continued)

Table 1. (*continued*)

Authors/Method/level of evidence	Objectives	Results
Moore, Z., Cowman, S. and Conroy, R. M. (2011) [15] **Method:** RCT **Level of Evidence:** 1	- To compare the incidence of PI in elderly people using a repositioning every 6 h with lateralization at 90° (control group) and a repositioning every 3 h with lateralization at 30° (experimental group)	- In this study the authors identified among the different components of the Braden Scale, that mobility and activity were the main responsible for the development of PI - The incidence of PI in the control group was higher (11%) than the incidence in the experimental group (3%). Thus, it was possible for the authors to conclude that positioning with a 30° slope every 3 h is more effective in reducing PI. These results were in line with previous studies. It should be noted that for the support surface used in these individuals, an alternating pressure device was used for chairs of 99% of the population and beds of 86% of the population in the control group and 96% of the population in the experimental group
Rich, S. E., Margolis, D., Shardell, M., Hawkes, W. G., Miller, R. R., Amr, S. and Baumgarten, M. (2010) [18] **Method:** Cohort study **Level of Evidence: 3**	- To compare the benefit of repositioning every 2 h and repositioning at intervals longer than 2 h in elderly patients undergoing hip fracture surgery, bedridden	- In this study the authors found that repositioning every 2 h in elderly patients with hip fractures does not effectively prevent PI. When compared with other studies, it was possible to realize that the ideal repositioning interval is inconclusive and that it should be selected according to the mobility characteristics and general clinical status of the patients - The risk of developing PI identified by the Braden Scale may also have influenced the effect of repositioning in this study, as high-risk patients repositioned every 2 h during visits of the first 5 days of hospitalization had a lower incidence of PI compared to those repositioned less frequently. Low risk patients had a higher incidence of PI repositioning every 2 h during the first 5 days of hospital stay compared to those repositioned less frequently. These differences were not very significant, so more studies focused on this topic are needed - In addition, the authors also found that the adherence of nurses to the most frequent repositioning was not much, because only in 53% of the days the repositioning every 2 h was accomplished. In patients with pressure redistribution support surfaces there was a higher prevalence of repositioning compared to patients on standard surfaces. Thus, the authors could verify that the use of pressure redistribution mattresses allow reminding professionals of the need for more frequent repositioning

(*continued*)

Table 1. (*continued*)

Authors/Method/level of evidence	Objectives	Results
Gaspar, S., Peralta, M., Marques, A., Budri, A. and Matos, M. G. (May 2019) [10] **Method:** Systematic Literature Review (RSL) **Level of Evidence:** 1	- To identify the most appropriate PI prevention strategies in a hospital context through the analysis of 26 studies, with the following inclusion criteria: publications during the period of 2009 to December 7, 2018, regarding the effectiveness of PI prevention; cross-sectional, prospective and retrospective, comparative, pre-test and post-test studies, almost experimental, experimental, RCT and studies with mixed design; studies with incidence of PI; studies with a population of adults admitted to hospital wards and acute units; language in English, French, Portuguese or Spanish	- The authors found that for the support surfaces, the low-pressure air mattresses and the alternating pressure air mattresses were more effective in preventing PI compared to the overlaps of alternating pressure air mattresses and add that the duration and intensity of the cycle of the support surfaces have a great influence on PI prevention. In addition, they concluded that dynamic surfaces, such as electric beds and hybrid air mattresses, reduce PI incidence more than standard hospital mattresses. Multi-phase alternating pressure air mattresses are effective for patients in geriatric wards and acute medicine, but for individuals in intensive care units the most effective are alternating pressure air mattresses. The authors state that it is difficult to define the ideal support surface because the development of PI depends on a set of associated risk factors. Therefore, they state that these should be selected based on the individual characteristics and needs of the users - Regarding the frequency of positioning, they found in some studies that positioning every two hours in association with pressure mapping technological devices can decrease the incidence of PI and consequently increase the comfort of individuals. The devices for mapping the heads of patients detect the pressures on the entire body surface and act as warnings, of the need for repositioning, for nurses However, they have also found in some studies that high frequency of positioning does not decrease the incidence of PI, but increases the adverse effects associated with clinical devices, as well as increases the workload of health professionals. The evaluation of the degree of position with an automatic positioning system helps to prevent PI. Additionally, these devices perform pressure relief in the sacrum area, control of skin temperature and humidity, prevention of sliding and preservation of the position with an angle of 30°. Also, these devices optimize the nursing team in the sense that it reduces the need of less personnel to perform this therapy

(*continued*)

Table 1. (*continued*)

Authors/Method/level of evidence	Objectives	Results
Meyer, D., Hecke, A. V., Varhaeghe, S. and Beeckman, D. (2019) [14] **Method:** RCT **Level of Evidence:** 1	- Compare the benefit between: experimental group 1 (application of a PROTECT - tool that evaluates the frequency and type of positioning required according to the individuals' risk factors and use of a bed positioning system); experimental group 2 (use of a bed positioning system, selection of the frequency and type of positioning according to the usual protocol); and, control group (positioning and frequency according to the usual protocols)	- In this study the authors found that when individuals were in bed, they were more often repositioned than sitting on chairs. The repositioning protocol resulting from the use of the PROTECT tool recommended that individuals should not be seated more than twice 4 h per day and in patients with Injury or erythema in the sacrococcygeal zone up to 3 times 1 h per day. However, these recommendations were based on literature reviews and expert opinions, and the authors may conclude that these cares can be difficult to integrate in practice - The use of the bed repositioning system managed to maintain the lateral positions from 30 to 45°, but there was no significant effect in reducing the pressure in the sacral zone. The authors could also see that this system provides comfort to the users and reduces the work of the nurses -Regarding the costs of the interventions, in the control group these were higher. This was due to the fact that in this group the repositioning time was longer. These results were in accordance with other studies
Lozano-Montoya, I., Vélez-Díaz-Pallarés, M., Abraha, I., Cherubini, A., Soiza, R. L., O'Mahony, D., Montero-Errasquín, B., Correa-Pérez, A. and Cruz-Jentoft, A. J. (2015) [12] **Method:** RSL **Level of Evidence:** 1	- Identify the most appropriate non-pharmacological strategies for the prevention of PI	- In this study it was found that pressure mattresses alternatively reduce the incidence of PI compared to standard foam mattresses. Constant low-pressure mattresses proved to be more suitable compared to standard foam mattresses for PI prevention. However, no differences were found between alternating pressure mattresses and constant low-pressure mattresses. The likelihood of PI risk reduction by medical sheep skin is like that of constant low-pressure mattresses In this way, the authors were able to conclude that new technology mattresses are more suitable than a standard hospital mattress - These results were in line with guidelines and recommendations from other institutions - Regarding repositioning, the authors concluded that there was no consensus among studies on the frequency and ideal techniques needed to prevent PI

(*continued*)

Table 1. (*continued*)

Authors/Method/level of evidence	Objectives	Results
Mateo, M. M. and Herrera, D. G. (2018) [13] **Method:** RSL **Level of Evidence:** 1	- Identify the support surfaces and repositioning that best prevent PI in the elderly, through the analysis of 3 articles	- The authors concluded that repositioning should be done every 3 h or every 4 h, instead of repositioning every 2 h. By increasing the repositioning time, it is possible to prevent PI, promote sleep and quality of life of the elderly and reduce the burden of the Nursing team - They also found that the inclination of the positioning of individuals in bed should be 30° as opposed to 90° - Regarding the support surfaces, they found that the most advanced in science and technology are better for PI prevention than the standard hospital mattress Although the pressure decreases on improved surfaces it is necessary to continue to reposition manually for PI prevention

4 Discussion

This Integrative Literature Review summarizes the contributions of position therapy addressing the PI prevention in the elderly population. Of the 7 studies analyzed, there was a general agreement among authors regarding the frequency and type of positioning, but with slight disagreements in the selection of support surfaces.

According to Lozano-Montoya et al. [12], the adequate frequency and technique of repositioning for PI prevention proved to be inconclusive. However, in the trial done by Moore et al. [15] the lateral position with a 30° slope every 3 h was identified as the most effective in PI prevention. Mateo and Herrera [13] corroborated this idea, stating that repositioning every 3 h or 4 h with a 30° slope is ideal to avoid tissue damage and, at the same time, promote a more peaceful sleep.

Regarding the repositioning of individuals every 2 h, this procedure was not proven to be beneficial for the prevention of PI in the elderly with limited activity. Rich et al. [18] were responsible for corroborating this idea, using as population the elderly with hip fracture. For Gaspar et al. [10], this repositioning is inadequate for prevention of PI, and may even potentiate the opposite effect. Furthermore, it increases the burden on the nursing team. In the study by Rich et al. [18], it was found that nurses adhere less to position therapy in the presence of very frequent repositioning. This author also concluded that the repositioning interval should be selected according to the mobility characteristics and general clinical status of the individuals.

Regarding the support surfaces, Lozano-Montoya et al. [12] found that the more advanced they are, provide a more effective PI prevention compared to standard hospital mattresses. Mateo and Herrera [13] proved the same idea in their study, adding that despite the presence of these improved surfaces it is essential to maintain repositioning by nurses.

In a study developed by Bergstrom et al. [4] the use of high-density foam mattresses proved the possibility of a longer repositioning period without increasing PI incidence. However, the use of electric beds or spring mattresses, associated with long periods of time in people with limited activity, may lead to the development of PI. In the study of Gaspar et al. [10], the authors concluded that even so, electric beds are more effective in preventing injuries compared to the standard hospital mattresses. Alternate pressure mattresses proved to be very effective in preventing PI in the studies published by Gaspar et al. [10] and Lozano-Montoya et al. [12]. The first authors state that this prevention is often influenced by the duration and intensity of the surface cycles. Although in the study of Rich et al. [18] there is no reference to PI prevention associated with alternating pressure mattresses, these worked as a reminder to professionals to reposition more frequently. The study developed by Gaspar et al. [10] also identified the use of pressure mapping devices with patients as a repositioning reminder. They work as alerts of the need for patient repositioning when pressure is high, being a fundamental aid for nurses.

Another alternative that makes nurses increase adherence to repositioning is the automatic positioning systems. These manage to maintain the position between 30 and 45°, increase comfort and decrease the costs of the nursing team, which consequently reduces costs in health services. The same is justified due to the manual positioning, in comparison with the automatic one, to demand more nurses available for that and more time spent by them on doing the positioning. These conclusions were verified in a study developed by Meyer et al. [14]. By analogy, the systematic review of Gaspar et al. [10] confirmed these results, adding that their prevention of injuries is related to maintaining the position at the desired angle, preventing sliding forces.

Furthermore, in the same study it was proved that the automatic positioning system allows a better control of skin temperature and humidity.

The support surfaces, together with the repositioning performed by the nurses and the clinical records are essential for PI prevention. The records additionally work as a reminder of all the care needed to be provided. This was the case in the Bergstrom et al. trial [4].

In this way it is possible to verify the acquisition of health outcomes resulting from position therapy. It prevents the development of PI, promotes the comfort of individuals vulnerable to this problem and, above all, improves the quality of life of the elderly. Moreover, it optimizes nursing teams and decreases costs in health services.

5 Study Limitations

The scientific publishing developed allowed the identification of the health outcomes of the position therapy to the elderly person at risk of developing PI, constituting an important contribution to the reflection on this problem, aiming at the implementation of professional intervention strategies in favor of the person's safety and compatible with excellence care. The therapy in question proved to be more economical in health resources and useful in promoting the quality of life of the elderly with limited activity. Future studies should be conducted adopting an empirical approach, to verify the effect of a repositioning program on elderly people at risk of developing PI. This experimental approach, involving the control triad, randomization and manipulation of the independent variable (repositioning program, with a structured protocol) is a methodological quality assurance of the study.

6 Conclusions

After analyzing the results and discussing them it was possible to conclude that the most appropriate repositioning for PI prevention is performed every 3 h, which can vary between lateral positions with a 30° of slant. However, it is always necessary that nurses take into consideration the needs of individuals and develop customized repositioning plans.

Another conclusion identified in this review was that the use of improved support surfaces, such as alternating pressure mattresses and high-density foam mattresses, becomes essential to increase repositioning time and, consequently, optimize the work of nursing teams.

Automatic bed repositioning systems should be increasingly implemented in health services because they bring long-term benefits to bedridden elderly and nursing care management. These benefits provided to individuals with limited self-repositioning are characterized by the control of humidity and skin temperature, as well as by the reduction of slipping forces, which are fundamental in preventing PI. In relations to the nurses, they become more available for other equally important care, as the time taken for repositioning is less with these devices.

Taking all these aspects into consideration, this Integrative Literature Review was able to answer both the objective and the PICO question initially proposed. The position therapy has proven to be quite useful in promoting the quality of life of the elderly with limited capability of self-repositioning and more economical in health resources.

References

1. Approval of the National Plan for the Safety of Patients 2015–2020 (2015) 28 DR 3882-(2) (Port)
2. Goes, M., Lopes, M.J., Oliveira, H., et al.: A nursing care intervention model for elderly people to ascertain general profiles of functionality and self care needs. Sci. Rep. **10**, 1770 (2020). https://doi.org/10.1038/s41598-020-58596-1
3. Balio, L.C.L.: Effectiveness of nursing care in preventing pressure ulcers. [Dissertation of Master's Degree, Escola Superior de Enfermagem de Coimbra]. Scientific Repository of Coimbra School of Nursing (2015). http://web.esenfc.pt/?url=2kHGzV99
4. Bergstrom, N., Horn, S.D., Rapp, M.P., Stern, A., Barrett, R., Watkiss, M.: Turning for ulcer reduction: a multisite randomized clinical trial in nursing homes. J. Am. Geriatr. Soc. **61**(10), 1705–1713 (2013). https://doi.org/10.1111/jgs.12440
5. Dealey, C.: Wound treatment: Guide for Nurses. Climepsi Editors (2006)
6. General Directorate of Health: Braden Scale: Adult and Pediatric Version (Braden Q) (2011). https://www.dgs.pt/departamento-da-qualidade-na-saude/ficheiros-anexos/orientacao_ulceraspdf-pdf.aspx
7. Duque, H.P., et al.: Manual of Good Practices. Pressure Leaders: A Strategic Approach. Formasau - Training and Health, Lda (2009)

8. European Pressure Ulcer Advisory Panel, National Pressure Injury Advisory Panel & Pan Pacific Pressure Injury Alliance. Prevention and Treatment of Pressure Ulcers/Injuries: Quick Reference Guide 2019 (2019)
9. Fernandes, T.S.H.: Influência do conhecimento dos enfermeiros sobre prevenção e tratamento de úlceras de pressão na prática clínica. [Dissertação de Mestrado, Instituto de Ciências da Saúde da Universidade Católica Portuguesa]. Repositório Institucional da Universidade Católica Portuguesa (2014). https://repositorio.ucp.pt/bitstream/10400.14/19732/1/TESE%20COMPLETA%205.pdf
10. Gaspar, S., Peralta, M., Marques, A., Budri, A., Gaspar de Matos, M.: Effectiveness on hospital-acquired pressure ulcers prevention: a systematic review. Int. Wound J. **16**(5), 1087–1102 (2019). https://doi.org/10.1111/iwj.13147
11. Jensen, K.: Evidence-Based Nursing Practice: 7 Steps to the Perfect PICO Search. Recuperado de EBSCO Health, 9 Janeiro 2018. https://www.ebsco.com/sites/g/files/nabnos191/files/acquiadam-assets/7-Steps-to-the-Perfect-PICO-Search-White-Paper.pdf
12. Lozano-Montoya, I., et al.: Nonpharmacologic interventions to heal pressure ulcers in older patients: an overview of systematic reviews (the SENATOR-ONTOP series). J. Am. Med. Dir. Assoc. **16**(6), 448–469 (2015). https://doi.org/10.1016/j.jamda.2015.01.083
13. Mateo, M.M., Herrera, D.G.: What is more effective in preventing pressure ulcers: postural changes or support surfaces? Gerokomos **29**(3), 138–140 (2018)
14. Meyer, D., Hecke, A.V., Varhaeghe, S., Beeckman, D.: PROTECT-trial: a cluster RCT to study the effectiveness of a repositioning aid and tailored repositioning to increase repositioning compliance. J. Adv. Nurs. **75**(5), 1085–1098 (2019). https://doi.org/10.1111/jan.13932
15. Moore, Z., Cowman, S., Conroy, R.M.: A randomized controlled clinical trial of repositioning, using the 30 tilt, for the prevention of pressure ulcers. J. Clin. Nurs. **20**(17–18), 2633–2644 (2011). https://doi.org/10.1111/j.1365-2702.2011.03736.x
16. Order of Nurses: Good practice guide - Caring for the person with mobility changes positioning, transfers and walking training (2013). https://www.ordemenfermeiros.pt/arquivo/publicacoes/Documents/GOBP_Mobilidade_VF_site.pdf
17. Pickenbrock, H., Ludwig, V., Zapf, A.: Support pressure distribution for positioning in neutral versus conventional positioning in the prevention of decubitus ulcers: a pilot study in healthy participants. BMC Nurs. **16**(60), 1–7 (2017). https://doi.org/10.1186/s12912017-0253-z
18. Rich, S.E., et al.: Frequent manual repositioning and incidence of pressure ulcers among bed-bound elderly hip fracture patients. Wound Repair Regeneration **19**(1), 10–18 (2011). https://doi.org/10.1111/j.1524475X.2010.00644.x
19. The Joanna Briggs Institute (2013). JBI Levels of Evidence. https://joannabriggs.org/sites/default/files/2019-05/JBI-Levels-of-evidence_2014_0.pdf

Barefoot and In-Shoe Plantar Pressure in a Portuguese Sample of Diabetic Patients: A Cross-Sectional Study

Liliana B. Sousa(✉), Rafael A. Bernardes, Inês Almeida, Filipa Ventura, Rosa Silva, João Apóstolo, Rui Baptista, Anabela Salgueiro-Oliveira, and Pedro Parreira

The Health Sciences Research Unit: Nursing (UICISA:E), Nursing School of Coimbra (ESEnfC), Coimbra, Portugal
baptliliana@esenfc.pt

Abstract. Background: Diabetes Mellitus (DM) is considered a metabolic chronic disease and global epidemic incidence in all age groups. One of the most common and severe complications of DM is diabetic foot ulceration (DFU), resulting in a high number of prolonged hospitalizations and limb amputations. Plantar pressure is considered an important predictor of the DFU development, along with contralateral temperature, shear forces, humidity and skin resistance. **Objective:** Characterization of barefoot and in-shoe plantar pressure in a sample of diabetic patients. **Method:** Observational cross-sectional quantitative study with 58 participants, aged between 28 and 84 years, diagnosed with DM. Relevant demographic and clinical data, as well as plantar pressure values were collected. **Results:** The mean values of barefoot (EMED) and in-shoe (PEDAR) plantar pressure evaluation showed increased values, with the majority of the sample having values above the proposed thresholds. **Conclusion**: In general, high plantar pressure values were identified, drawing attention to the need of prevention policies and the follow-up of this patients in primary health care. New solutions might also include the development of innovative footwear, innovative footwear that aims to reduce plantar pressure in critical regions of the foot, but also than enables the monitoring of plantar pressure values.

Keywords: Diabetes mellitus · Diabetic foot ulceration · Plantar pressure

1 Introduction

Diabetes Mellitus (DM) is a chronic metabolic disorder and a global epidemic that can affect a high number of persons in different group ages [1]. According to the International Diabetes Federation (IDF) [2], 537 million adults worldwide are living with DM. This number is predicted to increase to 643 million by 2030 and 783 million by 2045. In Europe, it is estimated that 61 million of adults are living with DM, with an expected increase to 67 million by 2030 and 69 million by 2045.

J. García-Alonso and C. Fonseca (Eds.): IWoG 2021, LNBE, pp. 257–266, 2022.
https://doi.org/10.1007/978-3-030-97524-1_24

Diabetic foot ulcers (DFU) are one of the most common and severe complication of DM [3]. It is estimated that 19% to 34% of diabetic patients are at risk of developing foot lesions, with ulceration secondary to progressive peripheral polyneuropathy being the most common cause of those diabetic foot lesions [4, 5]. Additionally, the presence of DFU in diabetic patients is considered the main precursor of lower extremity amputation in this population [6–8].

For the development of DFU, skin microclimate is a significant contributor, particularly plantar pressure [9], along with contralateral temperature, shear forces, humidity and skin resistance. In fact, several studies noted the relevance of plantar pressure parameters on DFU [10], recognizing that half of all DFUs occur on the plantar surface of the foot and are mainly caused by high levels of mechanical pressure during gait [11, 12].

The review by Patry et al. (2013) [13] effectively identified that peak plantar pressure in the shoe is a significant predictor of DFU development, establishing a pressure threshold value of 200 kPa as effectively preventing ulceration (appearing to be a safe value for patients with and without a previous history of DFUs). This 200 kPa cutoff point evaluated by PEDAR sensors was also identified in the review by Jones et al. (2020) [9]. In the EMED platform, for example, plantar ulcerations often occur in areas with plantar pressure greater than 500 kPa [14]. Despite this evidence, the pressure peaks demonstrate reduced sensitivity (63.5%) and specificity (46.3%) in predicting ulcer development in the DFU [9]. Indeed, despite the evidence of higher levels of plantar pressure in regions usually associated with DFUs (*hallux*, heel and metatarsals), only the metatarsal region and related plantar pressure values is significantly associated with higher risk of developing ulcers [15].

Thus, it is widely accepted in the literature that the therapeutic footwear is an effective measure to prevent ulcers in diabetic patients [16], especially for those with peripheral neuropathy [17, 18], since footwear personalization is usually designed to reduce plantar pressure during walking [19–21].

The *Science DiabetICC Footwear* project proposes the development of an innovative therapeutic footwear for the clinical condition of the diabetic foot. The proposed solution will consist of footwear and a removable insole, adding some important unique characteristics: new materials at the level of the insole and sole that allow greater impact absorption; shape adaptability and greater recovery after loading and less abrasion; ability to reduce the risk of developing infections associated with ulcers. At the same time, new material systems for the interior of the shoe will be investigated for greater ergonomic and thermophysiological comfort, as well as materials with shape adaptability and superior performance. In terms of design, decorative coatings for the exterior of the shoes will be studied, providing an appealing design for end users. Finally, the footwear will include self-sensing materials for monitoring and detection of plantar pressure, temperature and humidity.

This study is developed in the context of an initial stage of the project, namely consisting of an observational study that will be used to specify the user requirements and contexts of use. Specifically, the purpose of this paper is to characterize the values of barefoot and in-shoe plantar pressure in patients with DM.

2 Method

2.1 Design

Observational cross-sectional quantitative study.

2.2 Sample Recruitment

A total of 58 participants were randomly chosen from database of 919 patients diagnosed with DM from a Portuguese primary healthcare institution. The nurses were involved in the recruitment of the participants. The inclusion criteria were: (i) participants aged 18 years old or above; (ii) patients with the ability to fully communicate in Portuguese; (iii) participants able to consent; and (iv) diagnostic of DM type 1 or 2. The exclusion criteria were: (i) confused our disoriented participants; (ii) uncooperative participants; and (iii) participants with mobility limitations that compromise the pressure plantar assessment.

2.3 Material

A Case Report Form (CRF) developed by the research team and with the input of experts in the field was used to collect main demographic and clinical data according to the defined protocol. An informed consent term was also developed with a brief description of the study, the main purpose, and the voluntary nature of participation. To stratify the socioeconomic level of the participants the Portuguese version of the Graffar scale [22] was used. To assess plantar pressure both EMED (Novel GmbH, Munich, Germany) and PEDAR (Novel GmbH, Munich, Germany) systems were used, respectively for barefoot and in-shoe plantar pressure values.

2.4 Procedures

Before data collection, all relevant procedures were explained to the participants, which were also asked to sign the consent form. As predicted in the CRF, sociodemographic data (e.g. age, gender, education) was collected along with clinical data (mental *status*, physical impairment, smoking or alcohol habits, height, weight and body mass index, prior history of ulceration, amputation, Charcot foot, angioplasty or vascular surgery), considering important predictive risk factors for diabetic foot ulceration [16].

For the platform-based system used, participants were instructed to walk barefoot over a 3.6 m foam runway, with the EMED platform located in the middle. Participants were instructed to walk at their normal speed, and a minimum of three steps were taken per foot. For the insole-based system, the PEDAR insoles were fitted to each participant that wore their usual footwear. Participants wore a waist belt which contained a wireless telemetry unit for Bluetooth and a battery, and a zero-calibration was performed by unloading each measurement insole while inserted. Participants were instructed to walk a distance of approximately 10 m, before turning and returning to the initial start point, ensuring the collection of at least 20 midgait steps for each participant. For both systems, an initial familiarization time was allowed, where participants walked freely to simulate data collection.

2.5 Data Analysis

To analyze the pressure values, the PEDAR-X® software (Novel Electronics, St. Paul, MN, USA) was used. The first and the last footstep of each walking trial was removed automatically by the software to avoid acceleration and deceleration effects. Additionally, footsteps showing sensor errors or major deviances were removed manually, ensuring that 6 steps were selected for barefoot (3 in each foot) and 10 steps were selected for in-shoe (5 in each foot). Statistical analysis of the collected data was performed using the Statistical Package for Social Sciences (SPSS, IBM 24.0). Means, standard deviations, frequencies, and percentages were used as descriptive statistics.

2.6 Ethics

The overall research project was reviewed and approved by the Ethics Committee of the Health Sciences Research Unit: Nursing (UICISA:E) of the Nursing School of Coimbra (ESEnfC; Number P631/10-2019) and by the Ethics Committee of the Health Regional Administration (ACeS; Number 70/2020).

The eligible participants received written and oral information about the study and written informed consent was requested. Participants were assigned an ID number, which was used in all data collection instruments. All the documentation related to the study was saved in locked cabinets only accessible by the study members. In the same way, the data collected by plantar pressure were obtained and saved in a project computer only accessible by research team members. All collected data was exclusively used for this study, and confidentiality of participants was always ensured.

3 Results

3.1 Sample Characterization

Of the 58 participants, 63.6% ($n = 37$) were male, and ages ranged between 28 and 84 years old (M = 65.62; SD = 11.631). Regarding education, 44.83% ($n = 26$) participants completed the first cycle of basic education. With respect to current employment status, 55.2% ($n = 32$) were retired. Most of the participants (48.2%; $n = 27$) had a middle socioeconomically level (Table 1).

Table 2 presents some important clinical characterization for the participants. Only 3.45% of the participants ($n = 2$) were within normal parameters for BMI. All the participants presented a DM diagnostic, mainly type 2 (57.00%). The most prolonged diagnostic history with DM was 52 years (M = 12.18; SD = 11.837).

Table 1. Sociodemographic characterization of the sample (N = 58)

		N	%	M	SD	Min.-Max
Sex	Male	37	63.80			
	Female	21	36.20			
	Total	58	100%			
Age (years)				65.62	11.631	28.00 – 84.00
Education	4 years	26	44.83			
	6 years	6	10.34			
	9 years	11	18.97			
	12 years	9	15.52			
	University (>12 years)	6	10.34			
	Total	58	100%			
Occupation	Active	24	41.40			
	Unemployed	2	3.40			
	Retired	32	55.20			
	Total	58	100%			
Socioeconomic level	High	6	10.30			
	Middle-high	12	20.70			
	Middle	27	46.60			
	Low-middle	11	19.00			
	Missings	2	3.40			
	Total	58	100%			

M: mean; SD: standard deviation; Min: minimum; Max: maximum.

3.2 Plantar Pressure

Pressure peak average values are presented in Table 3, for barefoot plantar pressure in both right (M = 561.94; SD = 241.678) and left foot (M = 601.94; SD = 256.507). Considering both feet, only 25 participants (48.08%) had a plantar pressure peak average below 500 kPa.

Table 4 presents the pressure peak average values (M = 254.27; SD = 99.733 for right foot; M = 254.84; SD = 104.926 for left foot) and maximum pressure (M = 297.58; SD = 98.688 for right foot; M = 315.50; SD = 130.616 for left foot) for in-shoe plantar pressure in both right and left foot. Considering the maximum plantar pressure value on both right and left foot, only 5 participants (16.10%) had values under 200 kPa. When considering the plantar pressure peak average, a few participants had values below the 200 kPa: 10 participants considering the right foot (32.26%) and 9 in the left foot (29.03%).

Table 2. Clinical characterization of the sample (N = 58)

		N	%	M	SD	Min.-Max
Body Mass Index (BMI)	Normal Obesity Moderate obesity Severe obesity Morbid obesity	2 29 14 9 4	3.45 50.00 24.14 15.52 6.89			
	Total	58	100%			
Weight (kg)				83.53	10.943	63.00–109.00
Height (cm)				163.31	8.564	143.00–182.00
Type of DM	Type 1 Type 2	1 57	1.70 98.30			
	Total	58	100%			
Diagnosis time of DM				12.18	11.837	0.00–52.00
Diabetic foot consultation	Yes No	32 21	60.40 39.60			
	Missings	5				
	Total	53	100%			

M: mean; SD: standard deviation; Min: minimum; Max: maximum.

Table 3. EMED maximum pressure peak data (N = 52)

		Pressure peak average			
		Right foot		*Left foot*	
		N	%	N	%
Pressure peak (KPa)	<200	2	3.80	0	0
	≥200 < 300	2	3.80	2	2.80
	≥300 < 400	13	25.00	10	19.30
	≥400 < 500	8	15.5	13	25.00
	≥500 < 600	5	9.60	7	13.50
	≥600 < 700	9	17.40	5	9.60
	≥700 < 800	5	9.60	3	5.80
	≥800 < 900	4	7.70	3	5.80
	≥900 < 1000	0	0	5	9.60
	≥1000 < 1100	2	3.80	1	1.90
	≥1100 < 1200	1	1.90	1	1.90
	≥1200	1	1.90	2	3.80
Total		52	100	52	100
	M (SD) **Min - Max**	561.94 (241.678) 135.92–1200.00		601.94 (256.507) 215.00–1250.00	

KPa: kilopascal; SD: Standard deviation; Min: minimum; Max: maximum.

Table 4. PEDAR maximum pressure peak data (N = 31)

		Maximum pressure				Pressure peak average			
		Right foot		*Left foot*		*Right foot*		*Left foot*	
		N	%	N	%	N	%	N	%
Pressure peak (KPa)	<100	0	0	0	0	2	6.50	1	3.20
	≥100 < 200	5	16.10	5	16.10	8	25.80	8	25.80
	≥200 < 300	13	42.00	12	38.70	12	38.70	13	42.00
	≥300 < 400	8	25.80	9	29.00	6	19.30	7	22.60
	≥400 < 500	4	12.90	2	6.50	3	9.70	1	3.20
	≥500 < 600	1	3.20	1	3.20	0	0	0	0
	≥600	0	0	2	6.50	0	0	1	3.20
Total		31	100	31	100	31	100	31	100
	M (SD) Min - Max	297.58 (98.688) 112.50–502.50		315.50 (130.616) 152.50–670.50		254.27 (99.733) 85–452		254.84 (104.926) 75–612.5	

KPa: kilopascal; SD: Standard deviation; Min: minimum; Max: maximum.

4 Discussion

The '*Science DiabetICC Footwear*' project proposes the development of a new typology of therapeutic footwear for the clinical condition of the diabetic foot, which includes a removable insole with sensors for monitoring pressure, temperature, and humidity. This study is developed in the context of an initial stage of the project, and intended to characterize the in-shoe and barefoot plantar pressure values of participants with DM. So, for the plantar pressure assessment, it was used both EMED (barefoot) and PEDAR (in-shoe) systems from Novel (Munich, Germany).

As stated before, the analysis of the plantar pressure data included 6 steps for barefoot (3 in each foot; EMED) and 10 steps for in-shoe (5 in each foot; PEDAR). In fact, according to Kernozek, Lamott and Dancisak (1996) [23], to obtain a reliability coefficient better than 0.7 in in-shoe plantar pressure assessments, data from 2 steps is enough. With 10 steps, the reliability increases to 0.92, which is considered an excellent value of reliability.

Several studies intended to establish a plantar pressure threshold value to predict the risk for DFU, but this type of prediction remains problematic due to the multifactorial natures of the increased plantar pressure, such as tendon stiffness and fiber disorganization, decreased joint mobility and the degree of neuropathy [9]. Also, distinct cutoff points for plantar pressure has been pointed in scientific literature, depending on the platforms used to evaluate plantar pressure. Some authors suggest 1000 KPa as the pressure risk threshold in optical pedobarographs, recognizing, however, that this cutoff cannot be generalized to other devices. In the EMED platform, for example, plantar ulcerations often occur in areas with plantar pressure greater than 500 KPa [14], and a pressure threshold value of 200 KPa evaluated by PEDAR sensors is considered as preventing ulceration [9–13].

The mean values of barefoot plantar pressure evaluation in the EMED shows the increased values of the participants. In fact, considering both the right and left foot, only 25 participants (48.08%) had an average peak plantar pressure below the proposed threshold of 500 kPa. Similarly, the mean values of in-shoe plantar pressure evaluation in the PEDAR shows the increased values of the participants. In fact, considering the maximum plantar pressure value on both feet, only 5 participants (16.10%) had values under 200 kPa. When considering the plantar pressure peak average, a few participants had values below the proposed cutoff point of 200 kPa: 10 participants considering the right foot (32.26%) and 9 in the left foot (29.03%). This data highlights the need of monitoring the plantar pressure in diabetic persons and allows to agree with the findings of Moulaei et al. (2019) [24], which states that pressure was ranked as the most important variable to be monitored. Also, this study shows the major relevance of the therapeutic footwear for the reduction of plantar pressure and prevention of DFU [16–20].

Future studies should be performed with larger samples. In fact, an important limitation of this study was the loss of plantar pressure data in some participants, due to footwear characteristics (incompatible footwear designs with the PEDAR insoles) and time constraints. Additionally, future studies should also analyze plantar pressure data according to specific areas of the foot. Jones et al. (2020) [9] identified the hallux, heel, metatarsals and midfoot as most frequently targeted for monitoring of plantar pressure, which is in agreement with the study of Moulaei et al. (2019) [24]. In fact, Moulaei et al. (2019) concluded that the foot areas most frequently considered in the literature and identified by experts as a target for plantar pressure assessment were heel, metatarsal heads (1 to 5), hallux, 1st, 2nd and 5th metatarsal, and 1st phalange.

Also, future studies should analyze other important set of variables that have been consistently associated with the development of DFU, including age [25, 26], male gender [25], body mass index [26], smoking, hypertension [26], diabetic neuropathy, peripheral vascular disease, foot deformity, previous history of DFU or amputation [16–25], type 2 diabetes, longer duration of diabetes, diabetic retinopathy [26].

5 Conclusion

This study identified a small number of participants whose plantar pressure values were below the threshold for DFU development, thus having low risk. Despite the difficulty in the determination of a reliable plantar pressure threshold for the prediction of the risk for DFU, several studies emphasized the need of monitoring the plantar pressure in diabetic persons, as well as the importance of therapeutic footwear for the reduction of plantar pressure and prevention of DFU. It is important to follow-up of these patients from the health professionals, especially family nurses in the primary health care units. Also because of these abnormally high-pressure values, the development of innovations in the footwear industry are important to reduce and prevent DFU and related disorders, by reducing plantar pressure in critical regions of the foot, but also in monitoring important parameters such as plantar pressure, temperature and humidity.

References

1. Sarkar, S., Balhara, Y.P.S.: Diabetes mellitus and suicide. Indian J. Endocrinol. Metab. **18**(4), 468–547 (2014)
2. International Diabetes Federation. IDF Diabetes Atlas [Internet], 10th ed. (2021). www.diabetesatlas.org
3. Nehring, P., Makowski, A., Mrozikiewicz-Rakowska, B., Sobczyk-Kopcioł, A., Płoski, R., Karnafel, W.: Risk factors of diabetic foot of neuropathic origin in patients with type 2 diabetes. Endokrynol. Pol. **66**(1), 10–14 (2015). https://doi.org/10.5603/EP.2015.0003
4. Uçkay, I., Aragón-Sánchez, J., Lew, D., Lipsky, B.A.: Diabetic foot infections: what have we learned in the last 30 years? Int. J. Infect. Dis. **40**, 81–91 (2015)
5. van Netten, J., et al.: Diabetic foot Australia guideline on footwear for people with diabetes. J. Foot Ankle Res. **11**, 2 (2018). https://doi.org/10.1186/s13047-017-0244-z
6. NCD Risk Factors Collaboration: Worldwide trends in diabetes since 1980: a pooled analysis of 751 population-based studies with 4·4 million participants. Lancet, **387**, 1513–1530 (2016)
7. World Health Organization: Global Report on diabetes (2016)
8. American Diabetes Association: Consensus Development Conference on Diabetic Foot Wound Care: 7–8 April 1999, Boston, Massachusetts. American Diabetes Association. Diabetes Care, vol. 22, pp. 1354–1360 (1999)
9. Jones, P., et al.: Prediction of diabetic foot ulceration: the value of using microclimate sensor arrays. J. Diabetes Sci. Technol. **14**(1), 55–64 (2020). https://doi.org/10.1177/1932296819877194
10. Sutkowska, E., Sutkowski, K., Sokołowski, M., Franek, E., Dragan, S.: Distribution of the highest plantar pressure regions in patients with diabetes and its association with peripheral neuropathy, gender, age, and BMI: one centre study. J. Diabetes Res. **2019** (2019). https://doi.org/10.1155/2019/7395769
11. Pham, H., Armstrong, D.G., Harvey, C., Harkless, L.B., Giurini, J.M., Veves, A.: Screening techniques to identify people at high risk for diabetic foot ulceration: a prospective multicenter trial. Diabetes Care **23**, 606–611 (2000)
12. Prompers, L., et al.: High prevalence of ischaemia, infection and serious comorbidity in patients with diabetic foot disease in Europe. Baseline results from the Eurodiale study. Diabetologia **50**, 18–25 (2007). https://doi.org/10.1007/s00125-006-0491-1
13. Patry, J., Belley, R., Côté, M., Chateau-Degat, M.L.: Plantar pressures, plantar forces, and their influence on the pathogenesis of diabetic foot ulcers: a review. J. Am. Podiatr. Med. Assoc. **103**(4), 322–332 (2013). https://doi.org/10.7547/1030322
14. Cavanagh, P.R., Ulbrecht, J.S.: Clinical plantar pressure measurement in diabetes: rationale and methodology. Foot **4**(3), 123–135 (1994). https://doi.org/10.1016/0958-2592(94)90017-5
15. Chatwin, K.E., Abbott, C.A., Boulton, A.J.M., Bowling, F.L., Reeves, N.D.: The role of foot pressure measurement in the prediction and prevention of diabetic foot ulceration—A comprehensive review. Diabetes Metab. Res. Rev. **36**(4), 1–14 (2020). https://doi.org/10.1002/dmrr.3258
16. Monteiro-Soares, M., Boyko, E.J., Ribeiro, J., Ribeiro, I., Dinis-Ribeiro, M.: Predictive factors for diabetic foot ulceration: a systematic review. Diabetes Metab. Res. Rev. **28**(7), 574–600 (2012). https://doi.org/10.1002/dmrr.2319
17. Bus, S.A.: Foot structure and footwear prescription in diabetes mellitus. Diabetes Metab. Res. Rev. **24**, S90–S95 (2008)
18. Bus, S.A., et al.: Effect of custom-made footwear on foot ulcer recurrence in diabetes a multicenter randomized controlled trial. Diabetes Care **36**, 4109–4116 (2013)
19. Cavanagh, P.R., Bus, S.A.: Off-loading the diabetic foot for ulcer prevention and healing. Plast. Reconstr. Surg. **127**, 248S-256S (2011)

20. Bus, S.A., van Deursen, R.W., Armstrong, D.G., Lewis, J.E., Caravaggi, C.F., Cavanagh, P.R., International Working Group on the Diabetic Foot: Footwear and offloading interventions to prevent and heal foot ulcers and reduce plantar pressure in patients with diabetes: a systematic review. Diabetes Metab. Res. Rev. **32**(Suppl 1), 99–118 (2016). https://doi.org/10.1002/dmrr.2702
21. Lu, Y.C., Mei, Q.C., Gu, Y.D.: Plantar loading reflects ulceration risks of diabetic foot with toe deformation. BioMed Res. Int. **2015** (2015). https://doi.org/10.1155/2015/326493
22. Amaro, F.: Escala de Graffar Adaptada. In: Costa, A., et al. (eds.) (1996). Currículos funcionais. https://estudogeral.uc.pt/bitstream/10316/80863/2/Escala%20de%20Graffar%20Adaptada.pdf
23. Kernozek, T.W., Lamott, E.E., Dancisak, M.J.: Reliability of an in-shoe pressure measurement system during treadmill walking. Foot Ankle Int. **17**(4), 204–209 (1996). https://doi.org/10.1177/107110079601700404. https://doi.org/10.1080/07853890.2016.1231932
24. Moulaei, K., Malek, M., Sheikhtaheri, A.: Monitoring of external predisposing factors for diabetic foot: a literature review and physicians' perspectives. Med. J. Islam Repub. Iran **33**, 159 (2019)
25. Crawford, F., et al.: A systematic review and individual patient data meta-analysis of prognostic factors for foot ulceration in people with diabetes: the international research collaboration for the prediction of diabetic foot ulcerations (PODUS). Health Technol. Assess **19**(57), 1–210 (2015). https://doi.org/10.3310/hta19570
26. Zhang, P., Lu, J., Jing, Y., Tang, S., Zhu, D., Bi, Y.: Global epidemiology of diabetic foot ulceration: a systematic review and meta-analysis. Ann. Med. **49**(2), 106–116 (2017)

Health Interventions to Support Caregivers of Elderly People

Occupational Therapy Intervention Program for Post-COVID Users of an Elderly Care Home

Isabel Espino-Tato(✉), Sara Chimento-Díaz, Cristina Franco-Antonio, Esperanza Santano-Mogena, and Sergio Cordovilla-Guardia

University of Extremadura, Extremadura, Spain
isabelet@unex.es

Abstract. One of the significant global challenges today is the emergence of the pandemic derived from the SARS-Covid 19 virus, particularly affecting the most vulnerable population groups such as the elderly. This program aims to evaluate the changes that occur both cognitively and functionally after an occupational therapy intervention. From September to January 2021, a program was carried out with 30 users of the elderly care home in Arroyo de la Luz. Cognitive abilities were measured with the Lobo mini mental scale and the level of Independence with the Barthel index. Descriptive analyses were carried out to determine the percentages. Of the 30 people aged 74 to 95, 26.7% started with no cognitive impairment, which rose to 66.7% after the program. At the functional level, 60% started as independent and increased to 66.7% after the program. We could not find a significant association between cognitive and functional improvements and the effectiveness of the intervention program.

Keywords: Dependence · Quality of life · Covid-19 · Occupational therapy

1 Introduction

The SARS-Cov-2 virus causes the Covid-19 health crisis. It was first identified in December 2019 in Wuhan, the capital of Hubei province in the People's Republic of China [1], when a group of people came down with an unknown type of pneumonia. As a result, the World Health Organization (WHO) recognized it as a global pandemic on 11 March 2020. This situation has left more than 1.4 million dead and more than 18.1 active cases [2]. Among these data, although the methodology varies from country to country, the most vulnerable group affected by the current situation are people over 65 years of age. In Spain, more than 16,000 deaths of older people have been recorded in more than 5,000 residential homes [3], both public and private. Thus, the total number of deaths from the virus represents almost 70%. In addition to nursing homes, many older people are living alone at home for whom the government has restricted outings and any contact with other people to curb the pandemic. The experience of loneliness [4], which can be physical or emotional, accompanies many older people and has been aggravated by the pandemic. Family and friends, and neighbors play a crucial role here, being the most significant social protector they can have. One of the consequences of Covid-19 in older

J. García-Alonso and C. Fonseca (Eds.): IWoG 2021, LNBE, pp. 269–275, 2022.
https://doi.org/10.1007/978-3-030-97524-1_25

people is immobility syndrome [5]. Therefore it is vital to have an active life, to avoid lying in bed and sitting all day long. Being at home does not mean staying in pajamas. It is essential to follow daily grooming, dressing, housework, and hobbies and make an exercise plan according to their situation. Occupational therapy in geriatrics consists of a series of techniques that aim to enable older adults in their daily lives [6]. In other words, the aim is to ensure that these users can carry out daily activities as independently as possible. For all these reasons, an occupational therapy intervention program was carried out for older adults who have undergone Covid-19.

2 Material and Methods

The target population for which this program was designed was the users of the "Virgen de la Luz" Residence for the Elderly, located in a Spanish municipality in the province of Cá ceres. This residence, owned by the Regional Government of Extremadura, is managed by the Town Council of Arroyo de la Luz and subsidized by the Regional Government of Extremadura. The center's occupational therapy department selected the target group for the program because some difficulties had been perceived in the relationship with the activities of daily living of the center's users. The group is made up of 30 residents aged between 74 and 95 years old and predominantly female. All participants in the program have signed an informed consent form after approval from the center's management. The intervention program took place from September 2020 to January 2021, with five weekly sessions. The program was divided into two main parts, a block of physical content and cognitive content. The first block of physical content was carried out in two weekly sessions, one on Mondays and another on Wednesdays. We focused on joint mobility, postural hygiene, and recognition of the body schema. The second block with cognitive content was also developed in two sessions, one on Tuesdays and another on Thursdays. We focused on working on memory, comprehension, attention, and perception. Finally, Fridays, we worked on leisure and free time session to improve cognitive and functional skills.

The first week was a first contact with the residents to get to know their abilities and tastes and to approach the program to the needs that arose. Each session lasted approximately 50–60 min, depending on the activity we were doing that day. We did the physical and leisure sessions, but the cognitive sessions were divided into two groups. A pre-post design with a single intervention group was used to collect data for this activity. In addition, a retention measure was taken 20 days after the end of the program to verify whether the users had retained the information obtained. The program started in mid-September 2020 and ended in mid-January, and the retention measurement was taken in February 2021. Before the start of the program, dependent variables were collected for each resident. First, the Barthel index was used to measure the level of Independence of the users. The Barthel index [7] assesses the so-called basic activities of daily living, which are understood as the set of actions and activities that a person needs to do to maintain adequate self-care and stay active and safe. It has a maximum score of 100 points (90 in the case of wheelchair users), and each item can be scored with 0, 5, or 10 points. The 10 points are given when the subject is fully independent for the action, 5 when they need specific help or only supervision to act, and 0 when the subject is dependent on performing the activity. To measure cognitive impairment, we use the mini-mental Lobo scale [8] which is mainly used to detect and assess the progression of cognitive impairment associated with neurodegenerative diseases such as Alzheimer's disease. It is a simple structured scale, requiring no more than 5–10 min to administer. Its items explore five cognitive areas: orientation, fixation, concentration and calculation, memory, and language. The total score is 35 points, and cognitive impairment is considered present if the score is below 23 points. When analyzing a descriptive analysis, we made of the pre-and post-program measurements of the residents at both the cognitive and functional levels, and the post-program measurement was compared with the retention measurement was taken 20 days after the end of the program. To determine how the age was distributed, a box plot was used to obtain the median and interquartile range of the sample. In addition, we used frequency graphs to compare the scores obtained on both the Barthel scale and the mini-mental scale within the descriptive statistics. These will appear as grouped column graphs to see the changes in the three data collections more clearly. The sample was also divided into categories to know the status of each resident. The data were analyzed using SPSS statistics version 21 with a statistical significance of 0.05.

2.1 Inclusion Criteria

The exclusion criteria for this project were as follows:

- Users belonging to the center's day center.
- Residents who have been at the center for less than three months.

2.2 Exclusion Criteria

The exclusion criteria for this project were as follows:

- Users belonging to the centre's day centre.
- Residents who have been at the centre for less than 3 months.

3 Results

Thirty residents aged 74–85 years were included in the program. Ninety percent of the participants were women with a median age of 80 IQR [78-84], while the median for men was 89 IQR [84-92] (Fig. 1). All participants in the sample had passed the Covid-19.

3.1 Assessment of Cognitive Impairment

As we can see at the time of the pre-program data collection, the percentage of residents with mild cognitive impairment was 30% (n = 9), 43.3% (n = 13) with borderline impairment, and only 26.7% (n = 8) with no impairment. In the following graphs, we can compare how the percentages varied about the impairment of the participants (Fig. 2).

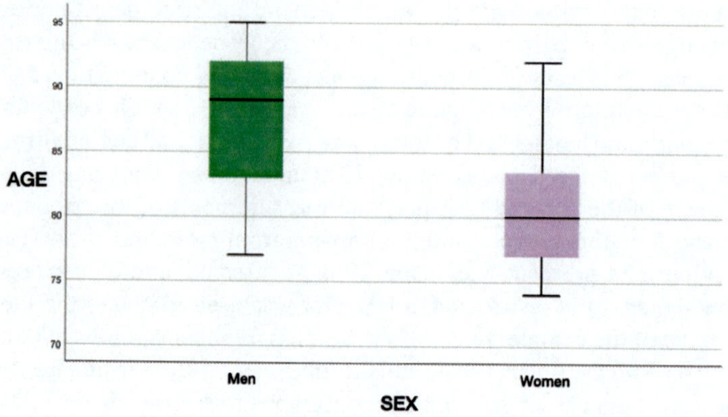

Fig. 1. Age distribution of the sample

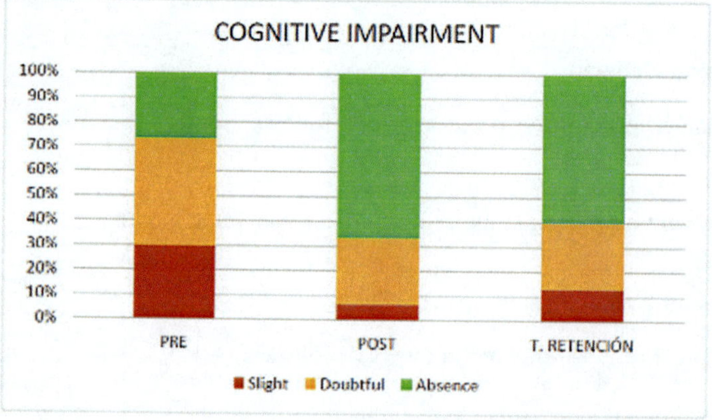

Fig. 2. Percentage of scores obtained in the Lobo Mini Mental Test

After the intervention program, 6.6% (n = 2) of the residents already had mild impairment, 26.7% (n = 8) had a borderline impairment, and 66.7% (n = 20) of the participants already had no impairment. Therefore, after visualizing these results, we found that the number of people with mild cognitive impairment decreased and those with doubtful impairment, but without doubt, the group where the difference was most apparent was in the group with absent impairment, which went from 26.7% to 66.7%. Finally, we took another measurement 20 days after the end of the program to see if the information they had received during those months had been retained. In this retention, we can see that the presence of mild cognitive impairment was 13.30% (n = 4), the presence of borderline cognitive impairment was 26.7% (n = 8), and 60% (n = 18) had no impairment as we can see the number of participants with mild cognitive impairment increased again from 6.7% to 13.3%. Participants with borderline cognitive impairment had remained the same, so the losses were from those in the absent cognitive impairment group from 66.7% to 60%.

3.2 Assessment of the Level of Independence

About the level of Independence of the residents, we can observe that in the initial data collection before the intervention program 3.3% (n = 1) were moderately dependent, 36.7% (n = 11) were mildly dependent, and 60% (n = 18) were independent. After implementing the intervention program, 3.3% of moderate dependency disappeared, the mild dependency group decreased to 33.3% (n = 10). Therefore the percentage of independent persons increased to 66.7% (n = 20). As can be seen in the graph, the data obtained (Fig. 3) at the end of the intervention program and the data obtained in the 20-day retention period show no difference. The moderate dependency group did not reappear in the last measurement, and the mild dependency group and the independent persons continued to show the exact percentages.

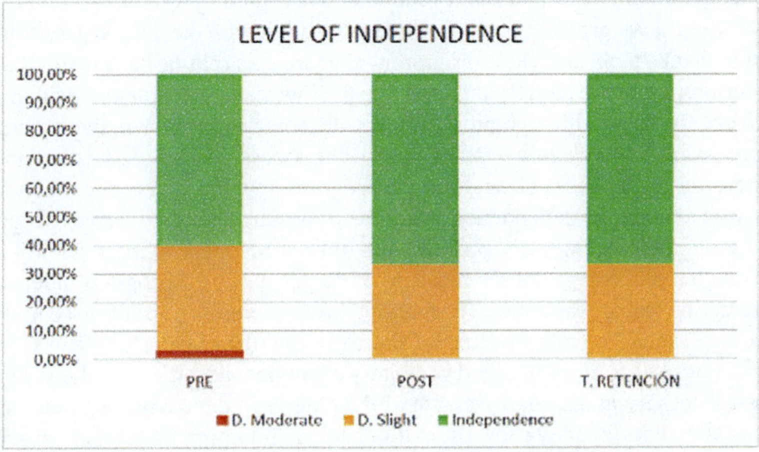

Fig. 3. Percentage of scores obtained in the Barthel Index

4 Discussion and Conclusions

The health of part of the population has been affected by the emergence of the pandemic derived from the SARS-CoV-2 virus. Which is one of the significant global challenges, not only in terms of physical health but also in terms of what we call mental health and particularly in the most vulnerable group such as the elderly [9]. Therefore, this project arose from the need to give back their physical and cognitive capacities to all these people. The main finding of this study was that the cognitive and functional improvements of the residents who participated in this project could not be associated with the efficacy of the intervention program, as we did not find statistical significance. However, based on the results obtained, although we cannot make inferences, we can observe a decrease in cognitive deterioration while the intervention program is being carried out. It is important to note that only 26.7% of the participants had no cognitive impairment at the beginning of the intervention program, which rose to 66.7% after the program was implemented. Let us compare the post-program measurement with the retention measurement was taken 20 days after the end of the program. We can see that the percentages of absent cognitive impairment had decreased by 6.7%, and it is essential to note that this percentage went directly from doubtful impairment to mild impairment. It should be noted that the literature on neurocognitive complications of the virus is limited. However, as shown in the article: "Psychosocial impact of the covid-19 pandemic on older adults with dementia and their caregivers" [10] by Moisés Schapira, patients with cognitive impairment usually present psychological and behavioral symptoms, which present as anxiety, depression, apathy. These have also been added to situations that have hurt their quality of life, such as the coronavirus. This virus has forced people with cognitive impairment to avoid continuing with their routines, being locked up most of the time in a room and without contact with their loved ones. Therefore, any stimulating activity and project that facilitates a particular routine and continuity promote the well-being of people with cognitive problems, which, if we compare it with the data we have obtained, we find that thanks to the activities programmed to create a routine have favored the cognitive deterioration of the participants. Despite the low statistical potential with a sample of 30, we observe how, although no significant differences are shown, their scores have been more positive at a cognitive level. About the assessment of the level of Independence, there are few chances throughout the program. In the initial data collection, only 3.3% showed a moderate dependence. After the program, where we carried out physical activity, among other things, disappeared and did not reappear in the retention period. We note that the percentages of the measure of the level of post-program Independence and the retention test are the same. Throughout the pandemic, one of the essential pillars has been to prevent the consequences of the isolation of our elderly. There is nothing better than physical activity to avoid sedentary lifestyles, according to the study: "virtual physical activity in the quality of life of the elderly in the covid-19 pandemic" [11, 12]. Physical activity is one of the alternatives for maintaining functional capacities in older adults. It is also one of the means that should be considered in comprehensive care programs as it has many benefits for both psychological and physical health. The practice of physical activity has been associated with a healthy lifestyle, improving health standards and quality of life. We can understand that physical exercise is an effective strategy to prevent cognitive decline by improving quality of life and mood. The present study has limitations that prevent us from extrapolating the results. Firstly, the small sample size did not allow us to make two groups to compare the data with a control group that did not do the program. On the other hand, the characterization of the sample has not been fully detailed because, although the main variables have been collected, we could have included some extraneous variables such as attendance at the physiotherapy department. The present study has significant limitations that prevent us from reaching clear conclusions. Due to the small sample size of this project, the possibility of conducting one with a larger sample size that includes a more significant number of characteristics and variables should be considered. There is no standardized definition of what an occupational therapy intervention for post-Covid older adults should be, nor how many sessions it should contain, so there is no external validity. Therefore, efforts should be made to define and compare possible approaches to this type of intervention.

Acknowledgments. This work has been partially funded by 4IE+ Project (0499-4IE-PLUS-4-E) funded by Interreg V-A Espan˜a-Portugal (POCTEP) 2014-2020.

References

1. WHO: Listings of WHO's response to COVID-19 (2020). https://www.who.int/news/item/29-06-2020-covidtimeline
2. Rogers, K.: Pandemic — Description, Preparedness, Historical Pandemics — Britannica (2020). https://www.britannica.com/science/pandemic
3. Ronkko, R., Rutherford, S., Sen, K.: WIDER Working Paper 2021/46-The impact of the COVID-19 pandemic on the poor: insights from the Hrishipara diaries. United Nations University World Inst. Dev. Econ. Res. **2021**(46), 1–36 (2021). https://doi.org/10.35188/UNU-WIDER/2021/984-6
4. PAHO: The Impact of COVID-19 on Mental, Neurological, and Substance Use Services in the Americas: Results of a Rapid Assessment. Technical report, Pan American Health Organization (2021). https://iris.paho.org/bitstream/handle/10665.2/54784/PAHONMHMHCOVID-19210018_eng.pdf?sequence=5&isAllowed=y
5. Anisa, L., Ahadi, A., Casman.: Vista de Las poblaciones vulnerables enfrentando los desaf´ıos durante la pandemia del covid-19: una revisi´on sistem´atica. Enfermerí a Globla **63**, 601–611 (2021). https://revistas.um.es/eglobal/article/view/456301/306061
6. WFOT: Occupational Therapy Response to the COVID-19 Pandemic—WFOT. Technical report, World Federation of Occupational Therapists (2020). https://wfot.org/resources/occupational-therapy-response-to-the-covid-19-pandemic
7. Cid-Ruzafa, J., Damián-Moreno, J.: Valoración De La Discapacidad Física: El Indice De Barthel. Re Esn Salud Pública **71**, 177–137 (1997)
8. Lobo, A., et al.: [Revalidation and standardization of the cognition mini-exam (first Spanish version of the Mini-Mental Status Examination) in the general geriatric population] - PubMed. Medicina Clínica **112**(20), 767–774 (1999), https://pubmed.ncbi.nlm.nih.gov/10422057/
9. Fernandez-Lasquetty Blanc, B., et al.: Clinical medicine quality of life and autonomy in patients with intermittent bladder catheterization trained by specialized nurses. J. Clin. Med **10**, 3909 (2021)
10. Schapira, M.: Psychosocial impact of the COVID-19 pandemic in demented older adults and its caregivers. Revista Argentina de Salud Pu´blica 12 (2020). http://www.scielo.org.ar/pdf/rasp/v12s1/1853-810X-rasp-12-s1-04.pdf
11. WHO: WHO guidelines on physical activity and sedentary behaviour. Technical report, World Health Organization (2020). https://www.who.int/publications/i/item/9789240015128
12. Díez Gutiérrez, E.J., Gajardo Espinoza, K.: Educar y evaluar en tiempos de Coronavirus: la situacion en España. Multidisc. J. Educ. Res. **10**(2), 102 (2020)

Nursing Interventions to Informal Caregivers of the Dependent Elderly People to Prevent Overload

Sofia Fonseca[1] and Helena Arco[2,3](✉)

[1] Centro Social e Paroquial de São Tiago, Urra, Portugal
[2] Instituto Politécnico de Portalegre, Portalegre, Portugal
helenarco@ipportalegre.pt
[3] Comprehensive Health Research Centre (CHRC), Évora, Portugal

Abstract. Objective: Caring is not always easy. In this sense we propose to identify the most appropriate nursing interventions in providing care to the Informal Caregiver of the dependent elderly people in order to prevent overload.

Method: The method used was an integrative literature review, carried out in the established databases: EBSCO Host Web - CINAHL Plus, MEDLINE and BOn, using the descriptors "caregivers", "need assessment", "burden" and "nursing", helping the search with the Boolean character "and". The integrative literature review followed the methodological procedures and arose from the following central question: What are the most appropriate Nursing interventions for the Informal Caregiver of the dependent elderly people in order to prevent overload?

Results: Fifteen articles were selected, whose results were grouped into four dimensions: definition and characterization of the informal caregiver, needs of the informal caregiver, burden of the informal caregiver and nursing interventions.

Conclusion: The importance of nursing interventions to meet the needs of informal caregivers of the dependent elderly people is evidenced and, consequently, to create security and confidence in the provision of care, reducing anxiety, preventing overload and improving quality of life.

Keywords: Informal caregiver · Needs assessment · Overload: community health nursing

1 Introduction

Aging is a global phenomenon, having social, economic and cultural repercussions. In Portugal, the sixth oldest country in the world, the elderly population plays a pivotal and significant role in the structure of Portuguese society. According to Pordata, the aging index has been increasing, with 165.1 people aged 65 and over for every 100 people under 15 years old [1]. The increase in this index is associated with a change in social roles, which may result in a decrease in social participation and also in a decline in the elderly person's functional, mental and physical capacity, which may lead to the development of diseases and disabilities [2]. This increase in comorbidities affects the

J. García-Alonso and C. Fonseca (Eds.): IWoG 2021, LNBE, pp. 276–285, 2022.
https://doi.org/10.1007/978-3-030-97524-1_26

elderly's self-care capacity, making them dependent. Dependence is a multidimensional concept and is related to a person's inability to meet basic human needs, as they are unable to adopt behaviors or perform tasks without the help of others. Dependence is not confined to aging. It can exist throughout the entire life cycle. However, the dependence of a young person, in so-called normal situations, is generally transitory, while in seniors, dependence often tends to worsen and even to be permanent. This dependence can be physical and/or psychological and is characterized by the situation the person is in, resulting from a chronic or incurable disease, disability, post-traumatic sequelae, lack of family support and who are unable to carry out life activities daily.

The activities of daily living influence all dimensions of the elderly population. The elderly's degree of dependence indicates their inability to take care of themselves in the context in which they live, allowing the definition of the types of care to be provided. It is therefore necessary to classify disability, using different scales that allow this classification. When there is functional incapacity, whether physical or mental, it becomes difficult to maintain self-care, the elderly people needing a formal or informal care provider [3, 4].

There is no uniformity in the terms informal caregiver/family caregiver; however, in this text, we understand as formal caregiver the professional who is hired and paid for this purpose, providing care at home or in institutions. In turn, informal caregivers are defined as family members, acquaintances, friends and neighbors who are not paid to provide care to the dependent elders.

Informal caregivers sometimes abdicate from working outside the home to take care of the dependent elderly people, interfering in their family and social life. In the case of the informal caregiver, this is often also sick, so they also need support. It is considered that informal caregivers are indispensable in the present, in helping the dependent elderly, with increased responsibilities in the future. However, for them to be able to play the role with quality and keep the dependent elderly person at home in order to fulfill their will, it is necessary to provide them with essential knowledge to take care of this, avoiding stress and overload and in order to reduce the inherent morbidity. Thus, it is necessary to find strategies so that informal caregivers are not forgotten when planning intervention activities in the home context.

To develop strategies for informal caregivers, we use Dorothea Orem's Self-Care Deficit Nursing Theory as a reference, in which individuals understand the capacity for self-care and where health status results from the knowledge and skills that individuals acquire. The theory dictates why people need nursing care [5].

According to the present Nursing Theory, nurses have experience for the practice they perform, having the ability to observe, reflect and reason, and should help and encourage the individual to self-care. When individuals do not have this ability, they need care to be provided by other people [5].

These caregivers can take on the role in a variety of ways, including guidance, surveillance, help, support and replacement whenever necessary. Regarding informal caregivers, it implies a change and a consequent transition to assume the new family role.

This change may cause the need to develop new skills, abilities and roles, with difficulty in adaptability. Thus, the nurse's intervention is essential, based on the needs felt by the informal caregiver, with the aim of developing appropriate nursing interventions. Consequently, overcoming these felt needs is one of the ways to prevent the informal caregiver's overload. This can also be prevented by applying the Caregiver Overload Scale.

Checking the relevance of the theme, an integrative literature review was elaborated whose main objective is to identify the most appropriate nursing interventions in providing care to the Informal Caregiver of the dependent elderly people, in order to contribute to the prevention of overload.

2 Methodology

An integrative literature review was produced as it constitutes a method of researching and making a critical diagnosis of publications cited in studies previously carried out by other authors [6].

Criteria for data collection, analysis and presentation of results were grouped, namely: a) Identification of the problem and formulation of the PICO question as a starting point; b) Designation of inclusion and exclusion criteria for studies, articles or guidelines; c) Selection of the phenomenon of interest to be extracted from the established research; d) Evaluation of the collected literature, according to the Joanna Briggs Institute® Manual [7]; e) Interpretation of results; f) Synthesis and presentation of the results obtained.

Subsequently, the research theme was reflected and discussed and the central question of this review was elaborated: What are the most appropriate Nursing interventions for the Informal Caregiver of the dependent elderly, in order to prevent overload?

Based on the central question, the search words "caregivers", "need assessment", "burden", "nursing" emerged, helping the search with the Boolean operator "and", thus combining the various established words. The referred words were selected considering the indexing bases and the MeSH and DeCS descriptors. The bibliographic research was carried out between September and October 2021, using studies in Portuguese, English and Spanish, from primary sources. The established databases were the EBSCO Host Web: CINAHL Plus, MEDLINE and BOn.

As inclusion criteria, the following were established: Informal caregivers of dependent elderly. Exclusion criteria are: Formal caregivers of dependent elderly. The exclusion was then made based on title/abstract/search criteria. The selected time interval was between 2014 and 2021, automatically excluding all articles prior to this interval and duplicate articles.

Two hundred and seven articles were identified from the bibliographical research, one hundred and seventy were excluded by the title/abstract/established research criteria and twenty were repeated, with seventeen having been selected for further reading. After reading and analysis, fifteen articles were selected in the final set for analysis.

During the preparation of the article, there was concern for ethical issues, making references and citations with respect for copyright.

3 Findings

The 17 selected articles were evaluated according to feasibility, adequacy, significance and efficacy, obtaining the level of evidence, according to the manual by Joanna Briggs Institute® [7].

Fifteen articles were selected for the acquisition of results, after performing the analysis and complete reading of them, we found that four had level 4b evidence, five

Table 1. Characteristics of selected articles

Id	Authors	Journal year	Method	Evidence level (JBI)	Recommendation Grade (JBI)
A [8]	Horseman *et al.*	BJCN (2019)	Qualitative Research	4b	A
B [9]	Becqué *et al.*	IJNS (2019)	Systematic Reviews	4a	A
C [10]	Cianfrocca *et al.*	ANR (2018)	Randomized Controlled Trial	1b	A
D [11]	Verbakel *et al.*	JESP (2014)	Analytical Cross Sectional Study	4b	A
E [12]	Rha *et al.*	EJON (2015)	Analytical Cross Sectional Study	4b	A
F [13]	Anker-Hansen *et al.*	JCN (2017)	Systematic Reviews	4a	A
G [14]	Melo *et al.*	RER (2014)	Systematic Reviews	4a	A
H [15]	Toye *et al.*	IJNS (2016)	Randomized Controlled Trial	1b	A
I [16]	Silva *et al.*	RBGG (2014)	Systematic Reviews	4a	A
J [17]	Hernández *et al.*	RC (2014)	Systematic Reviews	4a	A
L [18]	Martínez *et al.*	RC (2016)	Quasi-Experimental Study	2c	A
M [19]	Pino-Casado *et al.*	PLOS ONE (2019)	Systematic Reviews with Meta-Analysis	1a	A
N [20]	Bernal *et al.*	RC (2017)	Randomized Controlled Trial	1b	A
O [21]	Becqué *et al.*, 2020	JAN (2020)	Randomized Controlled Trial	1b	A
P [22]	Broekema *et al.*, 2020	SJCS (2020)	Qualitative Research	4b	A

with level 4a evidence, one with level 2c evidence, four with evidence level 1b and one with level 1a evidence.

Then, the respective Joanna Briggs Institute© checklist was applied, and articles that obtained a score higher than 75% of positive responses were accepted in the assessment of methodological quality. This assessment was carried out by the authors.

Subsequently, the articles were evaluated according to the degree of recommendation (Table 1).

After determining the levels of evidence and their methodological analysis, the results were extracted. After analyzing the content of the articles, reducing the data, grouping and categorizing, we identified four categories: definition and characterization of the informal caregiver (E, G, H, I, J, L, N, O, P), caregiver needs informal (A, C, F, G, I, J, L), informal caregiver burden (D, E, G, I, J, L, M, O, P) and nursing interventions (B, C, E, G, H, I, J, L, N, O, P).

4 Discussion

4.1 Definition of Informal Caregiver

Informal caregivers are understood as family members, acquaintances, friends and neighbors who are not paid to provide care for the dependent elderly people. For society, providing care is understood as a basic function of the family and the informal caregiver is responsible for the prevention and treatment of disease or disability and for organizing care [17, 18, 21]. This is responsible for the physical and mental care of the dependent elderly and for maintaining their autonomy, independence, integration and social and family participation [17].

The informal caregiver is mostly characterized by women, single, domestic or unemployed [14–18, 20]. They assume this role out of obligation, cultural reasons or gratitude. There are also informal caregivers who abdicate (due to incompatibility) from working outside the home to take care of the dependent elderly person. Associated with the provision of care, there is the daily domestic organization, the management of the family economy and daily routines [17], interfering in their family and social life.

Taking on a new role, namely the role of family caregiver, implies a transition that is a complex process and that can lead to the need to develop new skills and abilities [14, 22]. This transition is often assumed with little knowledge in the health area, without remuneration, with limited resources and with the need to make sometimes complicated decisions [12-18, 22].

Informal caregivers are sometimes sick themselves. They often have associated pathologies, predominantly arterial hypertension and other cardiovascular problems. They also have diabetes mellitus, gastritis, bronchitis, depression and musculoskeletal disorders [16–18].

Informal caregivers have several needs, the main one being the acquisition of knowledge. These must be the object of intervention by the nurse, through appropriate nursing interventions, with the objective of obtaining health gains [14, 21]. Better preparing caregivers to support the role of caregiver is essential for the success of caring for a population [15]. Thus, it is necessary to find strategies so that informal caregivers are not forgotten when planning intervention activities in the home context.

It is considered that informal caregivers are fundamental and indispensable in the present, in helping the dependent seniors, with increased responsibilities in the future.

4.2 Informal Caregivers' Needs

The care provided by informal caregivers is essential for the comfort and tranquility of the dependent elderly people. Thus, it is crucial that the intervention plan drawn up by health professionals aims to provide care to dependent elders, without forgetting informal caregivers. These must be informed and clarified about their main needs, so that the care provided is the most correct and preventive. Low health literacy can be associated with many problems, such as practice based on cultural knowledge, inappropriate self-management, inappropriate use of health services and mortality [10, 16].

Data collection through the identification of felt needs is the first step towards a nursing diagnosis and its subsequent interventions can collaborate in the transition process to the new role. One of the options to carry out effective data collection is through the application of the Carer Support Needs Assessment Tool (CSNAT), a tool that allows for a comprehensive assessment of the needs of the informal caregiver [8].

According to the literature, the main needs felt by informal caregivers are in the domain of information [13, 14, 18] namely on the mobilization and transfer of dependent people and their body mechanics. The communication and management of emotions, general care and medication management are also mentioned needs [13, 18]. Better access to health services, namely bureaucratic aspects, architectural barriers, reduced human resources, the lack of protocols for their articulation, are other needs [14]. Providing informal caregivers with specific knowledge is very important to take better care of the family member, but also of oneself, enabling them to make the best decisions and improve the quality of life for both of them [10].

These felt needs can generate an overload for the informal caregiver, if they are not addressed. Through the development of individual strategies such as effective communication, emotional, physical and economic support and empowerment to make decisions and plan for the future [10, 18], the informal caregiver can prevent overload, increase self-esteem, improve the integration of role care of the caregiver and, consequently, maintain a healthy relationship between dependent elderly-informal caregiver.

There is, then, the need for support in terms of information, training, training in personal competence and skills, where the most relevant problem is in the domain of information.

4.3 Informal Caregiver Overload

The term overload is the set of consequences that occur in the continuation of care for the dependent elderly, such as the overlapping of tasks and roles, accumulation of activities, lack of knowledge about the role performed, social isolation, inappropriate housing conditions and lack of care in health system [16].

This provision of care is often physically and emotionally draining, requiring availability and energy from the informal caregiver. In adapting to the new role of informal caregiver, this person is faced with new routines, feelings of loneliness, restriction of personal freedom, which can lead to emotional, physical, economic and social instability, manifesting as an overload of care [11–18]. Emotional instability occurs through stress, anxiety, irritability and guilt, while physical instability arises through headaches, insomnia, sleep disturbances and musculoskeletal pain. Regarding economic instability, this is evident through the loss of income source due to lack of employability or inflexibility of working hours due to dedication to the dependent elderly. Social instability occurs due to isolation, loneliness and lack of time for oneself.

When installed, this burden can be reduced through nursing interventions, such as the identification of the caregiver role, self-care, strategies for providing quality care, conflict management and communication [18–22]. Its application reduces depression and anxiety and increases the well-being of informal caregivers.

Knowledge about the degree of burden is important and demonstrates the informal caregiver's relationship with their quality of life. The level of burden can be assessed using the Caregiver Burden Scale, translated and adapted to Portuguese by Sequeira [2] from Zarit's Burden Interview Scale. It is a scale consisting of 22 Likert questions that allow the assessment of the objective and subjective burden of the informal caregiver. Subjective burden is a significant risk factor for depressive symptoms and can lead to clinical depression [4]. These questions analyze social life, personal life, financial situation, emotional situation and type of relationship [12, 18]. After summing up, a total score ranging between 22 and 110 is obtained. With a score lower than 46, the informal caregiver is not burdened. With a score between 46 and 56, the informal caregiver is in Slight Overload. With a score above 56, the informal caregiver is in Intense Overload.

The applicability of the burden scale allows planning and adapting care not only to the dependent elderly, but also to informal caregivers, allowing them to establish greater training for the provision of care and, at the same time, act towards prevention of caregiver burden.

4.4 Nursing Interventions

The articles highlight the importance of nurses, as qualified health professionals who are close to people, in helping informal caregivers to play their new role and acquire skills [17–22]. Nurses and the informal caregiver experience the various processes of change and demands for providing care and adapting to the new role. It is these professionals who support and prepare the informal caregiver for the new situation in which they find themselves, propose more interventions and develop more studies with the informal caregiver-dependent elderly dyad [17].

In order to support, train and achieve gains in health, nursing interventions are essential to meet the needs of informal caregivers and, consequently, create security and confidence in the provision of care, reducing anxiety, preventing overload and improving the quality of life [17, 21].

The main nursing interventions to be developed with the informal caregiver of dependent people are based on health education in the domain of the knowledge provided. Interventions can be developed through needs assessment, practical support, effective communication, active listening, family conflict management and decision-making guidance [17–21]. Multiple interventions have greater potential to meet the greatest number of needs of informal caregivers [9].

It is pertinent that nurses understand the complexity of transmitting knowledge to the caregiver. This knowledge must be transmitted based on the best scientific evidence available, transmitted clearly and in a calm environment [14–21]. This can be transmitted in groups, through health education sessions, or through individualized teaching in home visits. Individualized education allows the informal caregiver not to develop a feeling of abandonment by the dependent elderly person for traveling with the nurse and allows the nurse to have contact with the physical and social context of the dyad. Thus, it is possible to develop a more specific intervention, considering the attitude, family, environment, culture, spirituality, economy, lifestyle and understanding capacity [10, 17]. Orem argues that, allied to these factors, it is necessary to guarantee feelings of comfort, security, a feeling of being cared for, promoting affective and cognitive development and preventing the development of states of fear, anger and anxiety [5].

Clustering these factors, interventions are directed to the true felt needs of the informal caregiver and visualized by the nurse, which makes an effective relationship between them possible. For these interventions to be effective, it is essential that the degree of functionality of home visits be increased.

The literature demonstrates, as an example, the intervention with a group of informal caregivers, led by nurses [17]. The development of skills, needs and stress management techniques are part of these interventions. After applying these group interventions, they concluded that there was a reduction in caregiver burden and emotional discomfort and an improvement in family dynamics.

It is essential that nurses, as part of a multidisciplinary team, carry out these interventions with the informal caregiver and the dependent elders, not separating them. The coordination of nurses from the different health services is essential [14, 15] in order to maintain the continuity of care provided to the dyad, through the preparation and delivery of the discharge letter.

Thus, we realize that the maintenance of the elderly population in the community often lacks the existence of an informal caregiver. If there are comorbidities and also anxiety disorders, depression, among others, a real identification of problems is needed, encompassing the physical, psychological, social and economic components, for a shared and participatory global decision-making, where care educational and systematic, meeting the preferences of the seniors and involving the family, is essential [4].

We must be attentive and mobilize resources, we also emphasize in Portugal the role of the National Network of Integrated Continued Care, namely the caregiver's rest service in the Long-term and Maintenance Units and the Continuous Care Teams Integrated in the Community, essential partners for this care that advocate centered on the person.

5 Conclusions

The informal caregiver has been the object of recent research studies. In order to make quality nursing interventions available to informal caregivers, it is necessary to identify their needs, in order to allow the dependent elderly person to remain at home.

Providing informal caregivers with knowledge is essential for successful care and to avoid stress and overload, reducing inherent morbidity. In adapting to the new role, the informal caregiver can develop emotional, physical, economic and social instability, manifesting as an overload of care. It was concluded that one of the most appropriate ways to assess the level of burden is through the application of the Caregiver Burden Scale, translated and adapted to Portuguese by Sequeira [2] from Zarit's Burden Interview Scale. This scale makes it possible to plan and adapt nurses' interventions to informal caregivers and dependent elderly people.

As this is an area in which nurses work, it is imperative that they are qualified, competent professionals who perform their function based on ethical, deontological principles and with the best scientific evidence available, with a view to providing effective interventions and obtaining gains in health.

It is essential that health professionals inform informal caregivers about their specific regulations in force, benefits, support and other services, facilitating the coordination of health services. In Portugal, it is essential to emphasize the support provided to informal caregivers in providing care, through the National Network of Continuous Integrated Care, in the responsibility of the caregiver in the Long-term and Maintenance Unit and in the Integrated Continuous Care Teams. This network makes it possible to implement a model of care delivery centered on the person and their needs and provides an indispensable service through inpatient and outpatient units.

We tried to contribute to the updating of knowledge in this area; however we are aware of the limitation that may constitute not extending the search to more databases. Therefore, it is suggested that, for future investigations, similar literature reviews be carried out, with research in other bases and including caregiver-centered strategies.

Acknowledgment. The authors are grateful for the financial support provided by the project 0499_4IE_4_PLUS_4_E – International Institute for Research and Innovation on Ageing, co-financed by the European Regional Development Fund (ERDF), under the Interreg V A Spain - Portugal (POCTEP) 2014-2020.

References

1. Pordata. Índice de Envelhecimento. Consultado em Outubro de 2021. https://www.pordata.pt/Municipios/%C3%8Dndice+de+envelhecimento-458
2. Sequeira, C.: Cuidar de Idosos com Dependência Física e Mental. Lidel, Lisboa, Portugal (2014)
3. Arco, H., Pedro, A., Pinho, L., Proença, A.: Aging and functionality of the institutionalized elderly people of Alto Alentejo: contributions to the diagnosis of the situation. In: García-Alonso, J., Fonseca, C. (eds.) Gerontechnology III: Contributions to the Third International Workshop on Gerontechnology, IWoG 2020, October 5-6, 2020, Évora, Portugal, pp. 253–261. Springer, Cham (2021). https://doi.org/10.1007/978-3-030-72567-9_24
4. Pinho, L.G., et al.: Patient-centered care for patients with depression or anxiety disorder: an integrative review. J. Pers. Med. **11**(8), 776 (2021). https://doi.org/10.3390/jpm11080776
5. Orem, D.: Nursing Concepts of Practice. (6th edição). Mosby, St.Louis (2021)
6. Grupo Anima Educação [GAE]: Manual Revisão Bibliográfica Sistemática Integrativa: a pesquisa baseada em evidências. Belo Horizonte, Brasil: Educação à Distância (2014). http://disciplinas.nucleoead.com.br/pdf/anima_tcc/gerais/manuais/manual_revisao.pdf

7. The Joanna Briggs Institute. The Joanna Briggs Institute Reviewers' Manual 2015 - Methodology for JBI Scoping Reviews. Adelaide: JBI (2015). http://joannabriggs.org/assets/docs/sumari/Reviewers-Manual_Methodologyfor-JBI-Scoping-Reviews_2015_v2.pdf
8. Horseman, Z., Milton, L., Finucane, A.: Barriers and facilitators to implementing the carer support needs assessment tool in a community palliative care setting. British J. Commun. Nurs. **24**, 284–290 (2019). https://doi.org/10.12968/bjcn.2019.24.6.284
9. Becqué, Y., Rietjens, J., Driel, A., Heide, A., Witkamp, E.: Nursing interventions to support family caregivers in end-of-life care at home: a systematic narrative review. Int. J. Nurs. Stud. **97**, 28–39 (2019). https://doi.org/10.1016/j.ijnurstu.2019.04.011
10. Cianfrocca, C., Caponnetto, V., Donati, D., Lancia, L., Tartaglini, D., Stasio, E.: The effects of a multidisciplinary education course on the burden, health literacy and needs of family caregivers. Appl. Nurs. Res. **44**, 100–106 (2018). https://doi.org/10.1016/j.apnr.2018.10.004
11. Verbakel, E.: Informal caregiving and well-being in Europe: what can ease the negative consequences for caregivers? J. Eur. Soc. Policy **24**, 424–441 (2014). https://doi.org/10.1177/0958928714543902
12. Rha, S., Park, Y., Song, S., Lee, C., Lee, J.: Caregiving burden and the quality of life of family caregivers of cancer patients: the relationship and correlates. Eur. J. Oncol. Nurs. **19**, 376–382 (2015). https://doi.org/10.1016/j.ejon.2015.01.004
13. Anker-Hansen, C., Skovdahl, K., Oxon, B., Tønnessen, S.: The third person in the room: the needs of care partners of older people in home care services—A systematic review from a person-centred perspective. J. Clin. Nurs. **27**, 1309–1326 (2017). https://doi.org/10.1111/jocn.14205
14. Melo, R., Rua, M., Santos, C.: Necessidades do cuidador familiar no cuidado à pessoa dependente: uma revisão integrativa da literatura. Revista de Enfermagem Referência. **2**, 143–151 (2014). https://doi.org/10.12707/RIV14003
15. Toye, C., et al.: Outcomes for family caregivers from inclusion in the further enabling care at home program when older people are discharged home from hospital: a single blind randomised controlled trial. Int. J. Nurs. Stud. **64**, 32–41 (2016). https://doi.org/10.1016/j.ijnurstu.2016.09.012
16. Silva, R., Santana, R.: Diagnóstico de enfermagem "tensão do papel de cuidador": revisão integrativa. Revista Brasileira Geriatria e Gerontologia **17**, 887–896 (2014). https://doi.org/10.1590/1809-9823.2014.13069
17. Hernández, N., Moreno, C., Barragán, J.: Necesidades de cuidado de la díada cuidador-persona: expectativa de cambio en intervenciones de enfermeira. Revista CUIDARTE. **5**, 748–756 (2014). https://doi.org/10.15649/cuidarte.v5i2.87
18. Martínez, R.; Cardona, E., Gómez-Ortega, O.: Intervenciones de enfermería para disminuir la sobrecarga en cuidadores: un estudio piloto. Revista Cuidarte. **7**, 1171–1184 (2016). https://doi.org/10.15649/cuidarte.v7i1.25
19. Pino-Casado, R., Cardosa, M., López-Martínez, C., Orgeta, V.: The association between subjective caregiver burden and depressive symptoms in carers of older relatives: a systematic review and meta-analysis. PLoS ONE **14**, 1–16 (2019). https://doi.org/10.1371/journal.pone.0217648
20. Bernal, N., Becerra, J., Mojica, C.: Intervención de enfermería para el bienestar de cuidadores de personas en cuidado domiciliário. Revista CUIDARTE **9**, 2045–2058 (2017). https://doi.org/10.15649/cuidarte.v9i1.479
21. Becqué, Y., Rietjens, J., Heide, A., Witkamp, E.: The effectiveness of a nurse-led intervention to support family caregivers in end-of-life care: STUDY protocol for a cluster randomized controlled trial. J. Adv. Nurs. **76**, 1266–1272 (2020). https://doi.org/10.1111/jan.14326
22. Broekema, S., Paans, W., Roodbol, P., Luttik, M.: Nurses' application of the components of family nursing conversations in home health care: a qualitative content analysis. Scand. J. Caring Sci. **34**, 322–331 (2020). https://doi.org/10.1111/scs.12731

Empowerment of the Person with Neurological Disorders and Caregiver at Home: Gains Sensitive to the Contributions of Rehabilitation Nursing Care - Systematic Literature Review

Ana Soares[1](✉), Isabel Nunes[2], and Celso Silva[3]

[1] Beja School of Health, Beja, Portugal
20660@ulsba.min-saude.pt
[2] UCC de Odivelas, ACES Loures-Odivelas, Odivelas, Portugal
isabel.m.fonseca@arslvt.min-saude.pt
[3] North Alentejo Local Health Unit, Portalegre, Portugal

Abstract. Neurological disorders bring about disabilities associated with increased dependence for self-care, placing the person in a vulnerable position. We live in a social context in which the family, namely wives and daughters, mostly assume the role of caregiver. The Rehabilitation Nursing Specialist Nurse (RNSN) establishes a partnership with the person and the caregiver, developing and implementing Rehabilitation Nursing (RN) intervention plans to empower and maintain their functional capacity, empowering them with knowledge and skills that ensure the person's self-care satisfaction with fewer burdens on the caregiver, thus promoting the quality of life of both. **Objective:** Identify the RNSN interventions that can contribute to the empowerment of the person with neurological disorders and their caregiver in the home setting. **Methodology:** A systematic literature review (SLR) was conducted on the EBSCO host platform. The research question was formulated based on the PICO methodology. **Results:** Sensitive outcomes of RN care for the person with neurological disorders and caregiver are identified, in the sense of improved self-care. **Conclusions:** The importance of RN care at home is justified, focused on empowering the caregiver and promoting health literacy, bringing benefits to both the person with neurological disorders and the caregiver, promoting the improvement of functional capacity and self-care, particularly in reducing the occurrence of adverse events and complications at home after hospital discharge, both for the person and the caregiver.

Keywords: Rehabilitation nursing · Training · Informal caregiver · Self-care · Home care

1 Introduction

We live in a social context in which many people with neurological disorders are in the care of their families. "It is estimated (by default) that about 110,000 families integrate a dependent person in self-care and of these, 50,000 integrate a "bedridden" dependent

J. García-Alonso and C. Fonseca (Eds.): IWoG 2021, LNBE, pp. 286–295, 2022.
https://doi.org/10.1007/978-3-030-97524-1_27

person. These data justify the need for growth in the scope of the National Continuous Integrated Care Network (NCICN), as a way to meet existing needs [1]. The reform of the National Health Service (NHS), more specifically of primary health care, gave rise to the creation of Community Care Units (CCU) that have their intervention focused on health gains, at home, of the most vulnerable people and at risk of physical and functional dependence, with the need to obtain higher levels of health literacy, making this their mission, through the provision of health care, psychological and social support [2]. Alongside this reform, the RNSN's intervention has been progressively increasing with the person at home.

"Nursing is the profession which, in the area of health, aims to provide nursing care to human beings, healthy or sick, throughout the life cycle, and to the social groups in which they are integrated, in order to maintain, improve and recover health, helping them to reach their maximum functional capacity as quickly as possible" [3].

Rehabilitation is directed to the person involving him/her in a global, dynamic and continuous process throughout his/her life cycle and social context [4]. The family and/or informal caregiver are the main social support of the person, there is an urgent need to establish a partnership between the RNSN, the person and the informal caregiver, in order to involve them in the rehabilitation process, empowering them with knowledge that ensures that the person continues the process of reintegration into the community, in order to "correct, conserve, improve or recover the skills and functional abilities", as a way to achieve their life project [4]. The continuity of care and the achievement of greater health gains is achieved through a multidisciplinary family-centered approach throughout the life cycle, allowing the person to maintain their health, maximize their functional capacity in case of disease and ensuring the same access to services and opportunities as well as to be active elements in the community/society [5].

The RNSN sees its intervention in the identification of problems, early, develops and implements plans for rehabilitation nursing intervention with the population, ensuring the maintenance of their functional capacity. It acts in advance of the onset of disabilities and complications, promoting the maintenance and recovery of independence in life activities, reducing the effects of disabilities [6].

Nursing-sensitive outcomes are considered to be those that are important in the area of nursing intervention, in which evidence relates a given nursing intervention to the result obtained. They are nursing care directed to the needs of people, with direct influence on their functional status, self-care, symptom management, patient safety, patient satisfaction, psychological changes, health care utilization, and mortality [7].

The general objectives of the RNSN are to improve function, promote independence, maximize the person's satisfaction and ensure self-esteem. To this end "designs, implements and monitors differentiated rehabilitation nursing plans based on people's actual and potential problems". Through early diagnosis, it intervenes in a preventive way to guarantee the preservation of functionality levels, avoiding the appearance of complications and stimulating the development of residual functions. This way it allows "to maintain or regain independence in life activities, and to minimize the impact of installed disabilities (either by disease or accident) namely at the level of neurological, respiratory, cardiac, orthopedic functions and other disabilities. Through the use of "specific rehabilitation techniques and technologies and intervenes in the education of clients and significant persons, discharge planning, continuity of care, and reintegration of people into the family and community, thus providing them with the right to dignity and quality of life" [6].

According to the importance that has been found to reside in the caregiver's action, in the sense of providing care to the person at home who presents self-care deficit, and the proven need to involve the caregiver in the rehabilitation process and promote their empowerment in order to ensure continuity of care in the absence of the nurse, the objective of this systematic literature review (SLR) was to identify the interventions of the RNSN that can contribute to the empowerment of the person with neurological disorders and their caregiver at home.

2 Methodology

For this study, we used the Systematic Literature Review (SLR) methodology, which Fortin [8] defines as an in-depth analysis of the documentation collected on a topic that describes the results of an investigation, identifies and analyzes the empirical or theoretical models used by the authors and recognizes the advances in knowledge in a given area. In this way, it takes stock of the current knowledge on the subject studied, allowing a comparison to be made in the interpretation of the results, since it is based on scientifically accepted knowledge and establishes a guideline for the discovery of new knowledge.

After defining the subject to be studied, the research question was formulated, based on the PICO methodology, in order to guide the research to the problem under study.

According to Fortin [8], "The formulation of the question constitutes an important part of the research and determines the angle from which the problem will be considered, the type of data to be collected, as well as the analyses to be performed".

In order to describe and correlate concepts, in this case interventions sensitive to Rehabilitation Nursing care, the quantitative method was used to formulate the following question: Which Interventions (Outcomes) are sensitive to Rehabilitation Nursing care (Intervention) (Context) of the Person with Neurological Disorders (Population) and their Caregiver (Population), at the level of self-care (Comparison) at home?

In order to answer the previous question an advanced search was made on the EBSCOhost platform, during the month of March 2021, in the following databases: Academic Search Complete; Business Source Complete; CINAHL Plus with Full Text; ERIC; Library, Information Science & Technology Abstracts; MedicLatina; MEDLINE with Full Text; Psychology and Behavioral Sciences Collection; Regional Business News; SPORTDiscus with Full Text. In this search and according to the starting question, the following descriptors were used: "neurology"; "neurological assessment"; "neurological rehabilitation"; "nursing"; "nursing care"; "outcomes"; "intervention"; "education" combined with the Boolean operators "OR" and "AND".

The inclusion criteria for this search were the selection of full-text articles related to rehabilitation nursing care provided to the person and caregiver with neurological disorders at home, for a target population aged over 65 years. Duplicate articles that did not answer the original question, that did not focus on the intended target population, and that referred to hospital settings were excluded.

For the classification of the level of evidence of the selected articles, the Melnyk & Fineout-Overholt [9] classification system was used, in order to rank the evidence found as well as to ensure its reliability, eligibility and the quality of the knowledge found.

3 Presentation and Discussion of Results

Seven articles were selected from a total of 281, according to the description made through the flow chart using PRISMA recommendations, followed by the evaluation of the level of evidence based on the Melnyk & Fineout-Overholt classification system [9], which allowed us to rank the evidence found as well as ensure the reliability, eligibility and quality of the knowledge found. Each of these articles was subjected to an in-depth analysis in order to find an answer to the previously formulated starting question. With the data found in each one of them, Table 1 is a summary table organized by sensitive indicators of RE care where the interventions directed to the person and caregiver are described, from the perspective of empowerment for self-care in the home setting. This systematization of knowledge facilitates the analysis and discussion of the results in the articles and thus answers the research question.

According to the research conducted, before the elaboration of the rehabilitation nursing intervention plan, a data collection focused on personal background, behavior, functional capacity, state of consciousness and collection of information about the caregiver should be performed in order to identify factors that may condition the rehabilitation process [10]. This evaluation will allow the elaboration of an intervention plan

Table 1. Person- and caregiver-directed interventions and caregiver-sensitive indicators in rehabilitation nursing

Sensitive indicators of rehabilitation nursing care		
	Person	Caregiver
Functional Status Physical Capacity	- Assessment of physiological functions (respiratory, motor [10–12] and ADL dependence assessment) [12, 13] - Assessment of the level of ADL dependence using the Barthel Index [10, 13] - Use of FIM to assess functional capacity [10, 14] - Promoting patient functionality as well as patient participation in the rehabilitation process [13–15] - Management of emotions [14] - Assessment of depression and anxiety [11] - Home-based motor functional rehabilitation: walking, functional exercises and electrotherapy (an average of 10 sessions) [13] - Training on technical aids [12, 13] - Respiratory functional re-education: an average of 10 sessions [13]	- Integrating and empowering the caregiver in the rehabilitation process [12–16] - Using scales to assess the level of quality of life and burden of the caregiver [14] - Management of emotions [14] - Assessing the functional capacity of the caregiver [12] - Performing functional training to the caregiver, can increase their functional capacity by making them more active [13]

(continued)

Table 1. (*continued*)

Sensitive indicators of rehabilitation nursing care		
	Person	Caregiver
Safety Adverse Occurrences	- Prevention of complications secondary to the occurrence of stroke [11, 13, 14, 16] - Education about risk factors and prevention of cardiovascular disease and stroke [11, 16] - Promoting healthy lifestyles [11]: healthy eating (reducing salt and fat intake and carbohydrates), exercising regularly, quitting smoking, moderating alcohol consumption, compliance with usual therapy [16] - Providing symptom self-management [11] - Promoting a safe home environment to prevent the occurrence of adverse events such as falls [12]	- Provide guidance on the prevention of complications after the occurrence of stroke [16] and recurrent complications of immobility [13, 14] - Instruct and raise the caregiver's awareness about healthy lifestyles, in order to help the patient to better manage and control risk factors for the occurrence of stroke [16]
Empowerment for Self-Care Symptom Control Therapeutic Adherence Professional-user relationship	-Instruction of the patient for self-care in the home setting to improve functional capacity, quality of life and lower incidence of morbidity [11, 14] - Mobilization of body segments for pain relief, caused by the recurrent immobility of a stroke [13] - Optimization of pharmacological therapy [11, 16] - Monitoring and controlling blood pressure (BP) values at home as a way to reduce morbidity/mortality in stroke patients [16] - Include the patient in the decision making of his rehabilitation process [11, 13, 15] - Promote a therapeutic relationship with the patient for the success of the rehabilitation process [13] - Promote patient autonomy: a dynamic process throughout the rehabilitation process between social and individual autonomy of the stroke patient [15]	- To develop interventions to empower the caregiver of stroke patients for self-care at home (after hospital discharge) in order to reduce the caregiver's burden and improve their quality of life [14] and decrease the incidence of adverse events (related to the caregiver and the patient), such as falls [12] -Instructing the informal caregiver to promote the social autonomy (in a phase of greater dependence) and individual autonomy (in a phase of independence) of the stroke patient [15] - The specialized intervention of Rehabilitation Nursing may contribute to reducing the caregiver's fatigue and overload as well as his/her quality of life [14] - Supporting, motivating, and providing support to the caregiver in his/her role [16] - Encouraging the caregiver to provide care for the family member [14] - Involve the caregiver in the caregiving process [14, 16] - Promote a therapeutic relationship with the caregiver for the success of the rehabilitation process [13]

(*continued*)

Table 1. (*continued*)

Sensitive indicators of rehabilitation nursing care		
	Person	Caregiver
Psychological Support Cognitive Function User Satisfaction	- Developing interventions for emotion management during the rehabilitation process [14] - Cognitive stimulation [11, 13]) - Individualizing the care process for the patient in rehabilitation [13]	- Support the caregiver psychologically, in managing emotions and in family reorganization after the integration of a family member with stroke at home [14]
Health Services Utilization Human Resources	- Encouraging the patient to participate in the development of his/her own care plan [11, 13, 15] - Provision of care by the multidisciplinary team [11, 13, 16] in the home setting, focused on empowering the caregiver and patient [14, 16] and promoting continuity of care after hospital discharge in order to reduce the burden on health services [11] - Coordination of the multidisciplinary team for patient care [11] in rehabilitation at home [13, 14, 16]	- Develop interventions of empowerment for self-care to stroke patients at home, (after hospital discharge) contributing to reduce the burden on health services and the number of hospital readmissions [11, 12, 14]
Protective Factors Health Literacy	- Use of guidelines and protocols in the provision of post-stroke preventive care to patients in rehabilitation [13] - Promotion of self-governance, self-regulation and effective autonomy throughout the rehabilitation process of a stroke patient [15] - Maintenance of a favorable social context for the stroke patient's rehabilitation process (formal and informal caregivers) [14, 15] - Stroke patient follow-up in home settings, including nurses and informal caregivers, contributes to a decrease in patient morbidity and mortality [16] - Nursing care at home reduces the incidence of adverse events, after hospital discharge, in stroke patients at home [12] - Teaching about the disease and its implications [11, 16] in the rehabilitation process [13, 14] - Teaching about the use of technical aids [13] - Provision of support material, e.g. pamphlet format [16]) - Guidance on nutrition and lifestyles [11, 16]	- Include the informal caregiver in the rehabilitation process [13, 15, 16] in the prevention of complications, after the occurrence of a stroke, at home [13, 14, 16] - Provide guidance on the disease and the rehabilitation process in the home setting to promote continuity of care, improved care, improved quality of life for caregiver and patient [16], reduced levels of caregiver burden [14]

directed to the person and his/her caregiver. The studies also highlight the need to assess the patient's physiological functions, particularly at the respiratory and motor levels, as well as to identify the functional status and physical capacity of each person through the use of instruments duly validated for the population in question, in order to determine the level of dependence for self-care [10–14]. Three of the articles refer that the promotion of the person's functionality through the encouragement of his/her participation in the rehabilitation process works as a factor that promotes the success of the rehabilitation process [13–15]. The emotional support for managing emotions, both of the person and the caregiver, and for family reorganization after the integration of the stroke patient at home is another factor that contributes to the success of the rehabilitation process. The same study is convinced that rehabilitation nursing support at home, in empowering the caregiver, reduces the caregiver's burden and improves the quality of life, not only of the person but also of the caregiver [14]. In this sense, there is a need to assess the levels of anxiety and depression throughout the rehabilitation process, so that they do not become negative factors in the person's rehabilitation process after a stroke [11]. An average of ten sessions of Functional Motor Rehabilitation together with Functional Re-education of Breathing at home, based on walking, functional exercises and electrotherapy improved the patient's functionality, and when it is directed to the caregiver, he becomes more active, improving his functional capacity for self-care [13]. In five of the seven articles, the importance of integration and empowerment of the caregiver in the rehabilitation process is mentioned [12–16]. The results presented are in line with other studies [17–19].

In order to promote safety and prevent complications as well as decrease the incidence of adverse events after a stroke, the rehabilitation intervention plan should include teaching the person and caregiver about risk factors and their influence on the prevention of cardiovascular and cerebrovascular diseases [11, 16]. For the promotion of healthy lifestyles such as: healthy diet (with reduced intake of salt, fats and carbohydrates), regular physical exercise, smoking cessation, moderate consumption of alcoholic beverages, compliance with the therapeutic regimen as well as self-management of symptoms contribute to decreased morbidity and mortality [11–16]. There is a relationship between a safe home environment and a decrease in the occurrence of adverse events, such as falls, for example, through nursing rehabilitation care at home for the empowerment of the person and caregiver [12]. Immobility is pointed out as the main cause of complications in the person after the occurrence of a stroke [13, 14].

The empowerment of the person with stroke and his/her caregiver for self-care at home, encouraging and involving the caregiver and the person in the rehabilitation process, promotes the reduction of the caregiver's burden, improvement in the quality of life of both and a decrease in the incidence of morbidity [11, 14, 16]. This type of intervention decreases the incidence of adverse events such as falls [12]. Throughout the rehabilitation process, the caregiver should be instructed to promote the patient's autonomy, knowing that this is dynamic, and should encourage the person to exercise their autonomy, reinforcing the importance of instructing the caregiver to promote the social autonomy (in a phase of greater dependence) and the individual autonomy (in a phase of independence) of the stroke patient [15]. The mobilization of body segments allows for the relief of recurrent pain from immobility after a stroke, thus relieving and managing symptoms [13]. In addition to pain relief, blood pressure control should also be targeted at home after a stroke, with benefits in reducing morbidity/mortality [16]. The optimization of the pharmacological therapy at home is of utmost importance to ensure the person's adherence during the rehabilitation process, promoting the control of existing comorbidities [11]. Another aspect of central importance to the success and benefit of RN care is the relationship established between nurses and patients. This is the driving force of the whole process, and the RNSN should develop an intervention that promotes the construction of a therapeutic and inclusive relationship towards decision making with the person and caregiver during the rehabilitation process [11, 13, 15].

The use of health services and the intervention of human resources can be optimized through the implementation of interventions for empowering the caregiver for self-care of stroke patients at home, thus contributing to reduce the burden on health services and the number of readmissions to hospital [11, 12, 14]. Therefore, the intervention should be coordinated and performed by a multidisciplinary team with the person at home, focused on empowering the person and his/her caregiver, in order to promote the continuity of care after the stroke patient's discharge from hospital [11, 13, 14, 16].

The promotion of health literacy of the person and caregiver, based on the use of guidelines and protocols, has benefits in preventing the development of complications after a stroke in the person undergoing rehabilitation at home [13]. By increasing the level of knowledge of the person and respective caregiver, we favor the promotion of the capacity for self-management, self-regulation and effective autonomy of the person with stroke throughout the rehabilitation process [15]. Thus, the maintenance of a social context that promotes the rehabilitation process is ensured, guaranteed by the coordination between formal and informal caregivers, contributing to reduce the morbidity and mortality of the person [14–16, 20].

4 Conclusion

In conclusion, and in response to the starting question, the approach to the person undergoing the process of rehabilitation at home should begin with data collection using validated instruments that allow for an initial assessment of the functional capacity and level of dependence. Data collection should also focus on aspects such as: personal background, behavior, state of consciousness, physiological functions, and collection of information about the caregiver, in order to identify factors that may condition the rehabilitation process, thus the planning of interventions will be more targeted to the needs of each person and caregiver. Having an initial assessment allows identifying health gains when compared to the final assessment (after applying a rehabilitation intervention plan).

It was also identified that maintaining an intervention of emotional support throughout the rehabilitation process, to the person and respective caregiver, in order to manage emotions and facilitate family reorganization, contributes to the optimization of functional capacity for self-care, encouraging the person and the caregiver to be an active element in their rehabilitation process.

This SLR also found that the home-based RN care focused on empowering the caregiver brings benefits to both the person and the caregiver. It contributes to reducing the caregiver's burden and anxiety levels, as well as improving their functional capacity, thus promoting the improvement of the person's self-care and the quality of life of both. Prevents the occurrence of adverse events and complications in the person with neurological disorders.

Promoting health literacy, based on guidelines and protocols, for the person and caregiver in the home setting contributes to reducing adverse events and the development of complications in the person with neurological disorders through a preventive approach. Namely teaching about healthy lifestyles, blood pressure monitoring and control, teaching about symptom self-management, ensuring a safe home environment, and decreasing the burden on health services.

Immobility is considered to be the main cause for the development of complications in stroke patients, and rehabilitation nursing should have a preventive attitude towards it. This SLR concludes that the implementation of RFM sessions focused on the mobilization of body segments, gait training (to encourage walking), RFR sessions and an intervention focused on empowering the person and the caregiver for self-care are a way to promote mobility and, consequently, reduce the development of complications in people with neurological disorders. It was specified that the mobilization of body segments, in addition to maintaining mobility, promotes pain relief and the monitoring and control of BP values, as well as the adherence to pharmacological therapy after a stroke, reduces morbidity/mortality.

For the success of the person's rehabilitation at home, it is essential to create a therapeutic relationship between the nurse, the patient and the caregiver, integrating, encouraging and empowering them to participate in the decision making of their rehabilitation process.

References

1. Martins, T., Peixoto, M., Araújo, F., Machado, P.: A pessoa dependente & o cuidador informal. Enfermagem.porto (2016)
2. Ministério da Saúde: Despacho n° 10143/2009 de 16 de abril. Diário da Republica, 2ª série, n° 74, 15438–15440 (2009). https://dre.pt/application/file/a/2216123
3. Ministério da Saúde: Decreto-lei n°161/96 de 4 de setembro. Diário da República, I Série-A. N°205, 2959–2962 (1996). https://dre.pt/application/file/a/241564
4. Pestana, H.: Cuidados de Enfermagem de Reabilitação. In Marques-Vieira, C., Sousa, L. (eds.) Cuidados de Enfermagem de Reabilitação ao Longo da Vida. 1ª ed. pp. 47–56. Lusodidacta, Loures (2016)
5. Associação Portuguesa de Enfermeiros de Reabilitação: Contributos para o Plano Nacional de Saúde 2011–2016: Maximizar os ganhos em saúde da população: os Enfermeiros Especialistas em Enfermagem de Reabilitação como agentes na obtenção de ganhos em saúde (2010). https://www.aper.pt/ficheiros/documentos/aper2.pdf
6. Ordem dos Enfermeiros: Regulamento n° 392/2019 de 3 de maio: regulamento das competências especificas do enfermeiro especialista em Enfermagem de Reabilitação, 2ª série, n°85, 13565–13568 (2019). https://dre.pt/application/file/a/122216820
7. Doran, D., Pringle, D.: Patient outcomes as accountability. In: Doran, D. (ed.) Nursing Outcomes: The State of the Science 2nd ed., pp. 1–27. Jones and Bartlett, Sudbury (2011)
8. Fortin, M.: Fundamentos e Etapas do Processo de Investigação. Loures, 1.ª ed. Lusodidacta, Portugal (2009)

9. Melnyk, B., Fineout-Overholt, E.: Box 1.3: rating system for the hierarchy of evidence for intervention/treatment questions. In: Evidence-Based Practice in Nursing & Healthcare: A Guide to Best Practice. 3.ª ed., p. 11. Wolters Kluwer Health, Philadelphia (2015). https://guides.lib.umich.edu/c.php?g=282802&p=1888246
10. Eijk, M., Buijck, B., Zuidema, S., Voncken, F., Geurts, A., Koopmans, R.: Geriatric rehabilitation of stroke patients in nursing homes: a study protocol. BioMed Central Geriatrics **10**(15) (2010). https://doi.org/10.1186/1471-2318-10-15
11. Pugh, J.D., McCoy, K., Williams, A.M., Bentley, B., Monterosso, L.: Rapid evidence assessment of approaches to community neurological nursing care for people with neurological conditions post-discharge from acute care hospital. Health Soc. Care Community **27**(1), 43–54 (2019). https://doi.org/10.1111/hsc.12576
12. Mingshan, Q., Xiaojuan, W.: Current status and influencing factors of adverse events in home care for elderly disabled patients. J. Mod. Med. Health **35**(4), 494–498 (2019). https://doi.org/10.3969/j.issn.1009-5519.2019.04.004
13. López-Liria, R., Vega-Ramirez, F., Aguilar-Parra, J., Padilla-Góngora, D., Trigueros-Ramos, R., Rocamora-Pérez, P.: Evaluation of the effectiveness of a nursing/physiotherapy program in chronic patients. Int. J. Environ. Res. Public Health **16**(12), 2236 (2019). https://doi.org/10.3390/ijerph16122236
14. Day, C., et al.: Nursing home care educational intervention for family caregivers of older adults post stroke (SHARE): study protocol for a randomised. Trials **19**(96) (2018). https://doi.org/10.1186/s13063-018-2454-5
15. Proot, I., Crebolder, H., Abu-Saad, H., Meulen, R.: Autonomy in the rehabilitation of stroke patients in nursing homes. A concept analysis. Scand. J. Caring Sci.**12**(3) (1998). https://pubmed.ncbi.nlm.nih.gov/9801636/
16. Mendyk, A.M., et al.: Controlled education of patients after Stroke (CEOPS)- nurse-led multimodal and long-term interventional program involving a patient's caregiver to optimize secondary prevention of stroke: study protocol for a randomized controlled trial. Trials **19**, 1–8 (2018). https://doi.org/10.1186/s13063-018-2483-0
17. Fonseca, C., Pinho, L.G., Lopes, M.J., Marques, M.C., Garcia-Alonso, J.: The elderly nursing core set and the cognition of Portuguese older adults: a cross-sectional study. BMC Nurs. **20**(1) (2021). https://doi.org/10.1186/s12912-021-00623-1
18. Lopes, M.J., et al.: Functioning and cognition of Portuguese older adults attending in residential homes and day centers: a comparative study. Int. J. Environ. Res. Public Health. Special Issue: Ageing Health: Funct. Psychol. Perspect. **18**, 7030 (2021). https://doi.org/10.3390/ijerph18137030
19. Silva, A., et al.: Indicators sensitive to rehabilitation nursing care: a functional and technological respiratory rehabilitation program for elderly people. In: García-Alonso, J., Fonseca, C. (eds.) IWoG 2020. LNB, pp. 87–98. Springer, Cham (2021). https://doi.org/10.1007/978-3-030-72567-9_9
20. Fonseca, C., et al.: Training proposal technology for the elderly with changes in self care and for their caregiver: rehabilitation nursing care contributions. In: García-Alonso, J., Fonseca, C. (eds.) IWoG 2020. LNB, pp. 69–80. Springer, Cham (2021). https://doi.org/10.1007/978-3-030-72567-9_7

Check for updates

Contributions to Rehabilitation Nursing Care for the Elderly with Hip Fracture

Helena Teixeira[1], Magali Palma[1], Patrícia Messias[1], Pedro Dias[1], César Fonseca[2], Manuel Fernandes[2], Luís de Sousa[2], and Rogério Ferreira[3](✉)

[1] CHUA, Faro, Portugal
[2] University of Évora, Évora, Portugal
[3] Polytechnic Institute of Beja, Beja, Portugal
ferrinho.ferreira@ipbeja.pt

Abstract. Hip fracture in the elderly leads to loss of functionality, with increased dependence. The Nurse Specialist in Rehabilitation Nursing emerges as a crucial element in this rehabilitation process. Objective: To identify the contributions of rehabilitation nursing in the elderly with hip fracture submitted to surgery. Methods: A Systematic Literature Review was carried out using the PICO methodology. The electronic scientific database EBSCOHost was used and three randomized controlled studies were selected, between 2014 and 2019. Results: The contribution of rehabilitation nursing was reflected in greater autonomy, improved performance of daily life activities, improved physical function, mobility, balance, pain control, improved cognition, and a 25% reduction in falls and a 10% reduction in the death rate. Conclusions: It demonstrates the beneficial results of the intervention of the Nurse Specialist in the improvement of the quality of life to the elderly with hip fracture submitted to surgery.

Keywords: Nursing · Rehabilitation care · Hip fracture · Quality of life

1 Introduction

The aging of the Portuguese population is transversal to all the regions of the country. This phenomenon potentiates the whole society for new challenges and changes at various levels, whether social, political, economic, cultural or in the health dimension, the latter being perhaps the most worrying and with greater emphasis on the elderly population [1].

Analyzing the concept of aging, Spirduso [2] evades the simplest definition, related to the increase of physical age, but not neglecting the chronological factor, refers to this phenomenon as a "process or set of processes that occur in living organisms and that over time lead to a loss of adaptability, functional disability and, finally, death" (pp. 6).

Due to the decline in physical abilities, the drop appears as a recurring event in the elderly population and, considering the statistical data presented by the World Health Organization [4], annually about 28 to 35% of people over 65 years of age suffer falls,

J. García-Alonso and C. Fonseca (Eds.): IWoG 2021, LNBE, pp. 296–306, 2022.
https://doi.org/10.1007/978-3-030-97524-1_28

increasing this proportion to 32 to 42% in elderly people over 70 years of age. The cause of the fall is a set of factors that, individually or concomitantly, predispose the elderly person to the loss of balance. These factors [2] correspond to changes in the neuro-skeletal-muscular system, visual system, cardiovascular system, cognition, use of medication and environmental conditions.

Falls are an important cause of hospitalization and mortality in the population above 70 years of age, because they can result in injuries that cause loss of functionality and consequent loss of independence, leading to a sharp decrease in quality of life (QoL) [4]. It is important to mention that the International System of Functionality approaches a unified and standardized language that allows the description of health and its related states, constituting a valuable tool for the practice of nursing. This model is based on and defines two major concepts: functionality and disability, which are conceived in a dynamic interaction between health states and contextual factors. In this way, functionality covers all functions of the body, activities and participation. On the other hand, disability refers to the set of disabilities, limitations in these activities or restrictions of participation of the person [5].

Taking into account the concepts mentioned above, it is considered fundamental to have a differentiated intervention in order to minimize the recovery time and promote the return to the abilities prior to the injury, or, when this is not possible, to contribute to the adaptation of the person to his/her recent limitations. Functionality and disability are central elements in rehabilitation, whose ambition is not necessarily the repair of the body, but rather the well-being of the person in the singularity of his existence. Thus, the Nurse Specialist in Rehabilitation Nursing, endowed with a set of specific skills, emerges as a crucial element in the whole rehabilitation process through the promotion of autonomy and independence for self-care [5].

According to Orem [6], self-care can be defined as "(...) the practice of activities that the individual initiates and performs for their own benefit in order to maintain life, health and well-being". (pp. 174). In this sense, Couto [7] states that self-care consists in the activity performed by one's self and that leads to the satisfaction of one's individual basic needs. Self-care is then highlighted in health care by the evident increase in population aging, and the consequent prevalence of chronic diseases, and this focus of attention is a constant concern of the Nursing profession [8]. With this in mind, the elderly, together with health professionals, should aim to live independently in their usual environment for as long as possible [9].

The progressive aging of the population leads to an increase in the levels of self-care dependency, which is also evident in situations of hip fracture (HF) in the elderly population, with serious repercussions in the decrease of their quality of life. After hip fracture, there is often a lack of recovery of the previous functional level, so there is an increase in the degree of dependence on performing Activities of Daily Living (ADL) [10].

Law 156/2015, in its Article 102, establishes that:

> The nurse, in his exercise, observes the human values by which the individual and the groups to which he belongs are governed, and assumes the duty to do so: (...) c) To safeguard the rights of the elderly person, promoting their physical, psychic

and social independence and self-care, with the aim of improving their quality of life. [11].

In this sense, the rehabilitation process during the post-operative period aims at maximizing the functional state, promoting mobility and independence in the satisfaction of the ADL's, in order to guarantee an adequate reintegration both at family, professional and community levels [12].

The Regulation of Specific Competencies of the Nurse Specialist in Rehabilitation Nursing, in its Article 4, establishes that this professional.

a) It takes care of people with special needs, throughout the life cycle, in all the contexts of the practice of care; b) It enables the person with disability, limitation of activity and/or restriction of participation for reinsertion and exercise of citizenship; c) It maximizes functionality by developing the person's capabilities [13].

Thus, the rehabilitation programs implemented and evaluated by the Nurse Specialist in Rehabilitation Nursing to people who have suffered injuries, such as hip fracture, have as main goal the recovery of functional capacity of the person and promotion of their quality of life for an early reintegration and participation in society. Also according to the above mentioned regulation, this professional evaluates the user's functionality, carries out and implements intervention plans with a view to self-care, namely through motor training programs and ADL's training, with the aim of a re-adaptation to mobility limitations and consequent maximization of autonomy and quality of life [13].

The rehabilitation programs developed by nurses specialists in the area include: the performance of therapeutic exercises, based on body and posture movements, aimed at minimizing deficits; increasing strength and improving balance and range of movement. Examples of this type of exercises are gait training, bridge training, balance training, strength training, ADL training, breathing awareness, abdominal-diaphragmatic exercises, costal reeducation and cough teaching [14].

It is thus recognized that rehabilitation interventions contribute to the improvement of physical condition, increased confidence and independence in carrying out one's own daily activities, reduction of dependence on caregivers and also a reduction in hospital stays [15].

In this sense, the fall in the elderly, which often results in hip fracture, is an important and current public health problem. The increasing aging of the population leads to an increase in the absolute number of hip fractures, with several associated complications, an increase in the number of hospitalizations and a proportional socio-economic impact. Thus, the Nurses Specialists in Rehabilitation Nursing present themselves as central in the whole process of recovery of autonomy and consequent social reinsertion, so it made sense the elaboration of a Systematic Literature Review (SLR) about the contributions of rehabilitation nursing care in the elderly with hip fractures submitted to surgery. Taking into account this last point, the present work intends to demonstrate that the use of scales and instruments that evaluate the intervention of the Rehabilitation Nursing Specialist reveal results and constitute an added value for the practice of care consolidated in scientific evidence.

2 Objective

Identify the contributions of Rehabilitation Nursing care in the elderly with hip fractures submitted to surgery.

3 Research Question

What are the contributions of Rehabilitation Nursing care in the elderly with hip fractures submitted to surgery?

4 Methodology

For the search of this SLR, the search engine EBSCOHost - Research Databases was accessed through the reserved area available on the website of the Order of Nurses. The following databases were then accessed: CINAHL Complete; MEDLINE Complete; Nursing & Allied Health Collection: Comprehensive; Cochrane Central Register of Controlled Trials; Cochrane Database of Systematic Reviews; Cochrane Methodology Register; Library, Information Science & Technology Abstracts; and MedicLatina.

The search was carried out using as criteria the Boolean/phrase search mode with the word "AND", in the English language and literature published in the last 5 years (2014–2019). The researches were carried out during the month of December 2019.

MeSH was used for the choice of controlled descriptors. Due to the excessively high number of studies and unspecific results, the need arose to use uncontrolled descriptors, which are key words and correspond to terms identified in the scientific community related to the research area. Thus, the following Boolean phrase was obtained: (nursing or rehabilitation) AND ("self-care" or self-care or self- management or "self-management" or "activities of daily living" or "quality of life" or "health related quality of life" or independence or autonomy) AND ("hip fractur*" or "femural neck fractur*" or "intertrochanteric fractur*" or "subtrochanteric fractur*" or "trochanteric fractur*" or "proximal femur fractur*" or "subcapital fractur*") AND (aged or elder) AND (surgery or surgical) AND (program).

As a limiter, the option "Analyzed by experts" was selected and 13 articles were obtained. After reading the title and abstract, ten articles were excluded, thus obtaining a total of three Controlled Randomized Studies, used to perform this SLR.

Considering that specific rehabilitation nursing interventions are not clearly defined in other countries, the need arose to resort to articles that addressed rehabilitation interventions or programs adopted by other health professionals, whose intervention referred to competencies that are within the domain of the Nurse Specialist in Rehabilitation Nursing and accepted by the Portuguese Order of Nurses.

The following criteria are accepted as criteria for inclusion of studies for the elaboration of this SLR:

- Type of Participants: elderly people (aged 65 years or more) who have suffered hip fractures and have undergone surgery;

- Type of interventions: the study interventions include rehabilitation programs at hospital level, in care institutions and/or at home, to elderly people with hip fractures, submitted to surgery. The rehabilitation interventions must be integrated in a multidisciplinary team, seeking to identify the contributions arising from them.
- Type of Outcomes: the main outcomes of the studies focus on identifying the contributions of rehabilitation nursing care.
- Type of Studies: Randomized controlled studies.

After obtaining the articles, they were submitted to an evaluation according to their level of evidence and strength of recommendation according to the Joanna Briggs Institute Manual. Questionnaires belonging to JBI Critical Appraisal Checklist were also filled out (Table 1).

Table 1. Level of evidence and results of the JBI Critical Appraisal Checklist for ERC application.

Study	Evidence levels according to JBI	JBI Critical Appraisal Checklist
E1	1.c.- Randomized Controlled Study	11/13
E2	1.c.- Randomized Controlled Study	9/13
E3	1.c. - Randomized Controlled Study	8/13

Source: Elaboration propria.

E1- *"Effects of a simple home exercise program and vitamin D supplementation on health related quality of life after a hip fracture: a randomized controlled trial"* [10].
E2- *"How balance task-specific training contributes to improving physical function in older subjects undergoing rehabilitation following hip fracture: a randomized controlled trial"* [16].
E3 - *"Should we provide outreach rehabilitation to very old people living in Nursing Care Facilities after a hip fracture? A randomised controlled trial"* [17].

5 Results

For a correct interpretation of the selected articles, Table 2 was elaborated, which synthesizes the data extracted from the studies relevant to SLR, namely, the identification of the study with its authors and design, the objective and participants of the study, the interventions or phenomena of interest, the results obtained and the respective conclusions.

6 Discussion

Taking into account that the objective outlined for this SLR is to identify the contributions of Rehabilitation Nursing care in elderly people with hip fractures submitted to surgery,

Table 2. Results of the integrative literature review

Identification and study design	Objective and participants of the study	Interventions or phenomenon of interest	Results	Conclusions
E1 [10] *Randomized Controlled Study*	To evaluate the effects of the administration of Vitamin D (vit.D) and the implementation of Home Rehabilitation interventions (HR), in the relation health-quality of life in the first 12 months after HF Triemli City Hospital, Zurich, with HF between January 1, 2005 and December 31, 2007, over 65 years of age (n = 173)	The participants were submitted to two variables (presence/absence of high doses of vit.D; presence/absence of HR) In the acute phase all participants had 30 min. of rehabilitation The randomized patients for HR had 1 h of intra-hospital rehabilitation and 30 min. daily at home HR consisted of exercises of balance, strength and functional components of mobility The evaluation was performed at the beginning of the study, at 6 and 12 months after surgery, through the application of EuroQol EQ-5D-3L index value, which comprises five dimensions: mobility, self-care, usual activities, pain/discomfort and anxiety/depression	The value of the EuroQol EQ-5D-3L index worsened significantly between the pre-fracture period (0.71) and after 12 months (0.57) In the period between 6 and 12 months after HF, the group with 800UI + semHR significantly decreased the EQ-5D-3L index compared to 800UI + HR ($p = 0.046$). This difference, although less marked, was also seen when comparing the groups of 2000UI + semHR and 2000UI + HR ($p = 0.29$) Participants with HR presented a slightly higher probability of living without assistance (greater autonomy) when compared to participants without HR ($p = 0.09$) Participants with HR presented a significantly higher MMSE score ($p < 0.001$) when compared to participants without HR There was a sharp decline in the EQ-5D-3L index after HF, however, between 6 and 12 months this decline was no longer significant HR shows a 25% reduction in falls	HR and vitamin D supplementation can prevent a further decline in the health quality of life ratio after the 6th month of HF

(*continued*)

Table 2. (*continued*)

Identification and study design	Objective and participants of the study	Interventions or phenomenon of interest	Results	Conclusions
E2 [16] *Randomized Controlled Study*	Assess whether a rehabilitation program with specific balance training improves physical function and has benefits in pain control, ADL's, balance and QoL in people with HF Elderly people over 70 years of age undergoing internal fixation for HF (n = 52)	Held to the 2 groups individual sessions of 90 min, 5 times a week, for 3 weeks Control group (n = 26): open chain exercises in supine position, for increased hip and lower limb muscle strength, improved hip range of motion and thigh tissue elasticity; and gait training with Canadians for symmetrical gait pattern Experimental group (n = 26): specific exercises for balance training and gait training with Canadians for symmetrical gait pattern	On the WOMAC scale, an improvement in physical function ($p = 0.005$) and pain control ($p = 0.483$) of the experimental group was obtained relative to the control group In the Berg Balance Scale, there was an improvement of balance in the experimental group ($p = 0.419$) There was an improvement in ADL (Functional Independence Measurement, $p = 0.799$) and in quality of life also in the experimental group Significant differences were also found in the mental domains of the SF-36 scale, demonstrating the importance of the interventions studied in terms of developing emotional role and social function There was a significant difference between the groups, as individuals in the experimental group felt that the rehabilitation intervention helped them, while individuals in the control group did not feel this improvement ($p < 0.001$, given the Global Perceived Effect Scale)	A program based on specific balance training, reveals a more effective and lasting recovery of physical function, balance and ADL performance, than a program that includes general exercises, in which hip deficits were trained in separate components The perception of pain decreases in both groups, which demonstrates the positive effects of synergy between surgery and active exercises

(*continued*)

Table 2. *(continued)*

Identification and study design	Objective and participants of the study	Interventions or phenomenon of interest	Results	Conclusions
E3 [17] *Randomized Controlled Study*	Assess whether the effects of a rehabilitation program improve the quality of life and mobility Elderly people over 70 who have undergone surgery after HF. (n = 240)	Two groups were created Control group (n = 121): usual treatment; Experimental group (n = 119): geriatric, nutritional and physiotherapy evaluation. The rehabilitation exercises include mobility exercises and task specific training, muscle strengthening exercises and family follow-up, for 4 weeks	Through the NHLSD scale there was an improvement in the mobility score in the experimental group (p = 0.0055), as well as its nutritional status (p = 0.0338). After 12 months, the experimental group obtained better scores on the DEMQOL scale relative to QoL (p = 0.0051) After 4 weeks there was an 8% death rate in the experimental group and 18% in the control group	The 4-week rehabilitation program has improved mobility, nutrition and reduced mortality, compared to the control group. These improvements did not continue one year later, there was only an improvement in the quality of life

after the analysis of the three primary studies on the subject, the following discussion of results was carried out.

In studies E1, E2 and E3 there was a significant improvement in the quality of life of participants subjected to rehabilitation programs, compared to those in control groups.

A multidisciplinary intervention based on a geriatric consultation, a rehabilitation program and discharge planning benefits the elderly by promoting their quality of life during the first year after discharge [10].

The three studies under analysis also show that through a rehabilitation program there is an improvement in the capacity to perform ADL's in a more autonomous way.

This aspect is corroborated by the following statement [12]:

> Rehabilitation care is of fundamental importance in the pre and post-surgery period of the patient undergoing total hip protection surgery, allowing the timely recovery of hip functions as an integral part of the lower limb kinetic chain as well as the acquisition of the capacity to perform ADL's with autonomy and satisfactory safety (pp. 155).

Using the literature on the subject, it is clear that ADL training is an integral part of rehabilitation programs aimed at improving physical function and training for self-care [14].

Regarding the E1 study, it was identified that, through a home rehabilitation program, it was possible to obtain a 25% reduction in the number of falls, which may be related, among several factors, to the performance of mobilization, balance and muscle strengthening trainings, which contribute not only to the improvement of physical function, but also to greater autonomy.

The E2 study shows that the main beneficial results achieved are: the improvement of physical function, balance and ADL's through a specific rehabilitation program. Thus, rehabilitation interventions aimed at improving physical function, consequently lead to improved postural balance and thus prevent future falls. It is still evident that one in four patients with hip fractures dies within a year, and the survivors often report a decrease in their physical capacity as well as intense pain [19].

The perception of diminished pain, which is present in the E2 study, stands out as one of the important results to be taken into account when implementing rehabilitation programs. The studies by Heiberg, Bruun-Olsen and Bergland, recognize the importance of early initiation of this type of programs to improve pain control, quality of life and physical function [19].

The reduction of mortality from 18% in the control group to 8% in the experimental group was important evidence in the E3 study. The recognition of this fact has as a consequence the institution of early rehabilitation programs in elderly patients submitted to surgery after hip fracture. These results are in line with other studies conducted in the same field, for example, the study directed by Lahtinen [20], which examines the effects of physical and geriatric rehabilitation on institutionalized people after hip fracture. This study proved that through physical rehabilitation there is a decrease in mortality.

In addition to the positive results of Rehabilitation Nursing care in physical training, it is important to mention the benefits present at the level of mental health. Both have great weight in the perception of the quality of life, as sustains the World Health Organization, when it defines this concept as an individual perception of the position in life, in the cultural environment and values in which the person lives and relates to its objectives, expectations, norms and concerns. Quality of life is thus a broad, subjective term, which includes in a complex way the individual's physical health, psychological state, level of independence, social relations, beliefs, personal convictions and relationship with the environment. Given this definition, it is important to highlight the improvement in certain components of the mental domain, such as the emotional role and social function, contained in the E2 study and, in the E1 study, the presence of higher scores obtained through the application of the MMSE scale to participants undergoing rehabilitation programs of the study in question.

Overall, it is notorious that all the studies analyzed show the benefits of rehabilitation programs in terms of promoting self-care, improvement of physical function and consequent quality of life in elderly people with hip fractures after surgery. The results obtained after the analysis of the scientific studies approached are in line with what is described in the literature consulted and referenced throughout this SLR.

7 Conclusion

The fall in the elderly often results in hip fracture, which is seen as a worldwide health problem. The increasing ageing of the population leads to an increase in the absolute number of hip fractures, with a proportional increase in economic, social and public health burdens.

In order to perform this SLR, only Randomized Controlled Studies were used, in order to answer the central question: "What are the contributions of rehabilitation nursing care in the elderly with hip fractures submitted to surgery?". Through the evidence found in the analysis of the selected articles, it can be affirmed that the realization of rehabilitation programs that involve specific interventions, both intra-hospital and at home, clearly promotes the acquisition and improvement of independence in the self-care of the elderly submitted to surgery after hip fracture, with strong influence on their quality of life.

Thus, it is concluded that the Nurse Specialist in Rehabilitation Nursing through the adoption of certain programs, integrated in the specificity of the surgical intervention to the hip fracture and based on an evaluation directed to the needs/potentialities of each individual, promotes the following contributions: improvement of physical function, with a consequent greater autonomy in performing daily life activities; improvement of postural balance which contributes significantly to reducing the risk of fall; improvement of cognition e of certain components of the mental domain (emotional role and social function), as well as the emotional role and social function), as well as the, which results in a improving the quality of life; and lastly, reduction of mortality rates.

In light of the conclusions of the studies previously analyzed, it is possible to affirm that the Rehabilitation Nursing Specialist contributes effectively to the recovery of the functional capacity of the person being cared for and to the promotion of self-care and consequent quality of life, in order to promote their reintegration and participation in society. In turn, the conclusions reached by these studies are precisely in line with the expectations of this type of professional, and which is set out in the Regulation of Specific Competencies of the Specialist Nurse in Rehabilitation Nursing. In this document, not only are the skills of these professionals listed, but also reflect the need and their importance in promoting the health of the population.

During the course of the research for this SLR, it was found that there were no primary studies on this topic at a national level, so the need arose to extend the research to international studies, whose rehabilitation interventions would be ensured by health professionals belonging to a multidisciplinary team, but at the same time would meet the skills recognized by the Order of Nurses for the Specialist Nursing Rehabilitation in Portugal.

Therefore, it is suggested that primary studies applied to the Portuguese population on this subject be carried out. This proposal arises in order to contribute to greater scientific evidence as to the relevance of Rehabilitation Nursing care in the patient after hip fracture in the national panorama.

References

1. INE: População residente em Portugal com tendência para diminuição e envelhecimento (2004). https://www.ine.pt/ngt_server/attachfileu.jsp?look_parentBoui=218948085&att_display=n&att_download=y
2. Spirduso, W.W.: Dimensões físicas do envelhecimento. Editora Manole, Barueri (2005)
3. Organização Mundial de Saúde: Relatório global da OMS sobre prevenção de quedas na velhice (2010). http://www.saude.sp.gov.br/resources/ccd/publicacoes/publicacoes-ccd/saude-e-populacao/manual_oms_-_site.pdf
4. DGS: Programa nacional de prevenção de acidentes 2010–2016 (2010). https://www.dgs.pt/ficheiros-de-upload-3/dast-programa-nacional-de-prevencao-de-acidentes-pdf.aspx

5. Fonseca, C., et al.: Training proposal technology for the elderly with changes in self care and for their caregiver: rehabilitation nursing care contributions. In: García-Alonso, J., Fonseca, C. (eds.) IWoG 2020. LNB, pp. 69–80. Springer, Cham (2021). https://doi.org/10.1007/978-3-030-72567-9_7
6. Fernandes, S., Silva, A., Barbas, L., Ferreira, R., Fonseca, C., Fernandes, M.A.: Theoretical contributions from orem to self-care in rehabilitation nursing. In: García-Alonso, J., Fonseca, C. (eds.) IWoG 2019. CCIS, vol. 1185, pp. 163–173. Springer, Cham (2020). https://doi.org/10.1007/978-3-030-41494-8_16
7. Couto, G.: Autonomia/independência no autocuidado: sensibilidade aos cuidados de enfermagem de reabilitação. Dissertação de mestrado da Escola Superior de Enfermagem do Porto, Porto (2012)
8. Teixeira, S.M.M.: Autocuidado: contributos para um modelo de supervisão clínica em enfermagem. Dissertação de mestrado da Escola Superior de Enfermagem do Porto, Porto (2012)
9. DGS: Programa nacional para a saúde das pessoas idosas (2004). https://www.dgs.pt/documentos-e-publicacoes/programa-nacional-para-a-saude-das-pessoas-idosas-pdf1.aspx
10. Renerts, K., et al.: Effects of a simple home exercise program and vitamin D supplementation on health-related quality of life after a hip fracture: a randomized controlled trial. Qual. Life Res. **28**(5), 1377–1386 (2019). https://doi.org/10.1007/s11136-019-02100-4
11. Portugal: Lei n. 156/2015, de 16 de setembro. Diário da República, 1.ª série - N.º 181
12. Tinoco, A., et al.: Enfermagem em Ortotraumatologia. Formasau, Coimbra (2009)
13. OE: Regulamento das competências específicas do enfermeiro especialista em enfermagem de reabilitação (2010). https://www.ordemenfermeiros.pt/arquivo/legislacao/Documents/LegislacaoOE/RegulamentoCompetenciasReabilitacao_aprovadoAG20Nov2010.pdf
14. Soares, M.J., Ferreira, R., Alcobia, A., Vieira, J.V., Fonseca, C.: Rehabilitation nursing in the elderly with mobility deficit due to fracture of the femur. In: García-Alonso, J., Fonseca, C. (eds.) IWoG 2019. CCIS, vol. 1185, pp. 292–303. Springer, Cham (2020). https://doi.org/10.1007/978-3-030-41494-8_29
15. Berggren, M., et al.: Effects of geriatric interdisciplinary on complications and readmissions after hip fracture: a randomized controlled trial. Clin. Rehabil. **1**(33), 64–73 (2019)
16. Monticone, M., et al.: How balance task-specific training contributes to improving physical function in older subjects undergoing rehabilitation following hip fracture: a randomized controlled trial. Clin. Rehabil. 1–12 (2017)
17. Crotty, M., et al.: Should we provide outreach rehabilitation to very old people living in nursing care facilities after a hip fracture? A randomised controlled trial. Age Ageing **48**, 1–7 (2019). https://doi.org/10.1093/ageing/afz005
18. Shyu, Y.I.L., Liang, J., Wu, C.C., Cheng, H.S., Chen, M.C.: An interdisciplinary intervention for older Taiwanese patients after surgery for hip fracture improves health-related quality of life (2010) https://bmcmusculoskeletdisord.biomedcentral.com/articles/10.1186/1471-2474-11-225
19. Heiberg, K., Bruun-Olsen, V., Bergland, A.: The effects oh habitual functional training on physical functioning in patients after hip fracture: the protocol of the HIPFRAC study. BMC Geriatr. **17**(23), 1–8 (2017)
20. Lahtinen, A., et al.: Geriatric and physically oriented rehabilitation improves the abilityof independent living and physical rehabilitation reduces mortality: a randomised comparison of 538 patients. Clin. Rehabil. **29**, 1–15 (2014). https://doi.org/10.1177/0269215514559423

Aging and Rural Depopulation in Extremadura. Analysis of Loneliness and Access to Services and Resources

Sara Chimento-Díaz(✉), Isabel Espino-Tato, Sergio Cordovilla-Guardia, César Fonseca, and Pablo Sánchez-García

University of Extremadura, Extremadura, Spain
schimento@unex.es

Abstract. The percentage of aging people has not stopped increasing. According to the National Institute of Statistics, in 2068, 29.4% of the population will be over 64 years old. In Extremadura, in 2019, more than 50,000 aging people were living alone. We reviewed a bibliographic review on the existing resources and services in a rural area of Spain. It was base on the promotion of the autonomy of aging people. We pursued to contextualize aging and loneliness in Extremadura and observe whether the portfolio of existing services in the region meets the population needs. Once we break down the portfolio of benefits, it is worth highlighting the heterogeneity of the services offered. We evaluated at requirements of the population of Extremadura too. However, the question is, are the resources accessible to the people living in rural areas?

Keywords: Services · Aging · Covid-19 · Personal autonomy · Loneliness

1 Introduction

Extremadura has a surface area of 41,634.50 Km2 and has historically been a sparsely populated region, conditioning its population and spatial distribution and with a very low population density, 26 inhabitants per Km2 [1]. Nevertheless, the percentage of aging people has not stopped increasing in our country. In 2068 29.4% of the population will be over 64 years old [2]. If we focus on rural Spain, the data on aging is even more worrying. In Extremadura, the percentage of the population over 64 years of age is higher than nationally, as currently, 20.7% of the total population is over this age [3]. In some localities of the region, the aging index even exceeds 500 points [4]. The percentage of people over 65 years of age in Extremadura has increased by almost 2 points in the last ten years. They are rising from 19.05% to 20.89%, with a more excellent representation in the province of Cáceres. This event makes it the oldest region in the Autonomous Community, with 23.02% compared to 19.64% in Badajoz [5,6]. An important fact to note is that, in 2012, the dependency ratio decreased in both

J. García-Alonso and C. Fonseca (Eds.): IWoG 2021, LNBE, pp. 307–317, 2022.
https://doi.org/10.1007/978-3-030-97524-1_29

Extremadura and Spain compared to 2000, with 64.03% compared to 72.66%, with women being the group that generates more dependency (69.40%). However, the dependency ratio of people over 65 years of age showed a slight increase in 2012 (31.50%) compared to 2000 (30.50%) [7]. In Extremadura alone, more than 50,000 people over 65 were living alone in 2019 [8]. One of the main factors to consider with the population living alone is the presence of unwanted loneliness, the absence of a close social network, and the presence of mental disorders (M.D.). These variables act synergistic in older adults. However, loneliness is not necessarily a consequence of social isolation [9]. Death may be another of the most extreme and definitive effects. Nevertheless, it is a slow process of dissociation that distances the individual from its support network, where feeling lonely is increasingly present [10]. The population group of people over 65 is overgrowing. That has become a significant focus of action for policymakers as they increasingly recognize that social isolation and loneliness are serious concerns [11]. Early in the aging process, people may perceive family and family contact as a vital part of the quality of their lives. Moreover, when progressive loss of personal autonomy occurs, they expect their family members to make critical decisions and provide the necessary support, either by living with the same relatives or arranging for residential resources. At older ages, it is more often women who live alone [12]. In addition, women living alone in rural areas are more likely to suffer from mental health problems such as depression and anxiety [11,13]. One of the services that are gaining more weight due to the current situation is the Anglo-Saxon model known as "Aging in Place" (A.I.P). This model advocates that aging in places favors the permanence in the person's usual environment for as long as possible as long as the conditions are adequate and dignified. The development of day rehabilitation services that favor family respite reduces the risk of overload and facilitates care in community environments. On the other hand, in cases where it is not feasible to remain in the family environment, Extremadura has a portfolio of residential services to respond to the absence of family support and promote care in specialized services that reduce the risk of deterioration. Great use of public and social care services was positively associated with both living alone and the A.I.P. update [14,15]. The aging process has a significant impact on all people, progressively eroding both the physical and mental capacities of the individual. One of the consequences of the aging process is the possibility of leading to the person living in unwanted loneliness, thus diminishing the person's quality of life. We understood the quality of life as "the individual's perception of his or her position within the cultural context and value system in which he or she lives and concerning his or her goals, expectations, norms, and concerns." Therefore, if the person understands the aging process as a detriment of their physical and mental capacities, it would lower their perception of the individual. Quality of life is a concept that encompasses physical health, mental health, degree of independence, social relationships, and personal beliefs [16].

2 Material and Methods

We reviewed a bibliographic carried out on the existing resources, programs, and services in the community of Extremadura based on the promotion of the autonomy of people over 64 years of age. The objective pursued was to create an X-ray of the current situation in the Autonomous Community of Extremadura. Furthermore, we want to relate the resources and services that the Regional Government of Extremadura and public bodies such as the Extremadura Service for the Promotion of Autonomy and Care for Dependency (SEPAD) make available to the people who deserve them. We analyzed various scientific journals, and we revised the data published on the web portals of the Extremadura Service for the Promotion of Autonomy and Care for Dependency. The review took place during the months of November-December 2020.

3 Results

In Extremadura, the most significant regulatory body for services is the Extremadura Service for promoting Autonomy and Care for Dependency (SEPAD). In this case, the analysis focused on the existing services and resources for the over-64s in Extremadura. To regulate the primary conditions and guarantee equality in exercising citizens' right to promote personal autonomy and care for dependent persons. Accordingly, SEPAD approved Act 39/2006 of 14 December 2006 to promote Personal Autonomy and Care for Dependent Persons. Act 39/2006 of 14 December 2006, based on a standardized scale, recognizes three degrees of dependency, varying according to each person's situation. The degrees recognized are three: severe dependency, known as Grade III. In this case, the person would have the highest degree of dependency recognized and would therefore have access to services to prevent situations of dependency. Furthermore, to benefit the Promotion of Personal Autonomy, we can find telecare, Home Help Services, which could have access to both day and night centers and access to residential centers. Furthermore, people have the right to receive a financial benefit for care in the family environment if they so wish and a financial benefit linked to respect in the family environment. In addition, it can assure access to residential centers with public or private places. Finally, they would have access to a benefit for the Promotion of Autonomy such as Occupational Therapy services, Early Care, Cognitive Stimulation, Promotion, maintenance, and recovery of functional autonomy and psycho-social rehabilitation. The intermediate level of dependency is Grade II or severe dependency. If the person has this degree of dependency recognized, they may have access to the same resources mentioned above, except for the personal assistance benefit. Finally, Grade I dependency is the lowest level of recognized dependency. In this case, the person would have a moderate dependency and would only have access to services for the promotion of personal autonomy, teleassistance, home help service, access to day and night centers, and could benefit from the places linked to the economic benefit related to a service and the economic benefits for care in the family environment. Lastly, they could also apply for the personal assistance allowance [17].

We should be noted that cash benefits are incompatible with the services in the catalog, except for services for preventing situations of dependency, promoting personal autonomy, and telecare. Cash benefits are also incompatible with each other [18]. If we look at the portfolio of services, we can see all the resources available depending on the pathology or condition that causes the situation of dependency. According to whether they are resources aimed at the population, we can see different categorizations: elderly, people with disabilities, people with mental health problems, people with cognitive impairment, and, due to the current situation caused by the health crisis, resources for home support in the face of the Coronavirus. We can access the list of available services and resources updated every month. In this case, we will describe exclusively the resources offered for people over 65 years of age. The resources including home help companies (316), of which 131 are in the community of Cáceres, day centers (101), with more than 42 companies in the province of Cáceres, social centers for the elderly (40), 14 of which are in the northern part of Extremadura, and night centers (1) in Badajoz. Regarding residential centers (256), in the whole province of Cáceres, there are more than 140 with 4504 places. The last of the services offered by the billboard is the day residential units (167) [19]. As for the different places offered both in day/night centers and in residential centers, we find variants depending on the degree of assistance required by the person. For example, we can see: socio-healthcare places or T2, understood as health care units focused on dependent persons who require continuous health care but not curative or intensive care, i.e., they need supervision within a health care context. On the other hand, there are T3 places, in this case, for people who require residential resources for care and rehabilitation of dependency. Furthermore, finally, T4 places are known as residential places [20]. Residential centers, depending on who is the managing body, can be classified as follows: Direct Management Residences (D.M.R), which are residential centers managed directly by the SEPAD, as are the Direct Management Day Care Centers (D.M.D.C.), or private centers if a company operates the center. The confidential nature of the center does not limit access to people with a recognized degree of dependency, but as a difference is made the number of places available in the center. In addition, we can find from the Municipal Agreed Places (M.A.P). The Town council of each locality managed these places. Finally, Service-Linked Places (S.L.P) are subsidized places in Accredited Private Centers that have an agreement with SEPAD. In this way, if the person does not have a place in an D.M.R, they can access a private center. The following services are offered by the Extremadura Government, from the highest to the lowest level of assistance required by the person: the club homes for the elderly are public centers where a series of services are provided by the needs of the individual of older people, such as social, care, therapeutic and socio-cultural services. The aim is to prevent dependency, promote integration and social participation, improve quality of life, and encourage the elderly to remain in their familiar environment for extended periods [21]. In this case, the person attending the center lives independently at home and has a minimum of physical and cognitive abilities. In that case, it is necessary to meet the criteria in Article 9 of Decree 83/2000 of 4 April, which regulates the Statute of the Senior Citizen Centers of the Regional Ministry of Social Welfare in Extremadura. These criteria are being 60 years old or a pensioner and over 55 years old, having subscribed to a special agreement or receiving unemployment benefits until retirement age. In addition, not to suffer from infectious or contagious diseases or mental disorders likely to alter the everyday coexistence of the Center. Spouses or common-law partners of the above may also be admitted [21]. Only in Cáceres, there are 14 public senior citizen centers managed by SEPAD [22]. For people that are living at home, we can find home help services, too. This service can be classified as municipal, either under an agreement with SEPAD or with local councils and accredited private companies. This service is base on the actions carried out in the home of the dependent person to cover the basic needs of daily life and increase the person's autonomy, thus encouraging the person to remain at home most of the time and avoiding or delaying transfers to possible residential centers [17]. Furthermore, it constitutes the set of actions that can be carried out in the home of dependent persons to attend to their basic needs, and entities accredited for this function can provide this service. It comprises two modalities: on the one hand, services related to the care of household needs such as cleaning, washing, cooking, and others, and on the other hand, services related to the care of the person [21]. Another resource to which the dependent person could have access is day centers. These offer comprehensive care during daytime hours. The aim is to improve or maintain the best personal autonomy level and support families and carers [17]. The increase in the rate of aging of the population has become a social problem. Therefore, it deserves attention and the creation of projects capable of preventing the inevitable consequences of aging, both on a biological and mental level. Therefore, the objective is to cover the needs of people at risk of limiting their autonomy to prevent the appearance of situations of dependency. To this end, SEPAD implemented programs and services which, in a transverse manner, are oriented towards the prevention of cases of dependence, based on comprehensive care that fosters continuity of care, the promotion of healthy living conditions, and a preventive and rehabilitative nature [23]. We can talk about aging from different dimensions. One dimension that we often overlook is associated with life's social and cultural transitions, including retirement, moving to more appropriate housing, and the death of friends and partners. Therefore, it is essential to consider the loss-related events associated with old age and those that can reinforce recovery, adaptation, and psycho-social growth [24]. The image of old age has a psycho-social component related to the current stereotype, oriented towards youth, cultivation of bodily health to feel young, to look young. No one wants to grow old because it takes them away from their child and brings them closer to death; it carries a social stigma. That is why they must distance themselves from society and isolate themselves from perfect bodies because old age becomes an incurable disease. Psychology has studied the difficulty of adaptation, which can become a stressful situation [25]. This situation can trigger the patient to resort to internalization. The relationship between generations at the family and social level can fear the imbalance between the active and inactive population, thus collapsing welfare state [26]. It had estimated the prevalence among adults over 60 years of age at 11.5% in Spain, 20.1% in Poland, and 6.1% in Finland [27]. Although depressive disorders are less prevalent in older adults than in the younger population, the presence of significant depressive symptoms is familiar in the elderly [28]. Therefore, an essential factor to consider is the presence of loneliness. It is regarded as a public health problem that predicts low quality of life among older populations, understanding this loneliness as an undesirable situation [28]. Being able to age at home depends on many social indicators, such as the purchasing power of the older adult and the family. Therefore, unwanted loneliness and having a close and secure support network can act as either a protective or limiting factor.

4 Discussion

In Spain, almost 4% of single-person households are people over 65 years of age. Nevertheless, older people feel more satisfied with their lives and perceive themselves as healthier to the extent that they maintain their social relationships [29]. To this definition, it should be added that it is beginning to be understood as an emerging health problem influenced by socioeconomic and, therefore, cultural changes [30]. The presence of a situation of unwanted loneliness leads to mental pathologist that can generate a problem. For this reason, over the last few years, loneliness has had a multitude of definitions. The biomedical sciences could understand as a risk factor for both physical and mental health. It documented that the tendency to emotional isolation is a significant predictor of greater morbidity and mortality [31]. A relationship has begun to emerge between the increased demand for professional care due to increased dependency and vulnerability problems for the subgroup of people over 80 who live alone either because of isolation, loneliness or because families are unable to be present and meet the demands of the older person [32]. Above mentioned we can see in the LAPAD the recognized degree of dependency and the resources stipulated. The LAPAD assessed also refers to how the situation of dependency. Each Autonomous Community will determine the assessment teams in charge of determining the corresponding degree of dependence of the person. Based on the International Classification of Functioning, Disability, and Health (I.C.F.) made the categorization of the degree of dependency. The assessed criteria are the degree of autonomy of the person, the capacity to carry out different activities of daily living (A.D.L.). The scale will assess the person's ability to carry out A.D.L.s by themselves and the need for support and supervision for their performance by persons with intellectual disabilities or mental illness [33]. Once the portfolio of existing services and resources in the Autonomous Community can break down, the heterogeneity of the services offered is worth noting. It can seem that depending on the needs of the dependent person, one resource or another may be used. For example, are the needs of the population of Extremadura covered, is the cost of the service covered in total, are the hours granted to the person sufficient depending on the degree of dependency?

The variability of the services included in this portfolio of services has been due to the social and health demands of the population. Both the users of the resources and the families have played a fundamental role, especially in Spain. Where aging is becoming a social problem due to the exponential growth rate of this group. However, despite these resources and their accessibility, The current avalanche of demand from the population does not ensure a place will be available for the entire population requesting it. Moreover, several articles show that aging, especially in rural areas, is one of the most critical challenges. It affects the whole community and is higher than in urban areas. The rural environment has a higher proportion of people who live alone, have little knowledge of these resources, and have more difficulty accessing these services. After assessing the degree of dependency of the person, the assessment team presents them with the list of services and resources they can access depending on their situation. Depending on the degree of dependency, there are different services: The Home Help Service is a resource offered to people who live at home and need help. When we want to stipulate whether a person is eligible for this service, the frequency of the service must be taken into account. It will be assessed according to the degree of dependency of the person. For example, between 46-70 hours per month for people with recognized high dependence (Grade III), between 21-45 hours per month for people with severe dependency (Grade II), and a maximum of 20 hours per month for people with moderate dependence (Grade I) [17]. This service constitutes the set of actions carried out in the home of dependent persons to attend to their needs and increase their autonomy, making it possible to remain at home for as long as possible. It can be broken down into two parts. On the one hand, personal care referring to the performance of daily living activities and the coverage of domestic or household needs: cleaning, washing, cooking, and others. Moreover, on the other hand, services related to personal care in the performance of activities of daily living, accompaniment, psycho-social support, and the development of healthy habits [34]. Having differentiated between personal care and domestic care, it is worth relating the ratio of hours granted to the dependent person (Table 1) to the person's actual needs, often exceed the hours granted. The following resource that can be accessed is day centers. Regarding the service cost, as in the night centers, it will be 650 euros per month, not including food and transport. The agreed places have stipulated these same prices. The price for privately arranged areas may be increased by up to 25% if a higher intensity of care or attention is required [18]. People who grade III and grade II are recognized as the power of the Day Center Service will be subject to the services of the center required [17]. As for residential centers, out of a total of 4504 places offered by the more than 140 centers in the province of Cáceres, we find that there are 3454 places reserved for dependent persons, of which almost 2500 are subject to economic benefits linked to the service, i.e., they are private places. Still, despite not being directly managed by the Extremadura Government, access is facilitated using public aid [35]. At a regional level, the number of available places amounts to almost 8500. Nearly 6000 there are reserved for dependent persons.

Table 1. Relation between grants to the home help service and degree of dependence

I Grade 20 h.	
Personal Care (50%)	Home-Based Care (50%)
10 h.	10 h.
II Grade 21-45 h	
Personal Care (55%)	Home-Based Care (45%)
24.75 h	20.25 h
III Grade 46-70h	
Personal Care (75%)	Home-Based Care (25%)
52.50 h	17.50

5 Conclusions

One of the questions to be answered is whether the existing resources in Extremadura are sufficient and cover the population's needs. Even today, there are still disparities between regions in terms of average retirement pensions. For example, Extremadura and Galicia, with pensions below 1,000 euros, are higher than Murcia and Andalusia. This gap is even more marked when comparing the average benefit amounts by sex. Women's pensions are again lower than men's due to their different working careers, occupations, or other types of annuities (widowhood, single) [36]. In the first instance, a variable to consider to the hour for knows the type of services afforded is each older adult's capacity economy. In addition, it is worth noting the increase of almost 45% in the cost of maintaining the home where older people live [36]. The territory of Extremadura is mostly rural since, of more than 37,420.88 km2, agricultural activities occupy almost 54% of the land. It has some 400 municipalities, of which only four have more than 40.000 inhabitants: Mérida, Plasencia, Cáceres, and Badajoz [1]. Due to the large size of the autonomous community, it has been divided into eight health areas [7]. After studying the relationship between health areas and existing services, we observed that recourses distributed about 54.6% among the health areas belonging to Badajoz (Badajoz, Mérida, Don Benito-Villanueva de la Serena, Llerena-Zafra). However, despite having the highest percentage, the category that prevails is that of home help services, reducing the care resources' rate to less than 17%, increasing this percentage in the province of Cáceres with almost 30% of its resources oriented towards residential care. We studied the relationship between the degree of dependency of the user and the resources to which they can have access, as stipulated in the LAPAD. They set a financial item aside to cover the cost of the services required by the person, for example, residential centers. The budgets are set at between 1,100€ and 1,600€ per month as a reference for the cost of the residential service. However, they can be increased by up to 40% if this service involves a greater intensity of attention or care [18]. This is another of the problems we encounter. So much so that the speed with which the user can access the resource depends on whether the person can pay for the service themselves if they are solvent or whether the older person's relatives pay for the service, even if they are paid for it afterward [29]. From an occupational point of view, being part of a group and acquiring a role in society is an essential factor to consider in rehabilitation or social integration. Considering the positive effect that the feeling of permanence could have, we see how it justifies the existence of intergenerational projects or projects that give an essential role to those older adults whom society has already retired. Therefore, social relations can be considered as a critical variable when it comes to completing or replacing, if possible, the public care network. Studies have shown that this can reduce the need to access care resources and increase the likelihood of practicing and maintaining preventive health behaviors. Undoubtedly, the presence of a close support network, whether family or community, constitutes a social reference that assigns a greater relevance and sense of permanence to a group. It is perhaps in rural areas where we can best see the relationship between aging and loneliness. The main objective towards which social resources should be oriented is favoring relationships and improving people's social support and well-being with active aging. This service should be focused in to be a senior center accessible to the whole population. This senior center can be offered all kinds of training workshops and physical and cognitive activity regardless of their social condition.

Acknowledgments. This work has been partially funded by 4IE+ Project (0499-4IE-PLUS-4-E) funded by Interreg V-A España-Portugal (POCTEP) 2014-2020.

References

1. Porcel, M.A., Valpuesta, E.R.: Ageing in Spain: It's a challenge or social problem? Gerokomos **23**(4), 151–155 (2012). https://scielo.isciii.es/scielo.php?script=sci_arttext&pid=S1134-928X2012000400002&lng=es&nrm=iso&tlng=es. https://scielo.isciii.es/scielo.php?script=sci_abstract&pid=S1134-928X2012000400002&lng=es&nrm=iso&tlng=es
2. Abellán-García, A., Aceituno-Nieto, M.P., Ramiro-Fariñas, D., Castillo-Belmonte, A.B.: Statistics on residences: distribution of centers and residential vacancies by province. Technicall report, Informes Envejecimiento en red nº 27, Madrid (2021). http://envejecimiento.csic.es/documentos/documentos/enred-estadisticasresidencias2020.pdf
3. BOE: Law 39/2006, of December 14, 2006, on the Promotion of Personal Autonomy and Care for Dependent Persons (2006)
4. Cardona Arango, D., Peláez, E.: Population aging in the twenty-first century: opportunities, challenges and concerns. Barranquilla (Col.) **28**(2), 335–348 (2012)
5. Castellanos Pinedo, F., Cid Gala, M., Duque San Juan, P., Martín Zurdo, J., Toribio Felipe, R.: Integral plan for social and health care for cognitive impairment in Extremadura [Pidex] first part. Junta de Extremadura, junda de e edn. (2007)
6. Celeste, G.P.M.: Demographic aging and land-use planning in Extremadura. Ph.D. thesis, Universidad de Extremadura (2013)

7. Cobano-delgado, V., Llorent-bedmar, V.: Women's well-being and rural development in depopulated Spain. Int. J. Environ. Res. Public Health **17**(6) (2020). https://www.ncbi.nlm.nih.gov/pmc/articles/PMC7143739/pmc/articles/PMC7143739/pmc/articles/PMC7143739/?report=abstract
8. Cohen-Mansfield, J., Hazan, H., Lerman, Y., Shalom, V.: Correlates and predictors of loneliness in older-adults: a review of quantitative results informed by qualitative insights. Int. Psychogeriatrics, **28**(4), 557–576 (2016). https://pubmed.ncbi.nlm.nih.gov/26424033/
9. Government of Extremadura: RESOLUCIÓN de 3 de abril de 2014, de la Secretaría General, por la que se da publicidad al Convenio entre la Consejería de Salud y Política Social, el Servicio Extremeño de Promoción de la Autonomía y Atención a la Dependencia y el Ayuntamiento de Miajada (2014)
10. Government of Extremadura: ORDER of November 30, 2012 establishing the catalog of services and economic benefits of the System for Autonomy and Care for Dependency, the intensity of the services and the compatibility regime, applicable in the Community (2005)
11. Cordovilla, S.: Extremadura. Aging index by municipality (2020). https://datawrapper.dwcdn.net/17TbG/10/
12. DOE No 63: ORDER of March 24, 2010 establishing the catalog of services and economic benefits of the System for Autonomy and Care for Dependency in the Autonomous Community of Extremadura (2010)
13. Domènech-Abella, J., et al.: Loneliness and depression among older European adults: the role of perceived neighborhood built environment. Health Place **62**, 102280 (2020)
14. INE: Aging Index in Spain (2019). https://ine.es/jaxiT3/Datos.htm?t=1418
15. Fernández-Carro, C.: Ageing at home, co-residence or institutionalisation? Preferred care and residential arrangements of older adults in Spain. Ageing Soc. **36**(3), 586–612 (2016)
16. Galván, A., et al.: Extremadura Health Plan 2013-2020. Technical report (2013)
17. García, A.A., Del Pilar, M., Nieto, A., Fariñas, D.R.: Residential statistics: distribution of residential centres and places by province. Data from April 2019. Technical report (2019). http://envejecimiento.csic.es/documentos/documentos/enred-estadisticasresidencias2019.pdf
18. Giró-Miranda, J.: Aging and society: a multidisciplinary perspective. uniroja.es, La Rioja (2004)
19. Gonzalo-Plaza, N., Pérez-Melero, A.: Effects of loneliness on the health of the elderly population (2021)
20. Hassoun, H., Bermejo, J.C., Villacieros, M., Millán-Asín, M.Á., Arenas-Antúnez, A.: Relation between spiritual wellbeing, quality of life and sense of suffering in a population of eldery religious resident in Spanish centres. GeroKomao **30**(3), 124–129 (2019). http://scielo.isciii.es/pdf/geroko/v30n3/1134-928X-geroko-30-03-124.pdf
21. IMSERSO: Beneficiaries and grouping of benefits (2019). http://www.imserso.es/InterPresent2/groups/imserso/documents/binario/im_062034.pdf
22. IMSERSO: Program for the Promotion of Personal Autonomy and Care of People in a Situation of Dependence. Technical report (2019). https://www.imserso.es/InterPresent2/groups/imserso/documents/binario/iai2019_c5saad.pdf
23. IMSERSO: Grades and Levels (2020). https://www.imserso.es/InterPresent1/groups/imserso/documents/binario/im_061360.pdf
24. INE: Badajoz: Population by municipality and sex (2020). https://www.ine.es/jaxiT3/Datos.htm?t=2859

25. INE: Caceres: Population by municipality and sex (2020). https://www.ine.es/jaxiT3/Datos.htm?t=2863
26. INE: Aging Index by Autonomous Community (2020). https://www.ine.es/jaxiT3/Datos.htm?t=1452#!tabs-tabla
27. INE: Resident population by sex, age group and household status (2020). https://www.ine.es/jaxi/Datos.htm?path=/t20/p274/serie/def/p05/&file=03003.px#!tabs-tabla
28. INE: Proportion of people over a certain age by province (2020). https://www.ine.es/jaxiT3/Datos.htm?t=1488#!tabs-tabla
29. INE: Saldo vegetativo. Nacional (2020). https://www.ine.es/jaxiT3/Datos.htm?t=1416
30. Government of Extremadura: Who are we? (2017). https://saludextremadura.ses.es/sepad/quienes-somos#
31. Government of Extremadura: Services, Benefits and Programs for the Promotion of Personal Autonomy (2020). https://saludextremadura.ses.es/sepad/servicios--prestaciones-y-programas-para-la-promocion-de-la-autonomia-personal
32. Government of Extremadura: What do we mean by Autonomy Promotion? (2017). https://saludextremadura.ses.es/sepad/que-entendemos-por-promocion-de-autonomia
33. Government of Extremadura: Listado de Entidades Autorizadas y Acreditads (2020). https://saludextremadura.ses.es/sepad/detalle-contenido-estructurado?content=listado-de-entidades-autorizadas-y-acreditadas
34. Government of Extremadura: DECREE 83/2000, of April 4. Statute of the Senior Citizen Centers of the Department of Social Welfare in the Autonomous Community of Extremadura (2000). http://doe.gobex.es/pdfs/doe/2000/420o/00040093.pdf
35. Government of Extremadura: DECREE 7/2006, of January 10. Coordination Structures of the Social and Health Care and the Public Service of Social and Health Care in its modality Type Two (T2) and its Legal Regime is established (2006). http://doe.gobex.es/pdfs/doe/2006/70o/06040007.pdf
36. Government of Extremadura: Draft Decree. Regulation of Authorization, Accreditation, Inspection and Registration of Centers, Services and Care Entities for the Elderly of the Autonomous Community of Extremadura (2014)

Family Caregiver Rights and Community Resources Challenges

Fernanda Daniela Moura Silva[1], Maria de Fátima Mendes Carvalho Fernandes[1], Sónia Marisa Silva Teixeira[1], Andreia Costa[2,3](✉), and Maria Adriana Pereira Henriques[2,3]

[1] Mestranda do 11ºCurso de Mestrado em Enfermagem na Área de Especialização em Enfermagem Comunitária, Escola Superior de Enfermagem de Lisboa, Lisbon, Portugal
{fernandasilva,mariafatimafernandes, sonia.teixeira}@campus.esel.pt

[2] Centro de Investigação, Inovação e Desenvolvimento em Enfermagem de Lisboa (CIDNUR), Escola Superior de Enfermagem de Lisboa, Lisbon, Portugal
{andreia.costa,ahenriques}@esel.pt

[3] Instituto Saúde Ambiental (ISAMB) da Faculdade de Medicina da Universidade de Lisboa, Lisbon, Portugal

Abstract. Background: In Portugal there has been a marked aging of the population, enhancing chronic diseases and possible changes in individual capacity. The family is increasingly required to play the role of caregiver, changing their routines and priorities. Objective: To contribute to the empowerment of informal caregivers, improving their knowledge about their rights and duties, support and available resources. Methodology: Intervention was supported by the Health Planning Methodology. The diagnosis of the health situation was performed using a questionnaire resulting from the scoping review; the European Health Literacy Survey Questionnaire; the Zarit Scale; the WHO Wellness Index; the Barthel Index and the Lawton and Brody Scale to characterize the informal caregiver and the person being cared for. Resulting in a non-probabilistic sample. The theoretical framework used was that of Health Promotion by Nola Pender. Health Education, Empowerment, Health Marketing and Health Communication strategies were planned and implemented. Results: All the sample does not know how to be recognized as informal caregivers, 70% do not know their duties. 70% are unaware of the support available. As for community resources, 20% do not know about them. The overall literacy rate is problematic in 60% of the sample. The interventions implemented were the development of information products aimed at training informal caregivers and were evaluated with a satisfaction questionnaire.

Conclusion: Considering the important role of the informal caregiver and the limited resources, it is essential to know their needs in order to adapt future interventions.

Keywords: Informal caregiver · Health literacy · Nursing · Health promotion

J. García-Alonso and C. Fonseca (Eds.): IWoG 2021, LNBE, pp. 318–328, 2022.
https://doi.org/10.1007/978-3-030-97524-1_30

1 Introduction

Worldwide, there has been a demographic aging [1]. The World Health Organization [2] in 2015 reported that in every five people, one is over 60 years old. Portugal follows this trend. The aging index, between 2018 and 2080, will go from 159 to 300 elderly people for every 100 young persons and the number of elderly people (65 and over) will go from 2.2 to 3.0 million [3]. Aging leads to a gradual loss of physiological capacities, increasing the risk of contracting diseases, leading to people having more complex and chronic health needs. In addition to physiological losses, it also leads to changes in the individual's role and social position [2].

Elderly people are more vulnerable, making them dependent on third-party care [4]. The essential social support for the sociability, comfort and security of the elderly continues to be provided by family and friends, highlighting the importance of the informal system [5]. It is mainly the family, who provides care to the dependent person, thus becoming an informal caregiver, sometimes suddenly and unexpectedly.

In Europe there are about 100 million caregivers [6]. Portugal is the country with the highest rate of informal care provision at an European level (12.4%) and the lowest rate of non-home care (10.8%) [7]. Informal caregivers must be recognized and must have the appropriate conditions so as not to compromise their quality of life and well-being [8], thus needing support [9, 8, 10, 11]. Given that caregivers without adequate training are at greater risk of physical, emotional, social and financial burden [11], their training is crucial, so that they can deal with the situation, and provide continuity of care, in an autonomous way.

The promotion of health literacy in the empowerment of caregivers thus assumes an important role. Improving literacy is contributing to the promotion of individuals' health, thus enabling them to acquire the skills and knowledge necessary to achieve, understand, assess, and use information about their health, to make decisions, prevent diseases and lead healthy lives [12]. Regarding literacy in informal caregivers, it can be understood as referring to the knowledge, skills and abilities that caregivers have to take care of themselves and the person with dependency [13]. It is essential to adapt communication and information taking into account not only the social and cultural context but also the literacy levels [14].

Nurses have a fundamental role in adapting to transitions, aiming at health promotion and training [15]. Thus, we intend to contribute to the training of informal caregivers, improving their knowledge about their rights and duties, support and resources available in the community.

2 Methodology

This study is part of an extended project by the municipality of Lisbon on the profile of caregivers. The developed intervention was based on the methodology of health planning, comprising several steps: the diagnosis of the situation, which consists of defining priorities, setting objectives, selecting strategies, preparing programs/projects, preparing the execution; the execution, and the evaluation [16].

Step 1. Diagnosis of the Situation
To characterize the informal caregiver and the person being cared for, data collection instruments were used: a questionnaire for sociodemographic identification, and assessment of knowledge about rights and duties, support and resources that exist in the community. The European Health Literacy Survey, by Professor Dr. Kristine Sorensen, translated and validated for the Portuguese population by Professor Dr. Rita Espanha [12]. The Zarit Scale, translated and validated by Professor Dr. Carlos Sequeira [17], the WHO Well-being Index [18], the Barthel Index and the Lawton y Brody Scale, translated and validated by Professor Dr. Fátima Araújo [19].

The non-probabilistic sampling consisted of informal caregivers (people aged over or equal to eighteen years old, who provide care to dependent people at home). Data collection took place within the scope of monitoring these caregivers, in the context of nursing care at home, and took place from January 4th to 31st, 2021. Data were collected taking into account the preference, availability and safety of the participants, in view of the pandemic situation.

Step 2. Setting Priorities
After diagnosing the situation and taking into account the context, interventions were prioritized. A team of experts from the unit was involved and the classical criteria of magnitude, transcendence and vulnerability (Hanlon method) were used in order to obtain priority needs. From this prioritization, the Nursing diagnosis "Knowledge about the rights and duties, support and available resources compromised in informal caregivers" emerged.

Step 3. Goal Setting
To determine the objectives, using the Nola Pender's Health Promotion Model as theoretical support, it was considered that "contributing to the training of informal caregivers by improving their knowledge about the rights and duties, support and resources available" was the objective to achieve.

Step 4. Definition of Strategies
When defining the strategies, the particularities of the intervention, the nursing diagnosis, the characteristics of the group, the intended objectives, the existing resources, the pandemic situation, the theoretical nursing framework, the prediction of possible obstacles and how to overcome them were considered. Health Education, Empowerment, Health Marketing and Health Communication strategies were planned and implemented.

Step 5. Operational Planning/Execution
Once the strategies were outlined, activities were planned and executed. The implemented interventions were the development and distribution of information products aimed at training informal caregivers and subsequently evaluating them through a satisfaction questionnaire.

Three posters were prepared to make available to the population and three informational leaflets (one with information on rights and duties, another on support and another on the resources that exist in the community). The prepared guide, also available in digital format, with information on the support, resources and rights and duties of caregivers, is an instrument that, in the current pandemic context, was of particular importance.

Step 6. Evaluation
At this step, the satisfaction of the informal caregiver was assessed.

3 Results

The sample consisted of 10 informal caregivers. Data relating to the caregiver and the person being cared for were analyzed. Descriptive statistical analysis was used.

Regarding the informal caregiver, the ages vary between 58 and 87 years old, 50% were between 81 and 90 years old, mostly women (70%) retired (80%) caring for their spouse (60%) and living only with the person they care for (60%). Regarding educational qualifications, 40% have the 2nd and 3rd cycle, having developed different professional activities, and earn between €501–1000 (70%) monthly, as shown in Table 1.

As for Well-being, 40% reported having poor well-being and 60% feel intensely burdened (Table 2). In the context of the pandemic, it was not possible for us to act at this level, we only made caregivers aware of the resources that exist in the community that can minimize their burden. We also informed the health team.

With regard to the person being cared for (Table 3), the ages ranged between 75 and 100 years, evenly distributed by gender, of which 60% presented total dependency on ADLs, as for the IADLs they presented high levels of dependency.

Regarding health literacy, 60% of informal caregivers have a problematic General Index of health literacy, for each of the three health domains, 80% have a problematic level within the scope of healthcare, 30% within the scope of health promotion and 40% in disease prevention (Fig. 1).

Activity indicators were used to assess whether the expected outreach products were developed. And result indicators for assessing the satisfaction of informal caregivers, about the information transmitted, 80% of informal caregivers considered the available information useful or very useful and that it allowed them to increase their knowledge regarding their rights and duties, support and available resources.

The informal caregivers in the sample are not aware of being recognized as informal caregivers, 90% do not enjoy their rights and about 70% do not know their duties and 80% did not know about the law that defines them. Only 10% would add to financial aid to their rights. Regarding support, 90% are unaware of the law and 70% are unaware of the support available. Although 50% acknowledge that they need support, only 40% report benefitting from any support, namely from the national network of integrated continued care (25%) and from a community institution (75%) within the context of daily hygiene care. As for community resources, 20% do not know about them (Fig. 2). Those who know report having obtained information from health professionals, highlighting nurses and social service technicians. They consider that the main resource used is the health center (80%).

Table 1. Sociodemographic characterization of the informal caregiver

	Total	
	Nº	%
Caregiver age		
50-60 years	1	10%
61-70 years	2	20%
71-80 years	2	20%
81-90 years	5	50%
Sex		
Men	3	30%
Women	7	70%
Degree of kinship		
Daughter/Son	2	20%
Spouse	6	60%
Other	2	20%
Who they live with		
With only the cared-for person	6	60%
With other people	3	30%
Other	1	10%
Educational Qualifications		
1st cycle	3	30%
2nd and 3rd cycle	4	40%
Secondary	1	10%
Bachelor's degree	2	20%
Professional situation		
Full time	1	10%
Part time	1	10%
Retired	8	80%
Household monthly income		
<500€	1	10%
501-1000€	7	70%
1001-1500€	0	0%
1501-2000€	2	20%
2001-2500€	0	0%
Profession they have or had		
Cleaning lady	1	10%
Pastry helper	2	20%
Auto mechanic	1	10%
Teacher	1	10%
Administrative	1	10%
Hairdresser	1	10%
Cashier	1	10%
Religious	1	10%
Domestic	1	10%

Table 2. Characterization of informal caregivers regarding their well-being and burden felt

	Total	
	Nº	%
Wellness scale (WHO-5)		
Poor well-being	4	40%
Well-being	6	60%
Caregiver burden scale- Zarit Scale		
Absence of overload	2	20%
Moderate overload	2	20%
Intense overload	6	60%

Table 3. Characterization of the person being cared

	Total	
	Nº	%
Age of the person being cared for		
70-80 years	1	10%
81-90 years	6	60%
91-100 years	3	30%
Gender		
Male	5	50%
Female	5	50%
Index Barthel		
Total dependency	6	60%
Severe dependency	1	10%
Moderate dependency	3	30%
Total independence	0	0%

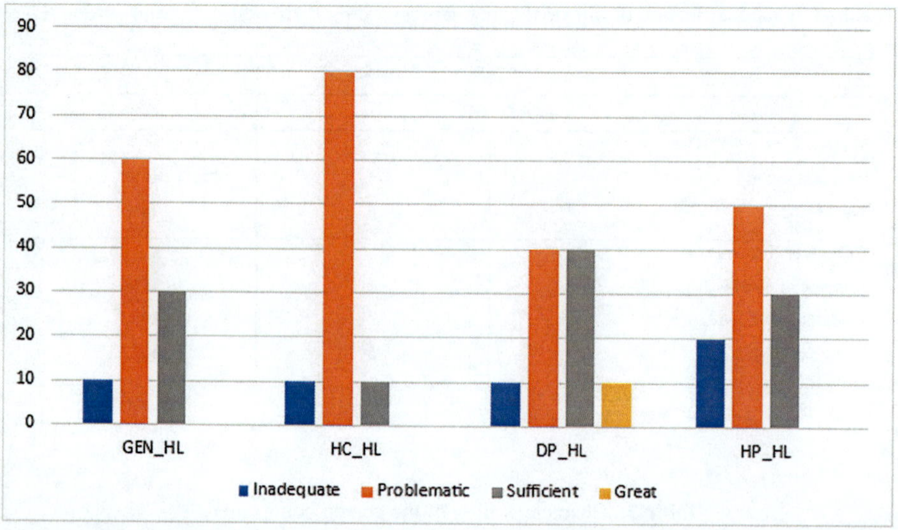

Fig. 1. Characterization of the informal caregiver regarding the level of literacy Subtitle: GEN_HL general health literacy index, HC_HL health care literacy index, DP_HL disease prevention literacy index, and HP_HL health literacy index in health promotion.

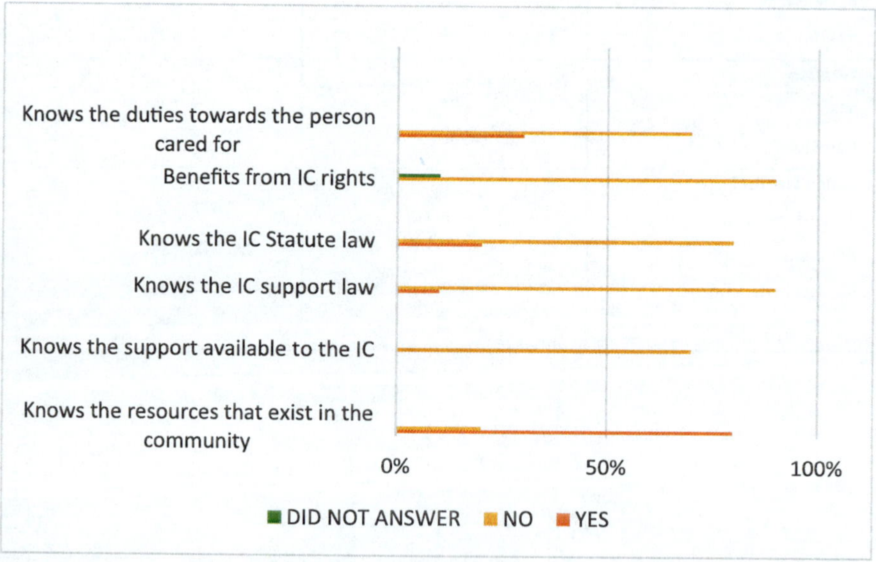

Fig. 2. Informal caregivers' knowledge of rights and duties, support and resources in the community

4 Discussion

Since 2016, several OECD countries have been developing strategies to recognize and protect the informal caregiver [6]. Health planning is essential, it can include an extensive set of activities to respond to the needs of communities [20]. In order to provide health gains [21].

It is essential that health services respond appropriately. Keeping in mind that home is the ideal place for care, promoting active and healthy ageing, person-centered care, valuing literacy, integrated and continuous care. The focus of care should be the dyad (caregiver and the person being cared for), the caregiver partner in care, the use of the individual care plan (PIC) and the creation of a network with partners [22].

Through the various stages of Health Planning, we were able to identify the informal caregiver's knowledge needs. Informal caregivers are unaware of their rights as caregivers [23]. The support available in each country is very divergent [24].

The caregiver role is predominantly played by women, daughters, with low educational level [25, 11, 26]. The general population uses direct contact with health professionals, when they need to obtain information about health, the use of patient associations is less frequent [12]. Caregivers have a lower perception of quality of life than the general population [27].

Nola Pender's Health Promotion Model provides relevant information on the factors that lead to people's participation in community health promotion activities, highlighting the individual's role in controlling their behavior, assessing motivation for behavior change [28]. The use of this model allows the creation of more specific projects to promote healthy lifestyles and identify the fundamental components of health-related behaviors [29]. The Health Promotion Model aims to train individuals, families and communities for self-care, decision-making and active participation in their own health [30].

Training can be acquired using information and communication technologies such as telephone and internet, through family meetings, individual or group sessions and community support groups [31–33, 25, 26].

5 Conclusion

This study aimed to contribute to improving the knowledge of informal caregivers about their rights and duties, support and available resources, which they considered to be useful to them. It also allowed the profile of informal caregivers and cared-for persons to be known. Based on the data found and using the health planning methodology, it was possible to target interventions to the detected needs. By increasing and strengthening informal caregiver's skills in the health and illness process, health literacy levels are raised.

The use of Health Planning should be a practice, as it leads to more appropriate decisions and the inclusion of various the sectors of society [21]. For continuous quality improvement, evidence-based practice is essential. It is necessary to carry out more studies and to create systems to identify and assess the needs of informal caregivers [34, 24].

We believe that the study may have contributed with relevant information so that other projects may emerge, taking into account the real role of the informal caregiver in today's society.

Author Contributions. FS and ST: methods, results and discussion. MF: methods and discussion. AC and AH: design and revision. All authors contributed to the article and approved the submitted version.

Ethics Statement. This study was carried out after approval by the Ethics Committee for Health of the Regional Health Administration of Lisbon and Vale do Tejo. Its participants (caregiver and cared-for person) provided written informed consent to participate in this study.

Financing. This research did not have any funding.

Conflict of Interests. The authors declare the absence of any situations that could be interpreted as a potential conflict of interest.

Study Limitations. This study was subject to some limitations, namely the pandemic situation and the time limitation. We also consider the low number of participants, although the use of such a broad assessment instrument, allowed the diagnosis of the situation to obtain results equivalent to those of the consulted bibliography, particularly in terms of health literacy and sociodemographic characterization.

Thanks. To all caregivers and cared-for people.

References

1. Centro Internacional de Longevidade Brasil. Envelhecimento Ativo: um marco político em resposta à revolução da longevidade. Centro Internacional de Longevidade Brasil (2015). http://ilcbrazil.org/portugues/wpcontent/uploads/sites/4/2015/12/Envelhecimento-Ativo-Um-Marco-Pol%C3%ADtico-ILC-Brasil_web.pdf
2. Organização Mundial de Saúde. Relatório mundial de envelhecimento e saúde (2015). https://apps.who.int/iris/bitstream/handle/10665/186468/WHO_FWC_ALC_15.01_por.pdf;jsessionid=DCDDAFFFBACBC7869E866AA27E3B1E9A?sequence=6
3. Instituto Nacional de Estatística. Projeções da população residente de 2018–2080. Instituto Nacional de Estatística (2020)
4. da Saúde, D.G.: Estratégia nacional para o envelhecimento ativo e saudável. DGS (2017)
5. Cunha, L.P., Pereira, F.A., Loureiro, A.: Educação para o suporte social e satisfação com a vida. In: Diálogos interdisciplinares do envelhecimento, pp. 47–65. Hipótese, São Paulo (2019). https://bibliotecadigital.ipb.pt/bitstream/10198/19574/3/EDUCAC%cc%a7A%cc%83O%20PARA%20O%20SUPORTE%20SOCIAL.pdf
6. Montgomery, A.: Advocacy and the global demographic age wave: What is being done to help family caregivers? Aging Today **39**(6), 8–10 (2018)
7. Barbosa, F., Matos, A.D.: Informal support in Portugal by individuals aged 50+. Eur. J. Ageing **11**(4), 293–300 (2014). https://doi.org/10.1007/s10433-014-0321-0
8. Reis, A.: O cuidador informal: Manual prático para cuidar dos que mais amamos. Mahatma (2019)

9. Paixão, C.: Desenvolvimento de competências sociais no cuidador informal. Cáritas (2017)
10. Romão, A., Pereira, A., Gerardo, F.: As necessidades dos cuidadores informais: Estudo na área do envelhecimento. Santa Casa da Misericórdia de Lisboa (2008)
11. Sequeira, C.A.: Cuidar de idosos com dependência física e mental. LIDEL (2010a)
12. Espanha, R., Ávila, P., Mendes, R.V.: Literacia em saúde em Portugal. CIES-IUL e FCG (2015)
13. Sequeira, C.: Cuidar de idosos com dependência física e Mental. LIDEL (2018)
14. da Saúde, D.G.: Manual de Boas Práticas Literacia em Saúde, Capacitação dos Profissionais. DGS (2019a)
15. Peixoto, M.J., Machado, P.P.: Programas de intervenção aos familiares cuidadores. In: Martins, T., Araújo, M.F., Peixoto, M.J., Machado, P.P. (Org.), A pessoa dependente e o familiar cuidador, pp.131–142. Escola Superior de Enfermagem do Porto (2016b)
16. Imperatori, E., Giraldes, M.R.: Metodologia do planeamento de saúde -Manual para uso em serviços centrais, regionais e locais. Escola Nacional de Saúde Pública (1993)
17. Sequeira, C.A.: Adaptação e validação da Escala de sobrecarga do cuidador de Zarit. Revista Referência, **12**, 9–16 (2010b). http://www.index-f.com/referencia/2010pdf/12-0916.pdf
18. World Health Organization: Medidas de Bem-Estar na Atenção Primária à Saúde: World Health Organization (1998)
19. Araujo, F., Ribeiro, J.L., Oliveira, A., Pinto, C.: Validação do Índice de Barthel numa amostra de idosos não institucionalizados. Revista Portuguesa de Saúde Pública **25**(2), 59–66 (2007). https://hdl.hendle.net/10216/15740
20. Crisp, N.: Planeamento em saúde - uma perspetiva global. Anais do Instituto de Higiene e Medicina Tropical. vol. 16 (suplemento nº1) (2017)
21. Simões, J.: Planeamento em saúde: da investigação à decisão política, na Europa, nas Américas e em África. In: Simões, J., Ferrinho, P. (eds.) Anais do Instituto de Higiene e Medicina Tropical. Planeamento em saúde, vol. 16 (suplemento nº1), pp. 7–8. Instituto de Higiene e Medicina Tropical (2017)
22. Lopes, M.: Desafios de inovação em saúde: repensar os modelos de cuidados (2021). https://doi.org/10.24902/uevora.24
23. Barber, C.: Carers legislation and the role of the HCA, AP and nurse. Br. J. Healthc. Assistants **7**(3), 125–128 (2013)
24. Courtin, E., Jemiai, N., Mossialos, E.: Mapping support policies for informalcarers across the European Union. Health Policy **118**(1), 84–94 (2014)
25. Schaller, S., et al.: Tailored e-Health services for the dementia care setting: a pilot study of eHeathMonitor. BMC Med. Inf. Decis. Mak. **15**(58), 1–9 (2015). https://doi.org/10.1186/s12911-015-0182-2
26. Yu, D.S., Li, P.W., Zhang, F., Cheng, S., Ng, T., Judge, K.S.: The effects of a dyadic stregth-based empowerment program and the health outcomes of people with mild cognitive impairment and their family caregivers: a randomized controlled trial. Clin. Interv. Aging. **14**, 1705–1717 (2019). https://doi.org/10.2147/CIA.S213006
27. Teixeira, A.R., et al.: Medidas de Intervenção junto dos Cuidadores Informais - Documento Enquadrador, Perspetiva Nacional e Internacional (2017). http://cuidadores.pt/sites/default/files/documentos/Doc_CI.PDF
28. Pender, N., Murdaugh, C., Parsons, M.: Health Promotion in Nursingpractice (7ªed.). Pearson (2015)
29. Chen, H., Hsieh, P.: Applying the Pender's health promotion model to identify the factors related to older adults' participation in community-based health promotion activities. Int. J. Environ. Res. Public Health **2021**(18), 9985 (2021). https://doi.org/10.3390/ijerph18199985
30. Murdaugh, C., Parsons, M., Pender, N.: Health Promotion in Nursing Practice (8ªed.). Pearson (2019)

31. Nieuwboer, M.S., Richters, A., Marck, M.V.: Collaborative primary care for community dwelling individuals with dementia: the DementiaNet approach. Int. J. Integr. Care. **17**(5), A22 (2017). https://doi.org/10.5334/ijic.3323
32. Etemadifar, S., Heidari, M., Jivad, N., Masaudi, R.: Effects of family-centered empowerment intervention on stress, anxiety, and depression among family caregivers of patients with epilepsy. Epilepsy Behav. **88**, 106–112 (2018). https://doi.org/10.1016/j.yebeh.2018.08.03
33. Deyhoul, N., Vasli, P., Rohani, C., Shakeri, N., Hosseini, M.: The effect of family- centered empowerment program on the family caregiver burden and the activities of daily living of Iranian patients with stroke: a randomized controlled trial study. Clin. Exp. Res. Aging **32**, 1343–1352 (2020). https://doi.org/10.1007/s40520-019-01321-4
34. Chen, Y., Hedrick, S.C., Young, H.M.: A pilot evaluation of the family caregiver support program. Eval. Program Plan. **33**, 113–119 (2010)

Public and Other Health Initiatives

Local Decision Making and Aging Policies During Covid-19

Luis López-Lago Ortiz(✉), Beatriz Muñoz González, and M. Ángeles Serrano Alfonso

University of Extremadura, Cáceres, Spain
luislopezlago@unex.es

Abstract. The municipal administration level plays a distinct role in managing and executing dependency policies and care for the elderly in Spain. Numerous services related to aging depend directly on the political leaders of the municipalities, a fact that is especially evident in towns of less than 2000 inhabitants in rural areas. In this article, we analyze the main elements in the decision-making process of mayors and councilors for aging policies in their municipalities. For this purpose, we have carried out fieldwork in 10 rural localities of Extremadura (Spain). The main results highlight the high level of knowledge of the environment that the mayors and councilors have when making decisions, although they state that their lack of knowledge of the pandemic is damaging. In addition, it is observed that other factors have influenced the decision-making process, such as the positioning of the party, the emotional impact of the pandemic, or neighborhood pressure. Finally, a proposal is made to improve decision-making processes in health crises in municipal policy as a result of the results obtained.

Keywords: Care · Covid-19 · Rural areas · Aging · Public policies · Decision making

1 Introduction

In Spain, the long-term care system and policies for the care of the elderly are primarily decentralized, with the regional and municipal levels playing a leading role in the management of resources [1, 2]. This recognition of the municipal administration in implementing policies related to aging has been reflected in numerous resources, services, and programs that depend directly on the municipalities. Since the 1980s, and with particular intensity since the 1990s, residences, daycare centers, telecare programs, home care services, active aging programs, etc. have become municipally managed or have been directly created by the municipalities, although always with the outstanding support of the autonomous community institutions [1, 3]. Likewise, this administrative decentralization has meant that mayors and councilors have a significant decision-making capacity over the form, duration, workers, and resources used in programs and services for the care of the elderly [4].

J. García-Alonso and C. Fonseca (Eds.): IWoG 2021, LNBE, pp. 331–340, 2022.
https://doi.org/10.1007/978-3-030-97524-1_31

In this context, and with the outbreak of the Covid-19 pandemic, municipal policymakers found themselves in the position of having to make decisions on municipal services for the care of the elderly, many of them of great importance for the lives of the elderly in their localities. Furthermore, while autonomy is not total[1], the immediacy required in many situations, or the fact that action protocols did not cover many others, meant that it was up to the municipal authorities to decide on the use of resources and services.

Because the pandemic struck the elderly particularly hard [5, 6], especially those of very advanced age, who lived in residences or shared spaces in day centers and other community resources, mayors and councilors of the rural municipalities studied recognize that the decision-making process regarding the operation of the resources was complicated and carried out under intense emotional stress.

In this article, we focus on one of the phases of the decision-making process: the choice of criteria. This paper aims to identify the main elements that have been significant for mayors and councilors in the decision-making process and develop a proposal to improve these processes in cases of crisis such as the Covid-19 crisis.

2 Materials and Method

The research was carried out in the autonomous community of Extremadura, located in the southwest of Spain. This region is characterized by marked aging of the population[2] [7] and the predominance of rural municipalities[3] [8]. Ten municipalities with a population of fewer than 2000 inhabitants were selected for the study. All of them were among the municipalities with the highest level of socio-aging in Extremadura [9]. On the other hand, a balance has been sought between the two major administrative divisions (provinces) of the region. Thus, of the municipalities studied, 5 belong to the province of Cáceres and 5 to the province of Badajoz. The subjects of the study were 14 mayors and councilors (8 women and 6 men) from the main political parties in the region, *Partido Socialista Obrero Español* -PSOE- (7) and *Partido Popular* -PP- (7). The interviews were conducted between May and July 2021, within the framework of the so-called "fifth wave" of the pandemic [10].

A qualitative methodology was selected as it provided the depth required by the research, which, beyond the data, aims to understand the criteria of mayors and councilors in decision-making densely. For this purpose, semi-structured interviews were conducted with political decision-makers. These were transcribed and reviewed by the research team members and examined with ATLAS.ti software (Scientific Software Development GmbH, v.8.4.24.0 for Windows), as were the other empirical materials were the object of collective reflection, the results of which are presented below.

[1] Municipal decision-makers for care services are in coordination with other provincial, autonomous, and state administrations.

[2] According to the Spanish National Institute of Statistics, the aging index of Extremadura in 2020 is 125.49.

[3] The Ministry of Agriculture, Fisheries and Food, in its 2020 Annual Indicators Report, states that in Extremadura, rural municipalities exceed 90% of the total, with a population of almost 50%.

Following the analysis of the empirical materials, the main elements that intervened in the decision-making of mayors and councilors about services for the care of the elderly during the pandemic are identified. Two main blocks identified by the aldermen stand out, which represented the priority corpus of information for decision-making: knowledge of the environment and the pandemic. In addition, we identified elements such as party positioning, the emotional impact of the pandemic, and community pressure, which had different degrees of influence on decision-making. Finally, we describe the actions that resulted from the decisions that were made.

3 Results

3.1 Knowledge of the Environment

Mayors and councilors recognize that they have a broad knowledge of their environment, of the situation of aging services, and the elderly and their caregivers.

Regarding municipal resources, when asked about existing services, most of them listed them accurately, and some were even able to identify the approximate number of users. In the smaller municipalities, there is even a direct relationship with the beneficiaries, with frequent visits to residences and homes for the elderly and even to private homes, which allows them to have first-hand information on the situation of the elderly served by the municipal services.

Likewise, all the councilors state that they always consider the training of the technical staff of the services (social workers, caregivers, nursing staff, occupational therapists, etc.), although the last word is left to them as political leaders. In addition, many of the politicians interviewed are professionally dedicated to caring about the resources and services of their locality, which means that they have a detailed knowledge of them. Thus, mayors and councilors recognize that this high level of knowledge of the situation of the services in their municipality was fundamental in assessing what actions had to be taken during the pandemic.

On the other hand, policymakers have extensive knowledge of the situation of the elderly and their caregivers. Concerning the former, a series of themes stand out during the pandemic that generally coincides in all the localities, and knowledge of these established to a large extent the parameters of the actions during the most challenging moments of the health crisis. In the first place, we find loneliness as a prominent theme. Through the direct information given to them by municipal workers or through their knowledge of the neighborhood, Mayors and councilors could locate people living alone in their municipalities. During their confinement, they often contacted them to keep abreast of their state of mind or home care needs. Secondly, the rulers were the recipients of the fears and concerns caused by the pandemic. Being conceived by the rest of the neighbors as the "authority figure", and the one who is "legitimized to solve problems" made them the recipients of a multitude of messages, many in the form of demands, which contained abundant information on the state of mind of the elderly of the town, including their state of mental health. Among these, those that stood out were those that emphasized the desire of the elderly to stay in their municipality at all costs, requesting mayors and councilors to expand services for the elderly so that they would not have to leave.

Finally, their extensive knowledge of the socio-economic situation of their neighbors, especially the elderly, and of the food and pharmaceutical supply systems in their localities enabled them to generate appropriate, even customized, solutions to supply difficulties during the pandemic.

In the case of the caregivers, the knowledge of the councilors about the situations is usually quite precise in the case of caregivers assigned to the dependent services of the municipality. In the case of private or family caregivers, the knowledge is less. In the smaller localities, the information they have on this subject is abundant due to the closeness of the relationships. Here the topics of interest also tended to coincide among those responsible for the different localities: the need for public resources due to the shortage of caregivers, the mental health of caregivers during the pandemic, care as a way of containing and attracting population, etc.

3.2 Knowledge of the Pandemic

Regarding the information that the councilors had about the pandemic, a clear differentiation is established between that which arrived through official channels from the provincial, autonomous, and state administrations and obtained through the media. Regarding the former, there are some discrepancies to its content and usefulness, and the attitude they have towards it is mediated by political positioning, being more positive if they are more sympathetic to the party in government (PSOE) and more critical if they are from the opposition party (PP). However, there is a consensus in considering official information as the main element for decision-making. This information took the form of legislation, different types of regulations, and circulars that normally arrived via e-mail from the state administration, through the Government Subdelegation, from the regional level, mainly from the Extremadura Health Service (*Servicio Extremeño de Salud*, SES) and the Extremaduran Service for the Promotion of Autonomy and Care for the Elderly (*Servicio Extremeño de Promoción de la Autonomía y Atención a la Dependencia*, SEPAD), of provincial administrations, *Diputación* of Cáceres y *Diputación* of Badajoz and from the Federation of Municipalities and Provinces of Extremadura (*Federación de Municipios y Provincias de Extremadura*, FEMPEX)[4]. Furthermore, while this body of official information is considered the main element for decision-making, there is also widespread dissatisfaction with the format among the aldermen. Most agreed that the legal language is complex, and it was sometimes problematic to interpret the instructions.

The information that reached them through the media was considered excessive, on numerous occasions expressed the sensation of saturation and considered it to be of little use. Generally speaking, they stated that the information provided by the media was spectacularized, often devoid of helpful content. In addition, several of the region's residents emphasized the urban nature of the information while stressing that the reality of the rural world was very different from what appeared in the media. They also pointed out their distrust of the information that reached them through social networks, suspecting it might be fake news.

[4] FEMPEX is an association composed by municipalities of the Autonomous Community of Extremadura that voluntarily decide to join it for the protection of their common interests [25].

Mayors and councilors also maintain that they had essential shortcomings in terms of knowledge of the functioning of the virus and protection measures. Beyond the basic instructions they received from the health administrations, in general, they demanded more in-depth training for themselves and their municipal workers that would prepare them more adequately to face the present pandemic or future health crises.

3.3 Other Elements: Positioning of the Party, Emotional Impact, and Community Pressure

The analysis of the material reveals other elements that influenced decision-making. In the first place, we observe that the political party positioning determined the relationship with other administrations. In the case of the PSOE councilors, this was reflected in a discourse of inter-institutional collaboration, while those of the PP were generally combative, expressing their discomfort with the management of the regional and state governments, which are of the opposite sign.

Secondly, the intense emotional impact that the management of the crisis had on mayors and councilors also influenced their decision-making. This was expressed on numerous occasions when they mentioned that, due to the stress, sadness, fear, lack of concentration, or irritability they experienced during the most challenging days of the pandemic, their decisions were sometimes hasty, lacking sufficient or at least adequate reflection because they were not in the best emotional conditions.

Finally, they allude to the pressure exerted by the community on their work. They point to the idea that in small communities, they are continually questioned by neighbors, which impedes the proper performance of their functions. In particular, respect for confinement, the closing or opening of businesses, or the observance of time restrictions was enforced by the municipal police. Thus, although the instructions on confinement or restrictions were the responsibility of other administrations, their application was a municipal responsibility, and the dissatisfaction of the disgruntled neighbors was focused on the local authorities.

3.4 The Actions

Although they are not the main object of study of this article, it is considered attractive to briefly describe the actions carried out by mayors and councilors to understand the dimensions of the decision-making process. These can be grouped into 3 categories: reinforcement, creation, and suspension of services.

The reinforcements were mainly in personnel, increasing the number of people hired in residences, daycare centers, home care, etc. On other occasions, the hours of contracted workers were increased, and some workers even voluntarily decided to be confined with users in various residences. Some services - such as home-delivered meals - significantly increased the number of users, for which more resources had to be made available. The widespread use of electronic devices in residences and day centers to combat isolation can even be seen as a reinforcement.

New services were also created, mainly aimed at supplying the elderly. These were generally aimed at the purchase of food, pharmaceuticals, and other essential products. In some cases, the government teams themselves made themselves available to users to carry out these services. In others, a municipal worker was assigned to these tasks, and in others, the municipalities organized brigades of volunteers to carry out the purchases and subsequent distribution. Mayors, municipal workers, and volunteers also organized mobility problems, transporting older adults requiring medical attention or vaccinations in municipal vehicles or independently.

Finally, the suspension of services mainly affected active aging programs, day centers, home-clubs for the elderly, and non-residential programs and spaces involving proximity between users. The suspensions began during the confinement, and many of these services had not resumed their activity at the time of the interviews. In some localities, home care services were also suspended, mainly because users were afraid of contact with staff coming from outside. With the end of the confinement, these services began to return to normal and were sometimes reinforced.

4 Discussion

Decision-making in the public sphere always impacts the lives of citizens, hence its relevance and the fact that it has a more significant consideration as an object of study than decisions in the private sphere [11]. Due to this impact on society, disciplines such as political science and sociology have addressed the processes that contribute to decision-making in the political arena. To this end, these disciplines have converged with other studies such as social psychology or organizational studies in business administration, generating an academic field with its entity [12]. In this field, the transcendence of the role of political leaders makes them the protagonists of the decision-making process [12, 13]. Therefore, this study focuses on the figures of those who hold municipal power.

Mayors and councilors understand that their knowledge of both the social dynamics of their community and the functioning of the services of their city councils was a very positive value, inadequately facing the decisions they had to make during the pandemic. In their testimonies, this assessment can be appreciated, establishing a distance from the decision-making in other political spaces of higher rank, at the autonomous and state level. Therefore, we are faced with a knowledge born of praxis and that the councilors value as optimal. As Daza [14] indicates, in politics, daily experience is a source of knowledge, which without being expert knowledge, if it is the product of common sense, and with the sieve of rational depuration, can be a valid element for the action of governing.

However, the mayors and councilors themselves recognized their limitations in terms of knowledge about the functioning of the virus and the measures that had to be taken. In this sense, they recognize the value of expert knowledge. In this regard, they affirm that a lack of specific training harmed decision-making and, personally, with pathologies such as anxiety or stress. A dynamic can be seen in other groups directly confronted with the virus, such as health care workers [15, 16]. In addition, in the face of the exponential increase in news reports about the pandemic [17], the aldermen show a saturation that they reflect with expressions such as "weariness", "fed up", "fatigue", concerning media work. To this must be added the distrust produced by the news that came through social networks, which, according to Aleixandre Benavent et al. [18], became a vehicle during the pandemic for unobjective or false news that could endanger the health of people.

Finally, the official information that arrived with regional and state instructions for action regarding the pandemic was not always easy to understand, as stated by many municipal policymakers. For this reason, it would be necessary to explore systems that bring the information closer to the users in a didactic and pedagogically adapted way. In this sense, the use of infographics, audiovisuals, and technologies such as smartphones and instant messaging applications open up interesting possibilities that public administrations can explore [19].

Regarding the role of the partisan political positioning of municipal decision-makers in decision-making, there is a contradiction between the neutrality expressed and the clear adherence of the discourses to the dominant narratives of the political parties to which they belong. During the interviews, the idea that in municipal politics in small towns, "people vote for the person, not for the parties" repeatedly appeared in the discourse of mayors and councilors. The idea that municipal electoral processes have an administrative character, where the management of the political response is mainly valued [20], or their potential capacity to manage resources since their life trajectory in the municipality is well known. In addition, the capacity to mobilize affection and personal family relationships play a fundamental role, where each councilor typically represents several votes coming from the close family environment [21]. However, in the course of the interviews, we found that the pandemic discourse of mayors and councilors was remarkably consistent with the state discourses of their parties. The narrative was highly polarized. Thus, the PSOE councilors maintained a confident attitude in managing the state and regional authorities, who are of the same political sign.

On the other hand, the political leaders of the PP maintained a very belligerent discourse, repeating some of the dominant ideas of that party at the national level: lack of freedom, lousy government management, referring to the government as social-communists with a derogatory tone, etc. Thus, the municipal narratives, which apparently appear to be more neutral, are influenced by the parties' discourses at the national level. This is mainly due to the process of "nationalization of local politics", where political discourses at the municipal level are gradually becoming more uniform with those developed by the parties at the State level, given the increasing importance of the State political parties in the local sphere [22]. This influence of national discourses somehow determines the relationship between administrations and affects the decisions made at the municipal level.

The emotional impact of the pandemic also influenced the decision-making of mayors and councilors. Traditionally, this process is considered a rational procedure where the best way to achieve an objective is calculated. Nevertheless, scientific evidence shows the decisive role of the mood of the actors and their emotional situation as fundamental elements in decision making [23]. This becomes even more evident in crises, where tension and stress alter the underlying mechanisms of decision-making [24]. Thus, while this tension could help us be more alert to the problems caused by the pandemic, it also distorted the rationality of the decision-making process.

Finally, mayors and councilors emphasize the pressure they feel when making decisions due to the proximity of personal relationships in small municipalities, where there is the possibility of being constantly questioned. As Fernández [21] points out, the neighbors expect solutions from the nearest administration, and they do such a demanding immediacy. Failure to comply with this generates a distrust expressed directly to local representatives who are perceived as being close and whose telephone number or address is known, or who can be found on the street or at their place of work and express their discontent. Furthermore, this context generates pressure because the aldermen feel continually watched and questioned [21]. This pressure was evident when they had to make decisions where health interests clashed with local businesses. Moreover, although it is advisable to follow the instructions of the health authorities, it is not always advisable to follow the instructions of the health authorities [5], the complexity of interests and the proximity of political power to the citizens in small municipalities clouds the decision-making process of mayors and councilors.

5 Conclusions

Mayors and councilors of rural municipalities in Extremadura have had to make decisions about resources and services for the elderly in a context of crisis. The lack of preparation for this type of situation complicated the development of their work and also had a strong emotional impact. To reduce this type of negative consequences detected in the decision-making process, it is proposed that the different administrations involved should have adequate uncertainty management systems in place, where the transfer of information is adapted to the different levels of understanding of the political actors and the need for immediacy in decision-making. For example, the legal texts that used to be sent to city councils and were difficult to understand for many political decision-makers should be accompanied by reading guides, infographics, or audiovisual material to facilitate their interpretation.

The knowledge of mayors and councilors of their environments, both of the situation of the services for the care of the elderly and the elderly in their localities, is particularly well-valued by their protagonists in the decision-making process. This detailed understanding of the reality can be very enriching for the regional and state administration when establishing solutions adapted to the rural world in contexts of health crises such as that of Covid-19 or to prevent these crises. To this end, it is recommended that spaces for reflection be created, with a preventive character, and consultative mechanisms, with the participation of the different administrations where the voice of the mayors of rural municipalities is taken into account.

Regarding the emotional impact of the pandemic and its negative repercussions on decision-making, it is proposed to intervene in several aspects. Firstly, sensitizing municipal authorities against the prejudices of psychological assistance and encouraging those affected by the current pandemic to receive professional treatment. Secondly, in prevention, the development of programs to prepare people psychologically to deal adequately with future crises. Furthermore, thirdly, creating a psychological care service in emergencies that contemplates the participation of mayors and councilors who need it in possible crisis scenarios. The intervention of psychology professionals can also provide the mayors with tools that will help them manage the pressure they suffer when their neighbors question them.

Likewise, training actions are proposed in the area of health crisis management for rural mayors, the preparation of contingency plans that contemplate the sustainability of health care services for the elderly, the supply of food, medicines, and other essential resources, as well as the availability of special budgetary allocations appropriate to the unforeseen events that have characterized the pandemic. All of this will contribute to better-informed decision-making and, therefore, to relevant and effective actions.

Finally, it is necessary to delve deeper into the political cultures of municipal councilors in order to understand the keys to the partisan positions that sometimes hinder decision-making. Once these are understood, different institutions can promote training courses for mayors and councilors to foster institutional collaboration regardless of political color.

Acknowledgment. This work was supported by the 4IE+ project (0499-4IE PLUS 4 E) funded by the Interreg V-A España-Portugal (POCTEP) 2014–2020 program.

References

1. Rodríguez Rodríguez, P., Sancho Castiello, M.: Envejecimiento y protección social de la dependencia en España: veinte años de historia y una mirada hacia el futuro. Psychosoc. Interv. **10**, 259–275 (2001)
2. López-Lago Ortiz, L., Arroyo Chacón, S., Cipriano Crespo, C., Luengo Polo, J., Muñoz González, B.: Technology in the face of the challenges of the long-term care system for the elderly in Spain. In: García-Alonso, J., Fonseca, C. (eds.) IWoG 2020. LNB, pp. 371–379. Springer, Cham (2021). https://doi.org/10.1007/978-3-030-72567-9_34
3. Puga González, M.D., Sancho Castiello, M., Tortosa Chuliá, M.Á., et al.: La diversificación y consolidación de los servicios sociales para las personas mayores en España y Suecia. Rev. Esp. Salud Publica **85**, 525–539 (2011). https://doi.org/10.1590/s1135-57272011000600003
4. Bellido Muñoz, M.D.C.: El papel de los ayuntamientos ante la Ley de Dependencia. In: Navarro, C. (ed.) La Ley de Dependencia: ¿qué papel juegan los municipios? Junta de Andalucía, Sevilla, pp 47–52 (2019)
5. Yanez, N.D., Weiss, N.S., Romand, J.A., Treggiari, M.M.: COVID-19 mortality risk for older men and women. BMC Public Health **20**, 1–7 (2020). https://doi.org/10.1186/s12889-020-09826-8
6. Fernández-Ballesteros, R., Sánchez-Izquierdo Alonso, M.: Impacto del Covid-19 en personas mayores en España: algunos resultados y reflexiones. Clínica Salud **31**, 165–169 (2020)
7. Spanish National Statistics Institute (INE), Instituto Nacional de Estadística (2020) Índice de Envejecimiento Por Comunidad Autónoma. https://www.ine.es/jaxiT3/Datos.htm?t=1452#!tabs-tabla. Accessed 29 July 2020
8. Ministerio de Agricultura Pesca y Alimentación: Informe Anual De Indicadores 2019. Madrid (2020)
9. Instituto de Estadística de Extremadura [IIEX]: Índice de sobreenvejecimiento. In: Padrón Munic. Habitantes 2020 (2021). https://ciudadano.gobex.es/web/ieex/publicaciones-tipo/-/publicacion-categoria/ficha/10091219. Accessed 1 May 2021
10. Iftimie, S., López-azcona, A.F., Lozano-olmo, M.J., et al.: Differential features of the fifth wave of COVID-19 associated with vaccination and the Delta variant in a reference hospital in Catalonia, Spain [Pre Print]. MedRxiv. Prepr. Serv. Heal. Sci. (2021). https://www.medrxiv.org/content/10.1101/2021.10.14.21264933v1.full.pdf. Accessed 7 Nov 2021
11. Gónzález Campos, C.H., Gómez Cárdenas, C.W.: El proceso de toma de decisiones en políticas públicas. Prospect. Rev. Trab. Soc. Interv. Soc. **12**, 75–104 (2007)

12. Mendieta, C.: La toma de decisiones en el sector público. Una mirada desde el dirigente. Rev. Científica Guillermo Ockham **3**, 31–48 (2005)
13. Joensuu, M., Niiranen, V.: Political leaders and public administrators: Interaction patterns and pictures in Finnish local government decision-making processes. Public Policy Adm. **33**, 22–45 (2018). https://doi.org/10.1177/0952076716673898
14. Daza, J.D.: El conocimiento saberes académicos, sentido común y acción política. Analecta Polít. **9**, 9–35 (2019)
15. Grupo Análisis e Investigación: Impacto del COVID en la enfermería. Informe de resultados. Madrid, April 2020
16. Fan, J., Hu, K., Li, X., et al.: A qualitative study of the vocational and psychological perceptions and issues of transdisciplinary nurses during the COVID-19 outbreak. Aging (Albany NY) **12**, 12479–12492 (2020). https://doi.org/10.18632/aging.103533
17. Lázaro-Rodríguez, P., Herrera-Viedma, E.: Noticias sobre Covid-19 y 2019-nCoV en medios de comunicación de España: el papel de los medios digitales en tiempos de confinamiento. El Prof. Inf. **29**, 1–11 (2020). https://doi.org/10.3145/epi.2020.may.02
18. Aleixandre-Benavent, R., Castelló-Cogollos, L., Valderrama-Zurián, J.C.: Information and communication during the early months of COVID-19: Infodemics, misinformation, and the role of information professionals. Prof. Inf. **29**, 1–17 (2020). https://doi.org/10.3145/epi.2020.jul.08
19. López-Lago Ortiz, L., Arroyo Chacón, S., Cipriano Crespo, C., Bonilla Bermejo, J., Muñoz González, B.: Technological solutions and informal care culture for the elderly: an intervention proposal for training actions. In: García-Alonso, J., Fonseca, C. (eds.) IWoG 2020. LNB, pp. 315–323. Springer, Cham (2021). https://doi.org/10.1007/978-3-030-72567-9_29
20. Capó Giol, J.: Elecciones municipales, pero no locales. Reis Rev. Española Invest. Sociol. **56**, 143–164 (1991)
21. Fernández, R.: El ayuntamiento es un rehén. Redes sociales y confianza en un municipio rural. In: Velasco, H., Díaz de Rada, Á., Cruces, F., et al. (eds.) La sonsrisa de la institución. Confianza y riesgo en los sistemas expertos. Editorial Universitaria Ramón Areces, Madrid (2006)
22. Carrillo, E.: La nacionalización de la política local. Polít. Soc **3**, 29–46 (1989)
23. Marki, O.: Rationality and emotions in decision making. Interdisc. Descr. Complex Syst. INDECS **7**, 54–64 (2009)
24. Starcke, K., Brand, M.: Decision making under stress: a selective review. Neurosci. Biobehav. Rev. **36**, 1228–1248 (2012). https://doi.org/10.1016/j.neubiorev.2012.02.003
25. Federación de Municipios y Provincias de Extremadura. Misión/Visión (2021). https://www.fempex.es/institucional/mision-vision. Accessed 5 Oct 2021

Prevention of Falls in the Elderly and in People with Mobility Changes

Magali Palma[1], Helena Teixeira[1], Pedro Dias[1], Patrícia Messias[1], Maria José Bule[2], Rogério Ferreira[3], and João Vitor Vieira[3](✉)

[1] Centro Hospitalar Universitário do Algarve, Faro, Portugal
[2] Universidade de Évora, Évora, Portugal
[3] Instituto Politécnico de Beja, Beja, Portugal
joao.vieira@ipbeja.pt

Abstract. Falls are a globally recognized health problem with harmful consequences, namely, restricted mobility, functional incapacity, reduced quality of life, institutionalization and consequent increase in costs associated with health. **Method:** Systematic review of the literature that used the PICO mnemonic to formulate the research question, which led to the search in the CINAHL Complete and PUBMED databases. Nine randomized controlled studies were selected. **Results:** The prevention of falls results from a multifactorial approach where the assessment and identification of the risk of falling, implementation of motor re-education programs, identification and control of risk factors for falls and health education are essential. **Conclusion:** Interventions that contribute to the prevention of falls in the elderly and/or those with mobility disorders include assessment and identification of the risk of falling, implementation of motor re-education programs, identification and control of risk factors, risk of falling intrinsic and extrinsic and health education.

Keywords: Elderly · Fall · Fall prevention · Nursing · Rehabilitation · Rehabilitation nursing

1 Introduction

Developed countries, particularly the countries of the European Union, have been experiencing a progressive population aging. According to the World Health Organization (2007), approximately 28% to 30% of people over 65 have falls each year, with an increase in the incidence of falls to 32% to 42% in people over 70 years old [1]. This phenomenon appears as one of the main causes of hospitalization, constituting a significant factor of morbidity and mortality, with serious consequences at a personal, family, social and financial level. The most frequent diagnoses resulting from falls are hip fractures, head injuries and injuries to the upper limbs. Its occurrence can lead to restricted mobility, functional disability, depression, loss of independence and autonomy, decreased quality of life and institutionalization. Falls represent 10 to 15% of episodes of admission to emergency services, with subsequent periods of hospitalization, which lead

J. García-Alonso and C. Fonseca (Eds.): IWoG 2021, LNBE, pp. 341–354, 2022.
https://doi.org/10.1007/978-3-030-97524-1_32

to an overload of health systems and increasing expenses with medication, consultations, treatments and rehabilitation with the population that suffers falls [1, 2].

The fall is identified as a condition of great complexity that has harmful consequences, constituting a great challenge for the population in general and for health professionals in particular. It is a problem of multifactorial etiology where intrinsic and extrinsic risk factors are identified. Intrinsic risk factors are related to the individual, such as hearing or visual impairment, changes in gait and mobility patterns, cognitive changes, neurological or other diseases, a history of falls, taking various medications. Extrinsic risk factors are related to the environment in which the person is inserted, such as poor lighting, difficult to access switches, wet or uneven floors, loose carpets, no handrail or safety bars, presence of obstacles, stairs, inappropriate footwear, among others [3]. Given the multifactorial nature of the fall, the intervention aimed at its prevention must involve not only the person at risk, but also the multidisciplinary team made up of nurses, doctors, pharmacists, physiotherapists, occupational therapists, nutritionists and psychologist, with the promotion of training, education, training, creating safe environments and establishing effective risk reduction policies.

The aging process occurs gradually, with multiple anatomical and physiological changes, sometimes associated with pathological processes, which lead to several deficits and losses of capacity directly related to the increased risk of falls in the elderly. These changes affect the most diverse organic systems, namely the vestibular system, central nervous system, cardiovascular system, musculoskeletal system, and it should be noted that the muscle weakness and atrophy that can lead to sarcopenia, appears as a cause of falls and fractures in the elderly [4].

Recent studies demonstrate that the early implementation of rehabilitation protocols based on progressive balance exercises, postural correction, resistance and gait training, contribute to prevent functional and cognitive decline associated with aging and/or immobility, with consequent decrease of the risk of falling [5]. Given the multifactorial nature of this type of incident, scientific studies show that an intervention that promotes the control of intrinsic and extrinsic risk factors is more effective when compared to the implementation of a single intervention, contributing to the reduction of the prevalence of falls in the elderly, either in context of hospitalization or in the community [1, 2, 6].

An approach centered on rehabilitation programs and control of risk factors for falls seems to contribute to several benefits, namely, increased autonomy and independence in carrying out activities of daily living, improving quality of life, lower incidence of isolation and depression, reduction length of stay, reduction of costs associated with medications, consultations, hospitalizations, rehabilitation processes [2, 6].

The rehabilitation nurse, a professional with a set of specific skills aimed at promoting health and preventing complications, is a fundamental health professional for the implementation of contributory programs to reduce the risk of falling for the elderly.

2 Method

Systematic literature review that included the formulation of a research question, research in scientific databases, the identification of inclusion and exclusion criteria, the selection of studies, the analysis and interpretation of the selected studies and the synthesis of the results obtained. For the formulation of the research question, the PICO mnemonic was used, (P) Population, (I) Intervention, (C) Comparison and (O) Results (outcomes). The research question formulated, which appears as a guide for this review, and which aims to answer the outlined objective, was the following: What are the rehabilitation nurse interventions (Interventions) that contribute to the prevention of falls (Results) in elderly people and/or with mobility changes (Population).

The research strategy, carried out independently by three authors, included the selection of studies published between January 2015 and December 2020 in the CINAHL Complete and Pubmed databases, and used the following keywords: fall, falls, fall prevention, falls prevention, rehabilitation, rehab, rehabilitation nursing, elder, elderly, seniors, old, older, hospitalized, hospitalization. Institutionalized, internment and interned. The descriptors were connected using the Boolean operators "AND" and "OR", in the following arrangement: "fall" OR "falls" OR "fall prevention" OR "falls prevention" AND "rehabilitation" OR "rehab" OR "rehabilitation nursing" AND "elder" OR "elderly" OR "seniors" OR "old" OR "older" AND "hospitalized" OR "hospitalization" OR "institutionalized" OR "internment" OR "interned".

The inclusion criteria defined for this review consisted of: Studies with people aged 18 years or older; Studies with people with contributory deficits for a greater risk of falling (elderly and/or with mobility changes); Studies that evaluate results of interventions recognized as rehabilitation nursing competence. The following studies were excluded: Studies whose methodology proved to be ambiguous and without correlation with the objective of the study; Studies with children under 18; Studies with people without contributory deficits for a higher risk of falls.

In the initial search, 2,048 results were identified, specifically, CINAHL Complete (n = 57) and PubMed (n = 1991), ordered by relevance or best match. Among these, there were 9 duplicates. The evaluation of the remaining 2039 results, carried out independently by three authors, was carried out in two phases. In the first, the titles and abstracts were read, which allowed the identification of 38 studies with potential interest

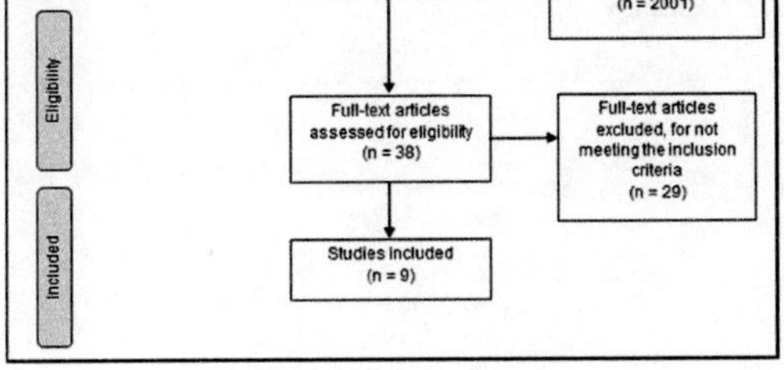

Fig. 1. PRISMA fluxogram

for the review. In the second phase the selected articles were read in full, the inclusion and exclusion criteria were applied, and the analysis of the levels of evidence and methodological quality was carried out, allowing the identification of 9 studies.

The evaluation of the levels of scientific evidence was carried out according to the levels of evidence of The Joanna Briggs Institute (2014) and the methodological quality was analyzed based on the Critical Appraisal Skills Program [7, 8]. The levels of evidence and methodological quality are shown in Table 1 (Fig. 1).

Table 1. Classification of selected studies according to the level of evidence and methodological quality

Study	Level of evidence	Methodological quality
Exercise for falls prevention in Parkinson disease A randomized controlled trial	1.c Randomized controlled trial	Level A
Fall rates in hospital rehabilitation units after individualized patient and staff education programmes: a pragmatic, stepped-wedge, cluster-randomised controlled trial	1.c Randomized controlled trial	Level A
Exercise and Vitamin D in Fall Prevention Among Older Women A Randomized Clinical Trial	1.c Randomized controlled trial	Level A
Reducing falls among older people in general practice: The ProAct65 + exercise intervention trial	1.c Randomized controlled trial	Level A
CoDuSe group exercise programme improves balance and reduces falls in people with multiple sclerosis	1.c Randomized controlled trial	Level A
A Randomized Controlled Trial of Screening, Risk Modification and Physical Therapy to Prevent Falls among the Elderly Recently Discharged from the Emergency Department to the Community: the Steps to Avoid Falls in the Elderly Study	1.c Randomized controlled trial	Level A

(*continued*)

Table 1. *(continued)*

Study	Level of evidence	Methodological quality
Dual-Task Exercise Reduces Cognitive-Motor Interference in Walking and Falls After Stroke: A Randomized Controlled Study	1.c Randomized controlled trial	Level A
Effect of Exercise Intervention on Functional Decline in Very Elderly Patients During Acute Hospitalization: A Randomized Clinical Trial	1.c Randomized controlled trial	Level A
Surface Perturbation Training to Prevent Falls in Older Adults: A Highly Pragmatic, Randomized Controlled Trial	1.c Randomized controlled trial	Level A

3 Results

The results obtained after analyzing the selected studies are presented in a table format (Table 2) to facilitate and simplify their reading and interpretation. For each study, a survey was carried out about the year, authors, country, participants, objective, interventions, results, conclusions and limitations. All selected articles are Randomized Controlled Trials, with an evidence level of 1.c., according to The Joanna Briggs Institute, and with level A methodological quality, according to the Critical Appraisal Skills Program for randomized controlled trials [8].

The nine selected articles are from different countries, namely Australia (Canning et al., 2015; Hill et al., 2015) [9, 10], China (Pang et al., 2018) [11], Finland (Uusi-Rasi et al., 2015) [12], Singapore (Matchar et al., 2017) [13], Spain (Martínez-Velilla et al., 2019) [14], Sweden (Carling et al., 2017) [15], United Kingdom (Gawler et al., 2016) [16] and United States of America (Lurie et al., 2020) [17]. Samples vary between 51 and 3606 participants, with the average age of participants included in the studies being above 65 years old (elderly population). Only exceptions are found in the study by Pang et al. (2018), in which the average age was 61.2 years [11], and in the study by Carling et al. (2017), in which the average age was 58 years, which includes participants with mobility deficits due to specific pathologies, respectively, Stroke and Multiple Sclerosis (MS) [15]. The study by Canning et al. (2015) also includes participants with a specific pathology, in this case Parkinson's disease [9]. Study shelves integrate interventions aimed at the elderly population, without specific associated pathology. It should be noted that despite the study by Hill et al. (2015) include people aged 60 or over, has an average age of 81.75 years and considers their conclusions to be generalizable to the elderly population [10].

Table 2. Synthesis of data extracted from selected studies.

Author's (year)/Sample	Objectives/Interventions	Results/Conclusions
Canning et al. (2015) [9] Patients with Parkinson's disease, aged ≥40 years, able to walk and live in the community (n = 231). Mean age: 71 years	Analyze if falls in people with Parkinson's disease can be avoided through a program of balance exercises, muscle strength of the lower limbs and strategies to reduce freezing gait Control Group: Usual care and fall prevention leaflet. Intervention Group: Program with 40–60 min personalized and progressive balance exercises, strengthening of the lower limbs and strategies to reduce gait freezing	There was a significant decrease in falls in the subgroup with mild disease in the intervention group ($p \leq 0.001$). The intervention group showed improvements in physical performance, sitting/standing, fear of falling and quality of life. A program of balance exercises, strength of the lower limbs and strategies to reduce freezing of gait, improves the physical and psychological health and reduces the fall in people with mild illness
Hill et al. (2015) [10] Patients admitted to a rehabilitation center, age ≥60 years (n = 3606). Mean age: 81.75 years	Evaluate the effectiveness of an individualized program for the prevention of falls of the elderly admitted to rehabilitation units Control Group (n = 1982): Usual care. Intervention Group (n = 1623): Individualized program based on behavioral changes, increased knowledge about the epidemiology of falls and fall prevention, alert for individual risk of falls, and prevention strategies	The intervention group had fewer falls and harmful falls The implementation of individualized education programs for the elderly admitted to hospital rehabilitation units, combined with training and feedback from health professionals reduces the rate of falls and falls with injuries
Uusi-Rasi et al. (2015) [12] Women between 70 and 80 years old, living in a household (n = 409). Mean age: 74.2 years	Determine the effectiveness of physical training and vitamin D supplementation in reducing falls and harmful falls in elderly women Control Group: Without exercise and taking a placebo. Exercise Group + Vit. D: 800 IU Vitamine D tablet + progressive training of balance, strengthening, bearings, functional and agility exercises, supervised twice a week (12 months), and then once a week (more 12 months) + home training program. Exercise Group: Same as the previous but taking a placebo tablet. Vitamine D Group: 800 IU Vitamine D tablet	The Exercise and Exercise + Vitamine D groups had a number of falls with significantly lower injuries The physical exercise group showed improvement in muscle strength and balance. The Vitamine D did not increase the benefits of exercise on physical ability. The rate of falls with injury decreased significantly through strength, mobility and balance training in elderly women living at home. When considering the number of falls, the result was not significantly different between groups Exercise improves physical capacity

(*continued*)

Table 2. (*continued*)

Author's (year)/Sample	Objectives/Interventions	Results/Conclusions
Gawler et al. (2016) [16] People aged ≥65 years, living in the community, inactive, with ≤3 falls in the last year and without significant cognitive impairment (n = 1256). Mean age: 73 years	Evaluate the effectiveness of a home exercise program (OEP) and a group exercise program (Fame) in comparison with usual care, in reducing falls and injuries resulting from falls Control Group (n = 458): Usual care. Grupo Fame (n = 387): Exercises aimed at improving strength and balance, for 1h with supervision, once a week, complemented with a home program of 30 min, twice a week. Implemented over 24 weeks. OEP Group (n = 411): Home exercise program for 30 min, 3 times a week, implemented in 24 weeks	Fame Group showed a significant reduction in the number of falls ($p = 0.04$) and harmful falls ($p = 0.04$) up to 12 months after the end of the intervention. The OEP Group showed a reduction in the number of falls that was not significant up to 12 months after the intervention ($p = 0.14$). These benefits were not seen at 24 months after the end of the intervention. Participants who maintained the exercises maintained the benefits of reducing falls ($p = 0.004$)
Carling et al. (2017) [15] People with Multiple Sclerosis, age ≥18 years, transfer capacity and gait up to 200 m (n = 51). Mean age: 58 years	Evaluate the effects of a group balance exercise program Control Group (n = 26): Usual care. Intervention Group (n = 25): Individualized program (small groups) and balance exercises that includes controlled leg movements, dual task (carrying something while walking) and sensory stimulation, with 2 sessions per week of 60 min, for 7 weeks; Home exercise program (2 to 5 exercises)	The intervention group showed significant improvements in balance ($p = 0.015$), gait ($p = 0.051$) and showed a statistically significant reduction in falls ($p \leq 0.01$) and near falls ($p \leq 0.04$) The implementation of the program has led to an improvement in balance and gait limitations, also contributing to the reduction of falls and near falls
Matchar et al. (2017) [13] Patients over 64 years who resorted to fall urgency or fall injuries, discharged home and expected recovery (n = 354). Mean age: 77.8 years	Evaluate the effectiveness of a personalized multifactorial physical activity program to reduce the occurrence of falls in high-risk elderly people Control Group (n = 177): Usual care and educational material for the prevention of falls. Intervention Group (n = 177): Personalized and progressive training of strength, balance (static and dynamic) and gait, for 3 months	The intervention group showed a statistically significant reduction in harmful falls ($p = 0.041$) and deterioration in physical functionality ($p = 0.029$). Although the intervention group had a lower number of falls, it was not statistically significant ($p = 0.146$). People with less than 2 severe comorbidities, there was a significant decrease in falls in the intervention group ($p = 0.002$) The difference in the number of falls was not significant between groups

(*continued*)

Table 2. (*continued*)

Author's (year)/Sample	Objectives/Interventions	Results/Conclusions
Pang et al. (2018) [11] People with stroke for more than 6 months, mild to moderate motor impairment, walking ability ≥10 m, age ≥50 years and living in the community (n = 240). Mean age: 61.2 years	Evaluate the effects of dual-task exercises on people with stroke Control Group: exercises of the upper limbs. Single Task Group: Balance training with single task mobility. Dual Task Group: Balance and mobility training with dual task. Mobility tasks (walking, time-up-and-go and crossing obstacles, timed) are associated with cognitive tasks (naming category words and sequential subtractions)	The double-task group showed improvement in walking capacity with double-task, reduced risk of falling ($p = 0.037$) and harmful falls ($p = 0.023$) during the entire follow-up. The single-task group had a lower number of falls than the control group, but it was not statistically significant. The benefits obtained in the intervention group were maintained after 8 weeks of intervention. The dual-task program improved mobility in the performance of several tasks simultaneously, reducing the risk of falls and injuries related to falls
Martínez-Velilla et al. (2019) [14] Elderly hospitalized over 75 years old, capable of walking and without cognitive impairment (n = 370). Mean age: 87.3 years	Assess the effects of an exercise-based intervention on the functionality of the target population Control Group: Usual care with rehabilitation when necessary. Intervention Group: Individualized resistance exercises, balance and moderate intensity walking, 2 daily sessions of 20 min., 5 to 7 consecutive days. Average duration of intervention: 5 days	Hospitalization led to a decline in the functional capacity of the elderly, which was less evident in the intervention group where there was a statistically significant improvement in functional capacity and quality of life ($p \leq 0.001$). There were no statistically significant differences in length of stay, number of falls and mortality in the 3 months after discharge ($p \geq 0.10$). The implementation of an individualized exercise program results in a significant benefit contributing to reverse the functional decline associated with hospitalization

(*continued*)

Table 2. *(continued)*

Author's (year)/Sample	Objectives/Interventions	Results/Conclusions
Lurie et al. (2020) [17] People over 65 years old, with a high risk of falling, indication of gait and balance training (n = 506). Mean age: 78 years	Compare the effectiveness of adding a surface disturbance training to gait and balance training, in reducing falls and injuries in high-risk elderly people Control Group (n = 253): Usual balance training. Intervention Group (n = 253): Treadmill training with surface disturbances integrated in the usual balance training. Individualized and progressive training of 45 min, 2–3 weekly sessions for 4–6 weeks Both groups with strengthening exercises, flexibility, postural correction, static and dynamic balance, mobility training, health education, indications for home training programs to be performed 4–5 times a week	Both groups showed significant improvements in balance, mobility and confidence in balance, with a reduction in the risk of falling and injuries associated with it. But without significant differences between them After 3 months, the intervention group significantly reduced the probability of suffering injuries associated with falling ($p \leq 0.01$) The addition of a surface disturbance training to gait and balance training significantly reduces falls injuries up to 3 months of treatment

4 Discussion

When analyzing the selected studies, it was found that balance training and gait training are fundamental in preventing falls, as these are part of all studies, with the exception of the study by Hill et al. (2015), where the effectiveness of health education is assessed [10]. The performance of lower limb strengthening exercises is also present in several studies [9, 12, 13, 16, 17]. These findings are corroborated by the American Geriatrics Society and British Geriatrics Society (2011) once in the guidelines for the prevention of falls in the elderly, it states that all interventions for this purpose must include balance, gait and training exercises of strength, such as rehabilitation, which can be developed in group or individual programs [18]. Cadore (2013) also found that balance, strength and gait training contribute not only to reducing falls in the elderly, but also to improve their balance and muscle mass [5].

According to the study developed by Alves et al. (2016), the main reason for falls in the hospitalized elderly is weakness and disturbances in balance and gait (46.7%), so interventions aimed at their improvement appear as essential to reduce the risk of falling [19].

American Geriatrics Society and British Geriatrics Society (2011) state that balance training can be applied as a single intervention when the number of falls is to be reduced [18]. On the other hand, resistance training [12, 14] and flexibility [17] may appear as a complement to the remaining exercises, but there is no evidence of their effectiveness as unique components of a program [18]. This was a factor taken into account in the aforementioned studies, given that their interventions integrate other types of exercises.

A study by Cadore et al. (2013), who intended to evaluate the effects of balance training, muscle strength and gait regardig the risk of falling and functionality in institutionalized nonagenarian elderly people, found a significant improvement in balance, strength, muscle mass, and execution capacity simple and double-task, and a reduction in the incidence of falls [5]. The studies by Pang et al. (2018) and Carling et al. (2017) ascertained the benefits associated with dual-task training, finding a reduction in the number of falls, harmful falls and near falls in the intervention groups [11, 15].

In the study Lurie et al. (2020), where all participants performed balance training exercises, muscle strengthening, flexibility, postural correction and health education, there was a significant reduction in the risk of falling and associated injuries, as well as a significant improvement in balance and confidence in balance [17]. In this case, the intervention group performed gait training with surface disturbances, obtaining a significant reduction in the probability of suffering injuries from falling, after 3 months of implementation [17].

In the studies Canning et al. (2015) and Matchar et al. (2017), when considering the entire population, there was no significant reduction in falls. However, when considering only participants with mild Parkinson's Disease [9, 13], and people with less than 2 severe co-morbidities [13], a significant reduction in the number of falls is observed.

The reduction in the number of falls in the intervention group, analyzed in all studies, was statistically significant in several studies [10, 11, 15, 17]. In addition to analyzing the number of falls, some studies assessed the number of harmful falls, with a statistically significant reduction in all intervention groups [10, 13, 16, 17]. In this sense, in the studies by Uusi-Rasi et al. (2015) and Matchar et al. (2017), there was a statistically significant decrease in harmful falls, although the same does not occur when considering the totality of falls, which may allow considering that a better physical condition prevents the occurrence of consequent injuries [12, 13].

When considering the study by Martínez-Velilla et al. (2019), where the interventions adopted were based solely on the physical component, there was no significant reduction in the number of falls among participants in the different groups [14]. Even so, it should be noted that the exercises included in this study (resistance training, balance and gait) contributed to a smaller decline in the functionality of the elderly associated with hospitalization, obtaining a better quality of life and cognitive function in the intervention group. The authors also found that bed rest, often related to hospitalization processes, is closely related to muscle atrophy, decreased strength and physical function, namely in the ascending/descending stairs, transfers and walking, with consequent impairment of functionality of the elderly [14].

In the study Uusi-Rasi et al. (2015), although there was a reduction in falls in groups with physical exercise, this value was not statistically significant; possibly this result may be due to the fact that the study only included people with a history of falling in the year prior to its realization, that is, it only included people already alone with a very high risk of falling [12].

Another possible justification for the statistically non-significant results obtained in the studies by Martínez-Velilla et al. (2019) and Uusi-Rasi et al. (2015) consists in the fact that they do not include a multifactorial approach to the fall [12, 14]. Given the multifactorial nature of the fall, many studies show that health education focused on the control of intrinsic and extrinsic risk factors, proves to be an asset [9, 10, 13, 16, 18]. Also, the National Institute for Health and care Excellence (2013), considers a multifactorial intervention fundamental, where the guidelines for the prevention of fall include not only strength and balance exercises, but also the assessment and control of environmental factors, visual acuity and habitual medication [20]. Teaching should be an integral part of hospital discharge planning, highlighting the importance of the health professional in contributing to the control of risk factors identified at home, in order to promote safety in performing daily life activities, and also a review of basic therapy, with special attention to people who take 4 or more medications, namely psychoactive medications or which may cause postural hypotension [2, 18].

The control of intrinsic and extrinsic risk factors for falls can be considered as a primary or secondary prevention, however they state that there is no evidence of their individual contribution in the prevention of falls [18]. On the other hand, when considering Hill et al. (2015) whose approach was based solely on health education, in which he intended to assess the effectiveness of an individualized education program for the prevention of falls, involving not only the participant but also the health professionals, with feedback occurring among them, there was a significant reduction in the number of falls and falls with injury [10].

The analysis of the nine selected articles also made it possible to verify that the benefits of implementing the interventions addressed are multiple, not restricted to the prevention of falls. In the intervention groups, there were gains in functional capacity [9, 13, 14], quality of life [9, 14], improvements in balance [12, 15, 17], mobility and gait [9, 11, 14, 17], Cadore (2013), when carrying out studies that aimed to determine the effectiveness and safety of the application of a protocol of strength and mobility exercises, found that the intervention group showed significant improvements in functional performance, balance, walking speed and ability to sit/stand [5].

The studies by Canning et al. (2015) and Lurie et al. (2020) also showed statistically significant improvements in the intervention groups regarding the fear of falling, and this is considered by itself only a risk factor for falling [9, 17]. American Geriatrics Society and British Geriatrics Society (2011) refer to the existence of several studies that reveal the benefits of balance training not only in reducing falls, but also in improving gait, balance and reducing the fear of falling [18]. However, it emphasizes the need to ensure safety in the implementation of exercises, given that other studies reveal an increase in the rate of falls in people with limited mobility [18].

With regard to the frequency with which rehabilitation programs are implemented, it appears that the majority of studies carried out have a minimum of 2 to 3 weekly sessions [9, 11, 13, 15, 17], sometimes complemented with exercises performed at home [12, 13, 15, 17]. This evidence is in accordance with the recommendations of the American Geriatrics Society and British Geriatrics Society (2011), which suggests carrying out training programs 2 to 3 times a week, with 3 sets of 8 to 12 repetitions per exercise [18]. These programs tend to be personalized and implemented progressively [9, 12, 17]. American Geriatrics Society and British Geriatrics Society (2011) advise the fitness and personalization of the exercises according to the physical condition and health of the people, to avoid increased health risks, namely the fall [18]. The implementation of personalized interventions that consider the needs, preferences and capacities of people, and that realistically integrate the available resources, can contribute to a better adherence to the program, further increasing the probability of continuing it [1].

The studies by Gawler et al. (2016) and Lurie et al. (2020) emphasize that only the continuity of physical activity allows to maintain the benefits achieved with the implementation of rehabilitation programs [16, 17]. When analyzing these studies, it appears that both intervention groups showed a reduction in the number of falls and/or harmful falls until a short period of time after the end of the intervention; after a long period (12 to 24 months), these benefits have not been maintained [17]. The study by Gawler et al. (2016) also found that the people who continued to perform the recommended exercises, maintained the gains obtained after 24 months [17]. WHO (2007) also warns of the need to continue the rehabilitation programs implemented, as their benefits in terms of improving quality of life and decreasing the risk of falling are only maintained if the elderly understand that the adoption of healthy behaviors will contribute to your independence and longevity [1]. These behaviors, which include physical activity and the control of intrinsic and extrinsic risk factors, must be incorporated into your routine, constituting a behavioral change in favor of your well-being and autonomy [1].

According to the National Institute for Health and care Excellence (2013), elderly people who report falls in the last year, who resort to health care due to falls, or who have changes in gait and/or balance, should be properly evaluated by a health professional with the necessary knowledge and skills, in order to obtain an individual and multifactorial fall assessment, looking for modification, improvement or control of risk factors [20]. It should be noted that any of the interventions previously identified as a way to prevent falls are in the domain of the rehabilitation nurse competences.

5 Conclusion

After analyzing the selected studies it was found that several interventions in the domain of rehabilitation nurse skills contribute to reducing the risk of falling in elderly people or those with mobility disorders. Among these interventions, the following stand out: the assessment and identification of the risk of falling, the implementation of motor re-education programs (based on balance training, gait training, muscle strengthening, and may also integrate other modalities such as double-task, disorders of the surface, resistance training and flexibility), identification and control of intrinsic and extrinsic risk factors for falls, health education for the person at risk and their significant persons.

The rehabilitation nurse, as a professional endowed with a set of specific skills with technical and scientific knowledge that allows the implementation of all the interventions, appears to be the professional of choice to carry out the assessment and identification of people at high risk of falling. The harmful consequences of the fall are multiple, namely limb injuries, fractures, the need for health care, hospitalization, increased levels of dependence and institutionalization, or even death. The fall is recognized as a public health problem with serious consequences both at a personal and family level, as well as at a social and financial level, with high costs associated with health. Thus, the involvement of health professionals in the search for a solution to this problem is fundamental.

The reduction of the risk of falling requires an intervention that involves several factors, and that a single factor approach does not allow to achieve the intended results. In this way, a motor reeducation program aimed at decreasing the fall and its consequences should involve the different types of exercises mentioned above, where balance training is essential. It is also up to the rehabilitation nurse to carefully analyze what type of exercises should prescribe for each individual according to their physical capacity and health status, given that their inadequacy may result in greater health risks and also an increased risk of falling. As such, the implementation of personalized and progressive interventions appears to be fundamental in the exercise of your profession.

Given the multifactorial nature of the fall, when it is intended to contribute to its reduction, there must be a thorough study of the intrinsic and extrinsic risk factors inherent to each individual, in order to identify those that can be controlled or changed by the health professional and/or person at risk. In several situations, this control or alteration, namely with regard to extrinsic risk factors, requires the commitment and acceptance on the part of the individual, so that the realization of health education sessions appear as a fundamental component. The aim of these sessions is to make people aware of the risks inherent to falls and to enable them to adopt strategies that contribute to their reduction, namely the use of appropriate footwear, avoiding places with low light or uneven floors, using bars support, use of glasses and hearing aid whenever there are visual or auditory deficits, adequacy of medication and respective schedules, among others.

With the implementation of the aforementioned interventions, it is expected not only to reduce the number of falls, harmful falls and near falls, but also to improve muscle strength, balance, walking capacity, with benefits in terms of functionality and autonomy in performing daily life activities. Improving the quality of life of individuals. It is also important to note that all these mentioned benefits only last in time if the person continues to perform the proposed training and maintains the care inherent in the control of intrinsic and extrinsic risk factors for falls.

References

1. World Health Organization: WHO global report on falls prevention in older age, pp. 1–47 (2007). https://extranet.who.int/agefriendlyworld/wp-content/uploads/2014/06/WHo-Global-report-on-falls-prevention-in-older-age.pdf
2. Falsarella, G., Gasparotto, L., Coimbra, A.: Quedas: conceitos, frequências e aplicações à assistência ao idoso. Revi. Lit. Rev. Bras. Geriatr. Gerontol. **17**(4), 897–910 (2014). https://doi.org/10.1590/1809-9823.2014.13064
3. Bittencourt, V., Graube, S., Stumm, E., Battisti, I., Loro, M., Winkelmann, E.: Fatores associados ao risco de quedas em pacientes adultos hospitalizados. Rev. Esc. Enferm. USP **51**, e03237 (2017). https://doi.org/10.1590/S1980-220X2016037403237
4. Esquenazi, D., Silva, S., Guimarães, M.: Aspectos fisiopatológicos do envelhecimento humano e quedas em idosos. Rev. HUPE **13**(2), 11–20 (2014). https://doi.org/10.12957/rhupe.2014.10124
5. Cadore, E.L., et al.: Multicomponent exercises including muscle power training enhance muscle mass, power output, and functional outcomes in institutionalized frail nonagenarians. Age **36**(2), 773–785 (2013). https://doi.org/10.1007/s11357-013-9586-z
6. Abreu, H., Reiners, A., Azevedo, R., Silva, A., Abreu, D., Oliveira, A.: Incidência e fatores preditores de queda em idosos hospitalizados. Rev. Saúde Pública **49**(37), 1–8 (2015). https://doi.org/10.1590/S0034-8910.2015049005549

7. Aromataris, E., Munn, Z.: Chapter 1: JBI systematic reviews. In: Aromataris, E., Munn, Z. (eds.) JBI Manual for Evidence Synthesis. The Joanna Briggs Institute (2020). https://doi.org/10.46658/JBIMES-20-01
8. Levels of Evidence of the Joanna Briggs Institute (2014). https://jbi.global/sites/default/files/2019-05/JBI-Levels-of-evidence_2014_0.pdf
9. Canning, C., et al.: Exercise for falls prevention in Parkinson disease: a randomized controlled trial. Neurology **84**(3), 304–312 (2015). https://doi.org/10.1212/WNL.0000000000001155
10. Hill, A., et al.: Fall rates in hospital rehabilitation units after individualised patient and staff education programmes: a pragmatic, stepped-wedge, cluster-randomised controlled trial. Lancet **385**(9987), 2592–2599 (2015). https://doi.org/10.1016/S0140-6736(14)61945-0
11. Pang, M., Yang, L., Ouyang, H., Lam, F., Huang, M., Jehu, D.: Dual-task exercise reduces cognitive-motor interference in walking and falls after stroke: a randomized controlled study. Stroke **49**(12), 2990–2998 (2018). https://doi.org/10.1016/S0140-6736(14)61945-0
12. Uusi-Rasi, K., et al.: Exercise and vitamin D in fall prevention among older women: randomized clinical trial. JAMA Intern. Med. **178**(5), 703–711 (2015). https://doi.org/10.1001/jamainternmed.2015.0225
13. Matchar, D., et al.: A randomized controlled trial of screening, risk modification and physical therapy to prevent falls among the elderly recently discharged from the emergency department to the community: the steps to avoid falls in the elderly study. Arch. Phys. Med. Rehabil. **98**(6), 1086–1096 (2017). https://doi.org/10.1016/j.apmr.2017.01.014
14. Martínez-Velilla, N., et al.: Effect of exercise intervention on functional decline in very elderly patients during acute hospitalization: randomized clinical trial. JAMA Intern. Med. **179**(1), 28–36 (2019). https://doi.org/10.1001/jamainternmed.2018.4869
15. Carling, A., Forsberg, A., Gunnarsson, M., Nilsagard, Y.: CoDuSe group exercise programme improves balance and reduces falls in people with multiple sclerosis: a multi-centre, randomized, controlled pilot study. Mult. Scler. **23**(10), 1394–1404 (2017). https://doi.org/10.1177/1352458516677591
16. Gawler, S., et al.: Reducing falls among older people in general practice: the ProAct65+ exercise intervention trial. Arch. Gerontol. Geriatr. **67**, 46–54 (2016). https://doi.org/10.1016/j.archger.2016.06.019
17. Lurie, J., et al.: Surface perturbation training to prevent falls in older adults: a highly pragmatic, randomized controlled trial. Phys. Ther. **100**(7), 1153–1162 (2020). https://doi.org/10.1093/ptj/pzaa023
18. American Geriatrics Society, British Geriatrics Society: Summary of the updated American geriatrics society/British geriatrics society clinical practice guideline for prevention of falls in older persons. J. Am. Geriatr. Soc. **59**(1), 148–157 (2011). https://doi.org/10.1111/j.1532-5415.2010.03234.x
19. Alves, A., Patrício, A., Albuquerque, K.: Ocorrência de quedas entre idosos institucionalizados: prevalência, causas e consequências. RPCFO **8**(2), 4376–4386 (2016). https://doi.org/10.9789/2175-5361.2016.v8i2.4376-4386
20. National Institute for Health and care Excellence. https://www.nice.org.uk/guidance/cg161/resources/falls-in-older-people-assessing-risk-and-prevention-pdf-35109686728645

Surveillance and Fall Prevention in the Elderly

João André[1], Maria Margarida Goes[2], Henrique Oliveira[2,3](✉), João Vítor Vieira[2], and Margarida Santos[4]

[1] Hospital José Joaquim Fernandes, Beja, Portugal
[2] Polytechnic Institute of Beja, Beja, Portugal
[3] Telecommunications Institute, Lisbon, Portugal
hjmo@lx.it.pt
[4] Salt Clinic Center, Póvoa de Varzim, Portugal

Abstract. Falls in the elderly are one of the main causes of death that occur in this population group and there are multiple factors that can contribute to this, greatly affecting their autonomy and quality of life. Therefore, nursing interventions are essential to prevent this type of event. **Objective:** Evaluate the efficiency of external hip protectors on preventing falls in the elderly people. **Methodology:** Integrative Literature Review, using the PICO methodology, which included the formulation of an initial research question, research in scientific databases, analysis and interpretation of selected articles, as well as the synthesis and presentation of the results obtained. This review also considered the PRISMA (Preferred Reporting Items for Systematic Reviews and Meta-Analyses) recommendation. The queries were performed under the "CINAHL Complete" database. **Results:** With the methodology applied, a final set of six studies were obtained, which do not sustain the efficiency of external hip protectors on the prevention of falls in the elderly. **Conclusion:** There is no scientific evidence that the external hip protectors are beneficial in reducing the number of falls in the elderly people. Focused interventions in many risk factors are more advantageous, comparatively to simple interventions. It is suggested the realization of more research studies relatively to this topic.

Keywords: External hip protectors · Falls · Prevention · Elderly · Nursing interventions

1 Introduction

Human aging corresponds to a slow, gradual and an inevitable process leading to several morphological, functional, biochemical and psychological changes, which can contribute to the increased vulnerability and incidence of chronic diseases. The chronic diseases can be silent or symptomatic, compromising the quality of life as well as the functional and cognitive capacity of the elderly, often leading to acute episodes of their health condition, usually associated with cardiac, respiratory and cerebrovascular problems or falls-related injuries [1]. Falls are one of the main causes of death in the elderly population. Falls are considered an unintentional movement of the body to a lower position than the initial one, with multifactorial causes, which affect postural stability and

J. García-Alonso and C. Fonseca (Eds.): IWoG 2021, LNBE, pp. 355–365, 2022.
https://doi.org/10.1007/978-3-030-97524-1_33

consequently the autonomy of the elderly, as well as their quality of life [2]. On the other hand, falls also has negative psychological effects on the elderly, causing them to feel ashamed, to lose confidence in themselves and, consequently, to potentiate their fears.

The family caregivers, in turn, also suffer from this event, as they start to ensure a significant part of the care that the dependents need, which of them are of great complexity and intensity. This entire situation requires some readjustment of the family dynamics, leading to an increase of its emotional, physical and economic burden.

In preventing falls, several risk factors must be considered, as the disability caused by the event will influence the family environment of the elderly, due to the levels of dependence that will arise when the functional limitations occur. This topic should be considered as a public health problem, and it will be increasingly necessary to implement measures aiming to reduce the occurrence of falls in the elderly population.

According to [3], to promote the prevention of falls, it is essential to consider the complexity of the several factors that involves this type of event and not to devaluate the independence capacity of the elderly to perform their activities of daily living (ADL). The same author also states that financial investments are the "engine" for preventive measures to be implemented in the context of falls, with the aim of preserving the functional capacity of the elderlies and allowing a better quality of their lives.

2 Objective

To evaluate the effectiveness of external hip protectors in the prevention of falls in the elderly.

3 Methods

3.1 Ethical Aspects

This is a secondary study for which the Ethics Committee has not been asked for an opinion. The formulation of the problem fulfilled the principles of clarity, precision, objectivity, allowing the results to be assumed as a contribution to nursing care, with benefits for the elderly in a hospital context. The extraction and analysis of data from the studies used were developed in defense of the principle of respect for the results obtained by these researchers. The referencing of the authors met the standards of good academic and scientific practice.

3.2 Type of Study

An integrative literature review was chosen, with the purpose of knowing the "state of the art", about the research topic and, therefore, to contribute to the understanding and incorporation of the findings of this study in clinical practice. The methodological procedures used involved the following steps: 1) formulation of the research question; 2) definition of inclusion and exclusion criteria of the studies; 3) definition of the information to be extracted from the studies; 4) evaluation of the included articles; 5) presentation and discussion of the results and 6) synthesis of the knowledge found.

3.3 Methodological Procedures

For the selection of articles and formulation of the research question, the PI[C]OD methodology was used: Target population (P); intervention (I); comparison (C); outcome - *outcome* (O); and type of study - *design* (D). The formulation of the research question serves as a guideline during the integrative literature review to achieve the previously established objective. For this reason, the following question was formulated: "In the *public hospital* patients, is there evidence to suggest that external hip protectors *(intervention)* can contribute to a reduction in the risk of falls *(outcomes)?"*.

The EBSCOhost platform was the chosen support platform for the implementation of the previously formulated question and subsequent collection of the respective scientific publications. The search terms used were: *"elderly", "aged", "older", "elder", "geriatric", "falls prevention", "preventing falls", "prevent falls", "reduce falls", "hip protectors", "hip pads", "hip savers"* and *"hip protective underwear"*. Using the use *Boolean operators "AND"* and *"OR"*, the descriptors (search terms) were organized as follows:

"[(elderly) OR (aged) OR (older) OR (elder) OR (geriatric)] AND [(falls prevention) OR (preventing falls) OR (prevent falls) OR (reduce falls)] AND [(hip protectors) OR (hip pads) OR (hip savers) OR (hip protective underwear)]"

As for the inclusion criteria, articles in which the methodology focused on the research theme considered in this article were chosen, in order to answer the formulated research question, those published in scientific journals and peer-reviewed, with availability of full text, written in full in English or Portuguese languages, published between January 2009 and March 2019, available in the CINAHL Complete database.

Twenty-six articles were identified, where 7 of them were eliminated from the list because they were considered duplicates, resulting in a total of 19 articles. For the selection of the articles, it was necessary to interpret the title and the respective abstract, to understand if they met the inclusion and exclusion criteria. Furthermore, if the subject of the article was not clear, it was read in full, so that no article on the list that answered the research question was excluded. Thus, the process of selecting the articles was organized according to two phases: (i) 1st phase, it was based on reading the titles and their abstracts, in which 8 articles were chosen, as the others were excluded because they did not present any relationship with the topic under discussion; (ii) 2nd phase, they were read in full, resulting in a final set comprising 6 scientific publications (see Fig. 1).

For an in-depth and critical analysis of the methodological quality of the selected articles, they were evaluated based on the levels of evidence of Centre for Evidence – Based *Medicine* [4].

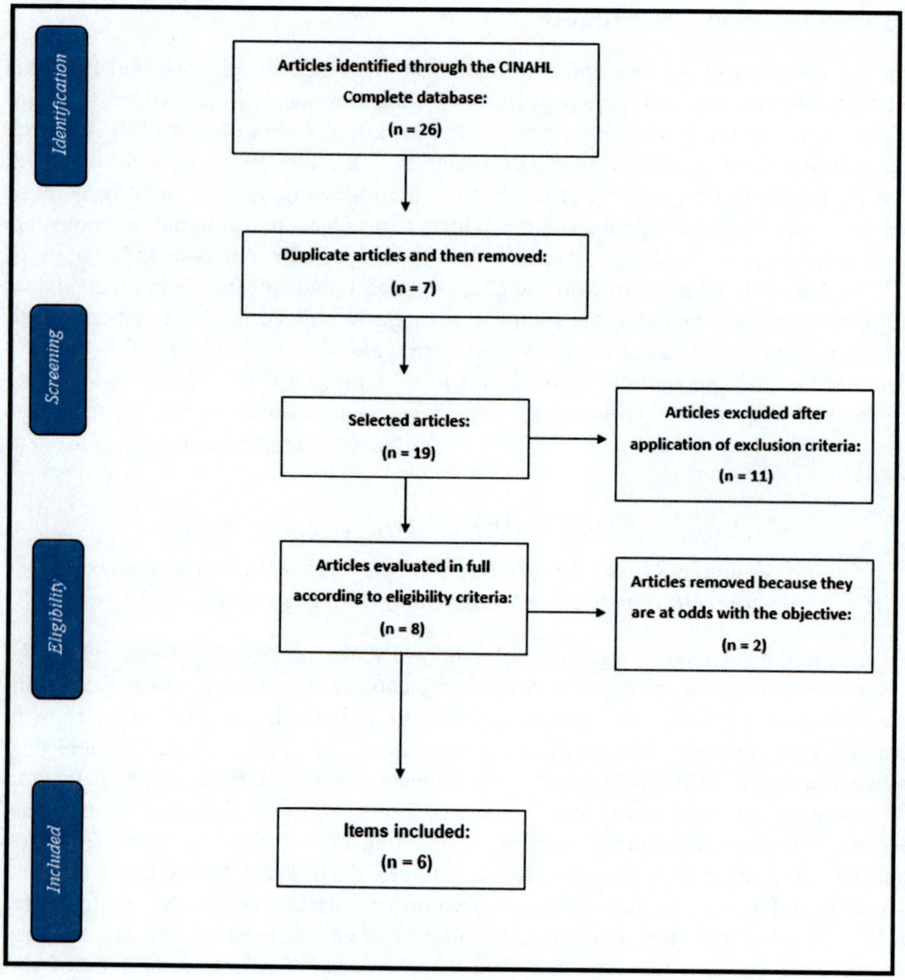

Fig. 1. PRISM flow diagram.

4 Results

After the analysis of the selected articles, the results of the integrative literature review are presented in Table 1.

5 Discussion

After analyzing the chosen articles, we highlight the lack of scientific evidence on which interventions that in fact prevent falls, in particular the one that addresses the use of external hip protectors. This topic has been studied by researchers and a right and uniform answer has not yet been found, so this topic should be the subject to further studies.

Table 1. Results of the integrative literature review.

References	Type of study/Population	Objectives	Results	Study limitations	NE/QM
[4]	Cohort Study/Health professional s (n = 37) and the elderly (n = 68) of a long-term care (LTC) residents	- Evaluate the attitudes of caregivers towards the use of PEQ at different times - Describe the elderly's support to protective equipment - Evaluate the differences in the characteristics of: (i) elderly who chose to wear the protector and elderly who refused to use; (ii) elderly who have joined and have not joined	• 85% of the elderly agreed to use the PEQ. After 8 months, only 29% continued to use the equipment • The health professionals considered that this withdrawal was caused by: pain, discomfort and lack of perception of the elderly about the usefulness of this equipment • This study reveals that nurses have a fundamental role: in the evaluation of the situation of the elderly and their characteristics and in education about the usefulness of using PEQ • Most of the nursing team, in both shifts, considers that the use of PEQ is feasible, important, beneficial and not time- consuming • The profile of the elderly is considered a determining factor in the equipment's adhering (if the elderly is disoriented, there is a greater probability of refusal) • PeQ had no beneficial effect in reducing the number of hip fractures • The study considers that the nursing team needs to have instructed for the appropriate use of the protector, because it influences their attitudes, and may have a clinical impact	- Small sample - The elderly was not asked about disadvantages of the use of PEQ - Requires further scientific validation of this equipment	2B/B

(continued)

Table 1. (*continued*)

References	Type of study/Population	Objectives	Results	Study limitations	NE/QM
[5]	SLR (included 20 ECAs)	- Assess the effectiveness of interventions in reducing the number of falls	• In 4 ECs that intervened multi-factorially and in 3 that acted in a risk factor: there was a significant reduction in the rate of fall, recurrent fall and percentage of elderly who suffered fractures at the femur level • Effective programs were considered: (i) individual assessment structured with safety recommendations; (ii) multidisciplinary program that includes strategies related to the context and specific for the elderly; (iii) intervention in multiple factors that predispose to the fall (education, adapted surrounding environment, balance, resistance training and PEQ); (iv) use of calcium supplements with vitamin D or just vitamin D; (v) review of prescribed medicines; (vi) multifactorial intervention (analysis of the evolution of the risk of fall and performance in general and specific interventions)	- Heterogeneous population in articles - Inconsistent results - Different nomenclatures - Cost versus efficacy was not assessed	1A/A

(*continued*)

Table 1. (*continued*)

References	Type of study/Population	Objectives	Results	Study limitations	NE/QM
[6]	Cohort Study/Health professional s (n = 39) and the elderly (n = 27) of two long-term care (LTC) residents	- Observe the perceptions of the population in the decision to use the PEQ - Identify the factors that influence their use	• The elderly expressed concern about the physical level of the equipment and questioned the need to use it • The elderly felt that they had no choice but to use the PEQ, being the cause of this, the concern and the insistence of health professionals to persuade the elderly to use the equipment • The study reveals that the decision-making capacity and the environment where the elderly are integrated influences the aid's	- More than 75% of the elderly had cognitive impairment	2B/B
[7]	SLR (included 10 MA)	- Identify the most beneficial intervention in the prevention of falls	• 9 MA included interventions in long-term care (LTC) resident and 2 include measurements at hospital level • In the units, scientific evidence is very inconsistent regarding physical exercise as a prevention of falls. Other interventions (vitamin D, PEQ, nutritional supplements or medication) also showed no benefit • There is evidence that a multifactorial intervention leads to a reduction in the number of falls	- Limited number of MAs analyzed - Results obtained through different evaluation methods - Possibility of data overlap	1A/A

(*continued*)

Table 1. (*continued*)

References	Type of study/Population	Objectives	Results	Study limitations	NE/QM
[8]	Cohort Study/Elderly (n = 62000) long-term care (LTC) residents	- Evaluate the effectiveness of the implementation of the program (gym classes, evidence on falls and their prevention, adaptation of the environment, review of chronic medication, prescription of vitamin D, PEQ and education) with reassessment after 3–9 years	• In general, the results were negative • The gym classes were only attended by elderly with adequate cognitive and physical status (only 13.5%), with variable efficacy according to physical status and exercise intensity • The PEQ had no benefit in reducing the fracture rate. These results may have been due to lack of adherence, uniform opinion about the benefit of these equipment and conflicts of interest between brands	- High turnover of health professionals - Reduced fidelity of training program components - Low standardization of employees' daily priorities - Little investment in the implementation of drop prevention	2B/B
[9]	Cohort Study/Elderly (n = 1923) long-term care (LTC) residents	- Evaluate the efficacy of PEQ in reducing the risk of fracture in institutionalize elderly (long-term care residents)	• PEQ scans were used about 60% of the times there were falls • There was a higher tendency to use these protectors in elderly males, with cognitive impairment, heart diseases, debilitated, under anxiolytics and with urinary and/or intestinal incontinence • PEQ led to an 18% reduction in fracture risk	- Limitation in the identification of the causes of falls - Uncertainty when determining data accuracy	2B/B

The scientific articles considered present some differences, namely in terms of the methodology used to assess the effectiveness of the interventions used. However, all assume common answers and highlight the lack of evidence about each intervention.

According to [5], nurses place external hip protectors and consider them important in preventing fall. On the other hand, in addition to the pain and discomfort they felt, the elderly did not believe in its effectiveness and considered it as a barrier in the performance of their ADL. After 8 months, there was no clear evidence that the external hip protector was effective in reducing the risk of hip fractures due to a fall event. In general, no benefit was identified in the incidence rate of hip fractures in relation to the use of this equipment. However, the use of these protectors should not be ignored, as it has resulted in the reduction of other types of injuries.

The authors in [8] state that there is no agreement regarding the physical exercise and vitamin D supplementation, as simple interventions, to reduce the consequences resulting from falls. In addition, there is no scientific evidence that the use of external hip protectors and medication are an option for the prevention of falls. Although the results are quite limited, multifactorial intervention is the ideal method for the prevention of falls in long-term care (LTC) resident and hospitals.

Corroborating the previous idea, the authors in [6] state that, due to the small number of studies included, there are inconclusive results in relation to multifactorial or individual interventions, as there has been no significant positive effect on the number of falls. Multifactorial intervention in people who are LTC residents seems more beneficial in preventing falls. The authors state that a careful approach is needed because programs that aim to reduce the number of falls can be ineffective or leading to some opposite effects.

The authors in [10] state that LTC residents with established risk factors for falls were more likely to accept and adhere to the use of hip protectors, e.g., those with wandering behavior, cardiac dysrhythmia, who presented some moderate to severe health cognitive impairment, or bladder incontinence, in which the use of these devices have been shown to be effective in preventing hip fractures. The research work also mentions the scarcity of research on dissemination and implementation strategies that promotes the adherence of external protective hip protectors by the elderlies.

For the authors in [7], adhering to external hip protectors is not a complex process. However, they state that it is very important to recognize the very fine balance between the elderly preferences and what are the most appropriate fall preventing measure that need to be adopted in each case. To accomplish this, they recommend that qualified people (social assistants, physiotherapists, occupational therapists, or psychologists) intervene with this target population, so that they accept their limitations and vulnerabilities and assume behaviors that protect them from possible injuries.

According to the authors in [9], the lack of resources was the main reason why the implementation of their program did not bring true benefits. They recommend a greater investment to ensure a real change in the measures and processes to be implemented in LTC residents, or even the adoption of an entirely new set of measures, about the use of hip protectors in the prevention of fractures caused by a fall event.

6 Conclusions

Fall prevention is a situation that involves caregivers, family members and health professionals. It is considered that the risk of falls is a diagnosis that must be made by the nursing team, which must adopt the necessary interventions aimed at preventing falls. From the assessment of the elderly regarding the risk of falls, nursing team should implement actions aimed at reducing or even avoiding fall events [11].

Considering the impact that falls can have, there is a need to develop a specific and appropriate plan for each elderly, which include associated preventive strategies. From the analysis of the articles published to date, it was noticed that the prevention of falls is a very complex and multifactorial process. The various authors concluded that there is no evidence (based on clinical practice) of the benefit in the prevention of falls, through interventions that act on only one risk factor.

After analyzing the results and methodological limitations of the studies presented, no significant scientific evidence was found that currently recommends the use of external hip protectors, since they do not have a significant impact on reducing the number of falls. This theme is extremely important, so it is necessary to carry out further studies, to create plans/protocols that are beneficial in the prevention of falls at hospital level.

References

1. Goes, M., Lopes, M.J., Oliveira, H., et al.: A nursing care intervention model for elderly people to ascertain general profiles of functionality and self care needs. Sci. Rep. **10**, 1770 (2020). https://doi.org/10.1038/s41598-020-58596-1
2. Sabino, L.: Prevention of the risk of fall in hospitalized elderly: contributions of the nurse specialist in rehabilitation nursing. Master's thesis, University of Évora (2018)
3. Luzardo, A., Junior, N., Medeiros, M., Wolkers, P., Santos, S.: Repercussions of hospitalization by fall of the elderly: health care and prevention. Braz. J. Nurs. **71**(2), 816–822 (2018). https://doi.org/10.1590/0034-7167-2017-0069
4. Centre for Evidence-Based Medicine: Oxford Centre for Evidence-based Medicine—Levels of Evidence (2009). http://www.cebm.net/index.aspx?o=1025
5. Milisen, K., et al.: Nursing staff attitudes of hip protector use in long-term care, and differences in characteristics between adherent and non-adherent residents: a survey and observational study. J. Am. Med. Dir. Assoc. **48**(2), 193–203 (2011). https://doi.org/10.1016/j.ijnurstu.2010.07.008
6. Neyens, J., et al.: Effectiveness and implementation aspects of interventions for preventing falls in elderly people in long-term care facilities: a systematic review of RCT's. J. Am. Med. Direct. Assoc. **12**(6), 410–425 (2011). https://doi.org/10.1016/j.jamda.2010.07.018
7. Sims-Gould, J., Mckay, H., Feldman, F., Scott, V., Robinovitch, S.: Autonomy, choice, patient-centered care, and hip protectors: the experience of residents and staff in long-term care. J. Appl. Gerontol. **33**(6), 690–790 (2014)
8. Stubbs, B., Denkinger, M., Brefka, S., Dallmeier, D.: What works to prevent falls in older adults dwelling in long term care facilities and hospitals? An umbrella review of meta-analyses of randomized controlled trials. J. Am. Med. Direct. Assoc. **81**(3), 335–342 (2015). https://doi.org/10.1016/j.maturitas.2015.03.026
9. Roigk, P., Becker, C., Schulz, C., Konig, H.-H., Rapp, K.: Long-Term evaluation of the implementation of a large fall and fracture prevention program in long-term care facilities. BMC Geriatr. **18**, 233 (2018). https://doi.org/10.1186/s12877-018-0924-y

10. Korall, A., et al.: Effectiveness of hip protectors to reduce risk for hip fracture from falls in long-term care. J. Am. Med. Direct. Assoc. **20**(11), 1397–1403 (2019). https://doi.org/10.1016/j.jamda.2019.07.010
11. Machado, T., Oliveira, C., Costa, F., Araújo, T.: Assessment of the presence of risk for fall in the elderly. Electron. J. Nurs. **11**(1), 32–38 (2009). http://www.fen.ufg.br/revista/v11/n1/v11n1a04.htm

The Care Provided by the Multi-professional Team to Institutionalized Aged: Integrative Review

Aline Ost dos Santos[2], Cenir Gonçalves Tier[1](✉), Silvana Bastos Cogo[2], Leticia Gonçalves Lira[1], Cindy Byane de Melo de Moura[1], Laura Neres de Melo[1], Melissa Frecero Consiglio[1], Jaime Coffi de Souza[1], Joana Jorge da Rosa[1], and Thayná da Fonseca Aguirre[1]

[1] Federal University of Pampa, Uruguaiana, Brazil
{cenirtier,leticialira.aluno,cindymoura.aluno,lauraneres.aluno, melissaconsiglio.aluno,jaimesouza.aluno,joanajorge.aluno, thaynaaguirre.aluno}@unipampa.edu.br
[2] Federal University of Santa Maria, Santa Maria, Brazil
aline.ost@acad.ufsm.br, silvana.cogo@ufsm.br

Abstract. Integrative literature review conducted in October 2021 by four independent reviewers. The guiding question was based on the Population/Patient/Problem - Interest - Context, Time strategy: What is the scientific evidence available on the care provided by the multi-professional team to elderly residents in LSIE in the last five years? Original articles were included, in Portuguese, English or Spanish, with a time frame of the last five years, in full and free of charge. Excluded: theses, dissertations, monographs, editorials, reflections, literature reviews, experience reports. Results: Fifteen studies were identified, which addressed care from the following perspectives: Care planning, Nursing diagnosis, Symptom management, Psychosocial support, Rehabilitation, Advance directive, Educational intervention, Person-centered care, Physical comfort of end-of-life patients, Promotion of rest, Educational program, Care planning meeting, Steps to care success program, and Advance care planning. Conclusion: It is necessary to deepen the theoretical and practical knowledge of this care for the teams that work in long-stay institutions to spread this care, as well as to provide opportunities for future teaching, research, and extension actions to qualify the care in the process of life, death, and dying of institutionalized elderly people.

Keywords: Advance directives · Homes for the aged · Health personnel

1 Introduction

With the increase in life expectancy, interventions focusing on the quality of life of the elderly are necessary. Such interventions should be focused on the autonomy and independence of the elderly [1]. Moreover, with aging there can be a gradual decrease in functional capacity, leading to functional impairment and dependence [2].

J. García-Alonso and C. Fonseca (Eds.): IWoG 2021, LNBE, pp. 366–377, 2022.
https://doi.org/10.1007/978-3-030-97524-1_34

From this perspective, in certain situations, some families decide to send their elderly to long-stay institutions due to the increase in the demand for elderly care, which implies in the context of nursing work [3]. Therefore, these institutions (LSIEs) can be public or private, and with or without financial help from the government [4]. Therefore, there is the need for care to be differentiated and provided by qualified professionals.

The institutionalized elderly, in general, present functional deficits, which are mainly evident in the dimensions of self-care, learning and mental functions, including cognitive impairments [5]. However, the challenges of multidisciplinary care to the elderly are to attend to their particularities, seeking to look at the elderly, i.e., in a multidimensional way [6].

According to the National Policy on the Health of the Elderly, to have an effective care practice for the elderly, it is necessary to have a multidimensional and interdisciplinary approach that considers the physical, psychological, and social factors that influence the health of the elderly, as well as the environment in which they live [7].

It is important to mention that health professionals working in homes for the aged need to understand how the aging process occurs to then define actions aimed at contemplating the institutionalized elderly in a comprehensive way, as well as assisting them with a focus on their autonomy [8]. In this sense, it is aimed to present, through scientific evidence, how the care for the elderly has been performed by the multi-professional team in long-stay institutions for the elderly.

2 Method

This is an integrative review, which presents a method that summarizes the scientific literature on a given topic to provide a greater understanding of the guiding question [9]. The development of this research followed the steps: formulation of the guiding question, sampling, extraction of data from primary studies, critical appraisal, analysis and synthesis of the review results, presentation of the integrative review [10]. We chose to adopt the referred Reporting Items for Systematic Reviews and Meta-Analyses (PRISMA).

The guiding question was formulated using the Population/Patient/Problem - Interest - Context, Time (PICoT) strategy: What is the available scientific evidence on the care provided by the multi-professional team to elderly people residing in LSIEs in the last five years?

It is worth noting that the acronym "P" (target population) multi-professional team of caregivers of older people in LSIE, "I" (interest) care of people in LSIE, "Co" (context) LSIE, "T" last five years. To survey the articles in the literature, we chose to search the electronic databases: Medical Literature Analysis and Retrieval System Online (MEDLINE) via PubMed; Web of Science; Latin American and Caribbean Literature on Health Sciences (LILACS) and the Nursing Database (BDENF) via the Virtual Health Library (VHL). No studies were found in SciVerse Scopus and Scientifc Eletronic Library Online (Scielo). These databases were chosen because they cover national and international databases. This search, selection, and extraction of primary studies occurred in October 2021 by four independent reviewers.

The capture of the studies was made through the use of search descriptors from the Descriptors in Health Sciences (DECS) and the Mesch Terms combined in sequence with

Boolean logic basis: AND or OR and by the following search strategy in all consulted databases: Elderly OR elderly person OR geriatrics OR, Long Stay Institution for the Elderly AND Patient Care Team OR Nursing Team OR nursing OR nursing care OR interdisciplinary communication OR patient care team AND patient comfort OR nursing care OR Comprehensive Health Care.

In this search step by using the descriptors, 43,776 articles were identified. Then, articles were selected according to the inclusion and exclusion criteria. Regarding the inclusion criteria, we considered original articles on the theme of care for the elderly in homes for the aged in Portuguese, English or Spanish, with a time frame of the last five years, available in full for free. Theses, dissertations and monographs, editorials, reflections, literature reviews (narrative, integrative, systematic, scoping, meta-analysis), experience reports as well as those that did not correspond to the theme of the study were excluded. From this perspective, duplicate studies were counted only once.

After applying these criteria, 43,005 articles were excluded due to not being written in Portuguese, English or Spanish, not having been published in the last five years, not being original research, not contemplating the care of elderly people in ILPI. Six duplicate articles were found. In this step, 771 articles were selected for title and abstract reading according to the guiding question, being inserted in the Endnote [11] reference manager.

Subsequently, the 771 identified articles were carefully read from the titles, abstracts, and keywords of the studies using the Rayyan tool without the researchers having access to the decisions of others to ensure the selection of publications related to the research question independently. In this step, the researchers were allowed access to the studies for the final consensus of the 101 titles and abstracts that presented divergences. After

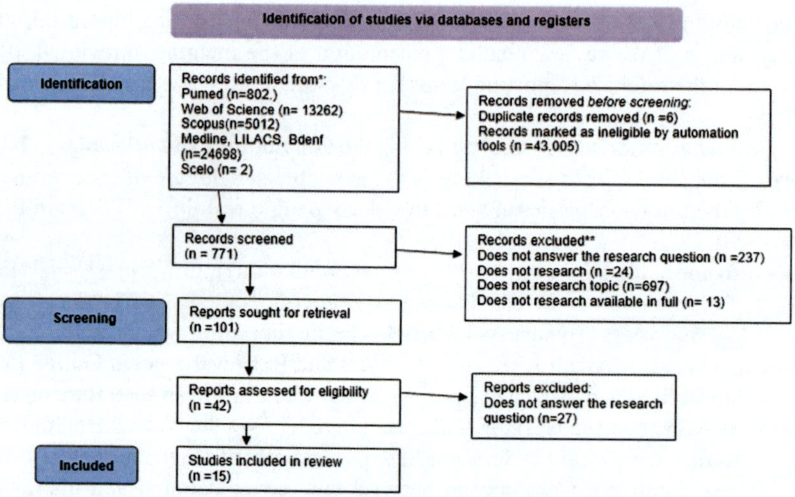

Fig. 1. Flowchart of article selection on the care provided by the multiprofessional team for residents of long-term care homes, Uruguaiana, Rio Grande do Sul, Brazil, 2021. Source: elaborated by the authors, 2021

the researchers met, 42 articles were selected to be read in their entirety. Of these, 15 studies were selected and made up the corpus of the analysis.

The interpretation of the studies and the presentation of the synthesis of the knowledge of the studies eligible for the corpus of this review will be by means of the synoptic flowchart in the PRISMA model as shown in Fig. 1:

For the extraction of the primary studies, a word table was used to construct the table containing article number, title, type of care, main results, and level of evidence. The critical evaluation of the primary studies was verified by the level of evidence, which establishes six categories: Level I - Evidence derived from systematic reviews or meta-analyses of relevant clinical trials; Level II - Evidence derived from at least

Table 1. Summary of primary studies on education and care technologies used by the multiprofessional team for residents of ILPIs, Uruguaiana, Rio Grande do Sul, Brazil, 2021

Title	Country, year	Objective	Care	Level of evidence
Nursing diagnoses for institutionalized elderly people based on Henderson's theory [12]	Brazil 2019	To develop nursing diagnostic statements for institutionalized elderly people	Nursing diagnoses for institutionalized elderly	NVI
Nursing home care trajectories for older adults following in-hospital palliative care consultation [13]	United States 2017	Analysis was to describe the care trajectories and experiences of older adults admitted to a nursing home following a Palliative care consultation during	Advance Assistance Planning Symptom Management Psychosocial support Spiritual Care Focus on Rehabilitative Care and Continuity of Comfort Care	NVI
Concordance Between Proxy Level of Care Preference and Advance Directives Among Nursing Home Residents With Advanced Dementia: A Cluster Randomized Clinical [14]	United States 2019	Examine concordance between advance directives and proxy care preferences among nursing home residents with advanced dementia and to determine the impact of an advance care planning video on concordance	Advance Directives and Advance Care Planning	NII

(*continued*)

Table 1. (*continued*)

Title	Country, year	Objective	Care	Level of evidence
The Impact of Nursing Homes Staff Education on End-of-Life Care in Residents With Advanced Dementia: A Quality Improvement Study [15]	Italy 2019	To compare end-of-life care in NH residents with advanced dementia before and after an educational intervention aimed to improving palliative care	Educational intervention to improve palliative care	NIV
How can a measure improve assessment and management of symptoms and concerns for people with dementia in care homes? A mixed-methods feasibility and process evaluation of IPOS-Dem. PLOS ONE [16]	United Kingdom 2018	To understand the mechanisms of action of a measure to support comprehensive assessment of people with dementia in care homes; and its acceptability, feasibility, and implementation requirements	Care planning and changes in care delivery and facilitated communication	NVI
Effectiveness of a Technology-Enhanced Integrated Care Model for Frail Older People: A Stepped-Wedge Cluster Randomized Trial in Nursing Homes [17]	South Korea 2021	To evaluate the impact of an information and communication technologies (ICT)-enhanced, multidisciplinary integrated care model, called Systems for Person-centered Elder Care (SPEC), on frail older adults at nursing homes	Person-centered care model	NII

(*continued*)

Table 1. *(continued)*

Title	Country, year	Objective	Care	Level of evidence
Comfort-Supporting Nursing Activities for End-of-Life Patients in an Institutionalized Environment [18]	Czech Republic 2018	To determine the utilization rate of comfort supporting nursing activities in end-of-life patients in an institutionalized environment in the Czech Republic in relation to the age of the registered nurses (RNs), length of work experience, education level, and type of workplace	Activities supporting the physical comfort of end-of-life patients such as pain monitoring, basic care and promotion of rest	NVI
No difference in effects of 'PACE steps to success' palliative care program for nursing home residents with and without dementia: a pre-planned subgroup analysis of the seven-country PACE trial [19]	Belgium 2021	To investigate whether the program effects differ between residents with advanced, nonadvanced, and no dementia	Educational program with six stages	NII
Level of Care Preferences Among Nursing Home Residents With Advanced Dementia. Journal of Pain and Symptom Management [20]	United States 2017	To describe and identify factors associated with level of care preferences among proxies of nursing home (NH) residents with advanced dementia	1) Intensive medical care; 2) Basic medical care; 3) Comfort care	NII

(continued)

Table 1. (*continued*)

Title	Country, year	Objective	Care	Level of evidence
An Advance Care Planning Video Decision Support Tool for Nursing Home Residents With Advanced Dementia [21]	United States 2018	To test whether an ACP video (vs usual care) has an effect on To document advance directives, level of care preferences, goals-of-care discussions, and burdensome treatments among nursing home residents with advanced dementia	Advance Directives A video about Advance Care Planning	NII
Staff experiences with implementing a case conferencing care model in nursing homes: a focus group study [22]	Norway 2019	To describe nursing home staff's experiences with an intervention consisting of comprehensive geriatric assessment and care planning in structured case conference meetings	Care planning meeting and Care plan recorded in the patient's electronic medical record	VI
Quality of dying and quality of end-of-life care of nursing home residents in six countries: An epidemiological study [23]	Belgium, Finland, Italy, Netherlands, Poland and England 2018	To determine the quality of dying and end-of-life care of nursing home residents in six European countries	The quality of death and the quality of end-of-life care in nursing homes in the countries studied are not ideal	VI
Dementia in institutionalized elderly: a nursing team's experiences and perceptions [24]	Brazil 2021	To understand nursing workers' experiences with the nursing care provided to elderly individuals with dementia living in a long-term care facility	Person-centered care, non-pharmacological measures, attachment, communication for the care of institutionalized elderly with dementia	NVI

(*continued*)

Table 1. *(continued)*

Title	Country, year	Objective	Care	Level of evidence
Evaluation of a Palliative Care Program for Nursing Homes in 7 Countries [25]	Belgium England, Finland, Italy, Netherlands Poland Switzerland 2020	To investigate the effect of the Palliative Care for Older People (PACE) Steps to Success Program on resident and staff outcomes	The Steps to Successful Palliative Care for the Elderly Program in Nursing Homes	NII
Advance care planning preferences in Chinese nursing home residents: results from two cross-sectional studies in Hong Kong and Taiwan [26]	Taiwan 2021	To explore and compare advance directive and end-of-life care preferences of nursing home residents in Hong Kong and Taiwan	Advance Directive and Advance Care Planning	NVI

Source: Researchers' production. Brazil, 2021

one well-designed randomized controlled trial, moderate evidence; Level III - Well-designed clinical trials without randomization; Level IV - Well-designed cohort and case-control studies; Level V - Systematic review of descriptive and qualitative studies, weak evidence; Level VI - Evidence derived from a single descriptive or qualitative study; Level VII - Authority opinion or expert committee report (Fineout et al., 2011). The fifteen articles included in the corpus of the analysis were synthesized in a synoptic chart containing the title, study objective, care provided, and level of evidence (Table 1).

3 Results and Discussion

The care identified in the corpus was performed by caregivers and nursing staff members to the institutionalized elderly, potentially triggering a small risk of bias in the included studies. The following were identified as care performed by the multidisciplinary team to the elderly person residing in a long-stay institution: advance directives [14, 21, 26], advance care planning [14]; supportive care for physical comfort of end-of-life patients such as pain monitoring, basic care, and promotion of rest [18]; advanced care planning, symptom management, psychosocial support, spiritual care, focus on rehabilitative care, and continuity of comfort care [13]; educational intervention to improve palliative care [15]; care planning and changes in care delivery and facilitated communication [16], person-centered care model [17]; educational program, Intensive medical care; Basic medical care; Comfort care [20]; Care planning meeting and care plan recorded in the patient's electronic medical record [22]; Person-centered care, non-pharmacological measures, person-centered care, bonding, communication for the care of the institutionalized elderly with dementia [24]. Nursing diagnoses for institutionalized elderly [12]. The Steps to Successful Caregiving Program and Advance Care Planning [26].

Advance Directives are a set of wishes, previously and expressly expressed by the patient, about care and treatment they wish to receive, when they are unable to express, freely and autonomously, their will [27]. From this perspective, advance care planning is associated with the fulfillment of advance directives of will. From this perspective, knowing the wills and recording the advance directives of the elderly helps in the planning of care for the elderly resident in LSIEs, since nursing homes are among the most common places of death in many countries [23].

A study of three hundred and twenty-two nursing homes in Belgium, Finland, Italy, the Netherlands, Poland, and England concluded that the quality of dying and quality of end-of-life care in nursing homes in the countries studied are not optimal [23]. End-of-life care can be planned with comfort measures. From this perspective, advance care planning and advance directives are presented as resources to optimize humanized patient-centered care [28] and safeguard the autonomy and dignity of the elderly.

Both the construction of advance directives and advanced care planning necessitate talking about end-of-life care with professionals and family members. To this end, a study developed in long-stay institutions with 238 elderly residents in Hong Kong and 87 in Taiwan found that 34 elderlies in Hong Kong and 16 in a study developed in long-stay institutions with 238 elderly residents in Hong Kong and 87 in Taiwan had participated in discussions about end of life. When drafting advance directives only seven in Hong Kong and eleven in a study developed [26].

In Boston, advanced care planning, construction, and compliance with Advance Directives requires knowing the wishes of seniors with dementia residing in long-stay institutions. Under this analysis, understanding the differences in intensive medical care, basic medical care, and comfort care for compliance and respect of wishes is necessary to talk about in addition to making it understandable to care seekers both formal and informal, and counseling of proxies that includes an explanation of this general poor prognosis, may shift the direction of care toward comfort [21].

Supportive care for the physical comfort of end-of-life patients such as pain monitoring, basic care, and promotion of rest are important care, but there is insufficient focus on the spiritual and psychosocial comfort of end-of-life patients [18]. It is worth noting that stubborn attempts to cure tend to lead to artificial prolongation of life, loss of personal autonomy and human dignity, triggering discussions about supposed rights of the patient to manifest their will in situations of incapacity [29].

New technological resources allow the adoption of disproportionate measures that can prolong the suffering of the patient with a disease considered terminal, without bringing him benefits, and these measures may have been rejected in advance by him [29]. In summary, the advance directives of the elderly in this study contained refusal to care that bar therapeutic obstinacy and the educational video content favored the acceptance of comfort care in the elderly who watched the video and increased the agreement between the wishes and the documentation of advance directives [14].

It is further complemented that comparing end-of-life care in long-term care facility residents with advanced dementia before and after an educational intervention aimed at improving palliative care concluded that effective in initiating a change in practices relevant to the quality of palliative care among patients with advanced dementia in Italy [15]. There is a gap in the care of the elderly person with dementia who resides in a long-stay institution [3]. Advance care planning has resolutive potential in older adults with advanced dementia. In this context, video had no effect on preferences, non-hospitalization, or costly treatments among residents with advanced dementia, but increased guidelines for withholding tube feeding [21]. There is a need for more studies on the needs and conditions of care in institutionalized elderly to allow, with greater precision, the development of models of care for the elderly [30].

The relevance of educational actions to modify care practices for the elderly in long-stay institutions is perceived. Under this approach, an educational program, in Belgium, with six stages: advance care, planning with residents and families; assessment, care; planning, and review of resident needs and problems; coordination of care via monthly multidisciplinary palliative care review meetings; high-quality palliative care with a focus on pain and depression; care in the last days of life and care after death [19].

4 Conclusion

The studies found focused on the care of the elderly person with a life-threatening illness. In view of the terminality of life, further studies are still needed on the wishes of the elderly who live in long-stay institutions about the process of death and dying well. To this end the advance care plan as well as advance directives must be recorded and applied in the multiple contexts that the elderly person goes through. The multidisciplinary team must be trained about palliative care, life threatening diseases, comfort care to avoid therapeutic obstinacy.

It is perceived that educational actions on action planning, management of complex cases, communication, bonding, person-centered model, use of the systematization of nursing care should be further encouraged since the teaching of health graduations. One should consider continuing education for formal and informal caregivers of the elderly in long-stay institutions.

Care focused on rehabilitation should be inserted to assist in active aging and comfort measures. In the context of the long-stay institution, no studies on active aging and care to maintain quality of life were found.

The results of this study should guide subsidies to deepen the construction of knowledge about human aging in the context of long-stay institutions in the world, considering cultural, social, physiological, psychological aspects in the construction of public health and social policies. All these considerations should have the potential to provide opportunities, in the future, opportunities for teaching, research and extension actions to qualify the care in the process of life, death and dying of the institutionalized elderly.

Therefore, this study is limited by the time frame of the last five years and the analysis and comparison of different cultures should be taken into consideration, since it was not possible to identify studies from all continents.

Acknowledgments. The Coordination for the Improvement of Higher Education Personnel (CAPES) for the financial support to master's student Aline Ost dos Santos, CAPES Social Demand Scholarship Holder.

References

1. Organização Mundial da Saúde (OMS) Relatório Mundial de Envelhecimento e Saúde [Internet], 28 p. OMS, Genebra (2015). https://sbgg.org.br//wp-content/uploads/2015/10/OMS-Envelhecimento-2015-port.pdf. Accessed 21 Out 2021
2. Ferreira, O.G.L., Maciel, S.C., Costa, S.M.G., Silva, A.O., Moreira, M.A.S.P.: Envelhecimento ativo e sua relação com a independência funcional. Texto Contexto Enferm. **21**(3), 513–518 (2012). https://doi.org/10.1590/S0104-07072012000300004
3. Siewert, J.S., Alvarez, A.M., Brito, F.A., Santos, S.M.A.D., Santana, R.F., Freitas, M.A.D.: Dementia in institutionalized elderly: a nursing team's experiences and perceptions. Texto Contexto - Enfermagem (2021). https://doi.org/10.1590/1980-265x-TCE-2020-0131
4. Piexak, D.R., Freitas, P.H., Backes, D.S., Moreschi, C., Ferreira, C.L.D.L., De Souza, M.H.T.: The perception of health professionals toward the care of institutionalized elderly. Rev. Bras. Geriatr. Gerontol. **15**(2), 201–208 (2012). https://doi.org/10.1590/S1809-98232012000200003
5. Arco, H., Pedro, A., Pinho, L., Proença, A.: Aging and functionality of the institutionalized elderly people of Alto Alentejo: contributions to the diagnosis of the situation. In: García-Alonso, J., Fonseca, C. (eds.) IWoG 2020. LNB, pp. 253–261. Springer, Cham (2021). https://doi.org/10.1007/978-3-030-72567-9_24
6. Carvalho Filho, E.T., Papaléo Netto, M.P.: Geriatria: Fundamentos, Clínica e Terapêutica. Atheneu, São Paulo (1994)
7. Brasil. Portaria nº 2.528, de 19 de Outubro de 2006. Dispõe sobre a Política Nacional de Saúde da Pessoa Idosa. Brasília (2006)
8. Lemos, J.C., Barros, J.D.C.: Equipe Multidisciplinar: essencial para o cuidado dos idosos em Instituição de Longa Permanência. Anais eletrônicos do 15º Congresso Brasileiro de Enfermagem (2021). http://apps.cofen.gov.br/cbcenf/sistemainscricoes/arquivosTrabalhos/I12375.E3.T1637.D3AP.pdf
9. Whittemore, R., Knafl, K.: The integrative review: updated methodology. J. Adv. Nurs. **52**(5), 546–553 (2005). https://doi.org/10.1111/j.1365-2648.2005.03621.x
10. Mendes, K.D.S., Silveira, R.C.C.P., Galvão, C.M.: Revisão integrativa: método de pesquisa para a incorporação de evidências na saúde e na enfermagem. Texto Contexto Enferm. **17**(4), 758–764 (2008). https://doi.org/10.1590/S0104-07072008000400018
11. https://endnote.com/
12. Fernandes, B.K.C., Clares, J.W.B., Borges, C.L., Nóbrega, M.M.L.D., Freitas, M.C.D.: Nursing diagnoses for institutionalized elderly people based on Henderson's theory. Rev. Esc. Enferm. USP (2019). https://doi.org/10.1590/S1980-220X2018004103472
13. Carpenter, J.G., Berry, P.H., Ersek, M.: Nursing home care trajectories for older adults following in-hospital palliative care consultation. Geriatr. Nurs. **38**(6), 531–536 (2017). https://doi.org/10.1016/j.gerinurse.2017.03.016
14. Cohen, S.M., Volandes, A.E., Shaffer, M.L., Hanson, L.C., Habtemariam, D., Mitchell, S.L.: Concordance between proxy level of care preference and advance directives among nursing home residents with advanced dementia: a cluster randomized clinical trial. J. Pain Symptom Manage. **57**(1), 37–46.e1 (2019). https://doi.org/10.1016/j.jpainsymman.2018.09.018
15. Di Giulio, P., Finetti, S., Giunco, F., Basso, I., Rosa, D., Pettenati, F., et al.: The impact of nursing homes staff education on end-of-life care in residents with advanced dementia: a quality improvement study. J. Pain Symptom Manage. **57**(1), 93–99 (2019). https://doi.org/10.1016/j.jpainsymman.2018.10.268
16. Ellis-Smith, C., Higginson, I.J., Daveson, B.A., Henson, L.A., Evans, C.J.: How can a measure improve assessment and management of symptoms and concerns for people with dementia in care homes? A mixed-methods feasibility and process evaluation of IPOS-Dem. PLoS One **13**(7), e0200240 (2018). https://doi.org/10.1371/journal.pone.0200240

17. Kim, H., Jung, Y.I., Kim, G.S., Choi, H., Park, Y.H.: Effectiveness of a technology-enhanced integrated care model for frail older people: a stepped-wedge cluster randomized trial in nursing homes. Gerontologist **61**(3), 460–469 (2021). https://doi.org/10.1093/geront/gnaa090
18. Kisvetrová, H., Vévodová, Š., Školoudík, D.: Comfort-supporting nursing activities for end-of-life patients in an institutionalized environment. J. Nurs. Scholarsh. **50**(2), 126–133 (2018). https://doi.org/10.1111/jnu.12341
19. Miranda, R., et al.: No difference in effects of 'PACE steps to success' palliative care program for nursing home residents with and without dementia: a pre-planned subgroup analysis of the seven-country PACE trial. BMC Palliat. Care **20**(1) (2021). https://doi.org/10.1186/s12904-021-00734-1
20. Mitchell, S.L., Palmer, J.A., Volandes, A.E., Hanson, L.C., Habtemariam, D., Shaffer, M.L.: Level of care preferences among nursing home residents with advanced dementia. J. Pain Symptom Manage. **54**(3), 340–345 (2017). https://doi.org/10.1016/j.jpainsymman.2017.04.020
21. Mitchell, S.L., Shaffer, M.L., Cohen, S., Hanson, L.C., Habtemariam, D., Volandes, A.E.: An advance care planning video decision support tool for nursing home residents with advanced dementia. JAMA Intern. Med. **178**(7), 961 (2018). https://doi.org/10.1001/jamainternmed.2018.1506
22. Nakrem, S., Stensvik, G.-T., Skjong, R.J., Ostaszkiewicz, J.: Staff experiences with implementing a case conferencing care model in nursing homes: a focus group study. BMC Health Serv. Res. **19**(1) (2019). https://doi.org/10.1186/s12913-019-4034-0
23. Pivodic, L., Smets, T., Van Den Noortgate, N., Onwuteaka-Philipsen, B.D., Engels, Y., Szczerbińska, K., et al.: Quality of dying and quality of end-of-life care of nursing home residents in six countries: an epidemiological study. Palliat. Med. **32**(10), 1584–1595 (2018). https://doi.org/10.1177/0269216318800610
24. Siewert, J.S., Alvarez, A.M., Brito, F.A., Santos, S.M.A.D., Santana, R.F., Freitas, M.A.D.: Dementia in institutionalized elderly: a nursing team's experiences and perceptions. Texto Contexto – Enferm. (2021). https://doi.org/10.1590/1980-265X-TCE-2020-0131
25. Van Den Block, L., Honinx, E., Pivodic, L., Miranda, R., Onwuteaka-Philipsen, B.D., Van Hout, H., et al.: Evaluation of a palliative care program for nursing homes in 7 countries. JAMA Intern. Med. **180**(2), 233 (2020). https://doi.org/10.1001/jamainternmed.2019.5349
26. Xu, X., Tu, S.W., Lin, C.C.: Advance care planning preferences in Chinese nursing home residents: results from two cross-sectional studies in Hong Kong and Taiwan. BMC Palliat. Care (2021). https://doi.org/10.1186/s12904-021-00820-4
27. Godinho, M.L.M., Barlem, E.L.D., Barlem, J.G.T., Rocha, L.P., Cogo, S.B., Dalmolin, G.D.L.: Diretivas Antecipadas de Vontade e a concepção do protagonismo do enfermeiro na visão de estudantes de Enfermagem. Rev. M. Estudos sobre norte mortos morrer **5**(9), 67 (2020). https://doi.org/10.9789/2525-3050.2020.v5i9.67-83
28. Leite, C.D.S.W., Fernandes, C.A.: Desfechos do planejamento antecipado de cuidado e diretivas antecipadas em unidade de terapia intensiva: revisão integrativa. Rev. SBPH **24**(1), 28–38 (2021). http://pepsic.bvsalud.org/scielo.php?script=sci_arttext&pid=S1516-08582021000100004&lng=pt
29. Cogo, S.B., Lunardi, V.L.: Diretivas antecipadas: uma análise documental do contexto mundial. Texto Contexto – Enferm. **27**(3) (2018). https://doi.org/10.1590/0104-070720180001880014
30. Morgado, B., Fonseca, C., Lopes, M., Pinho, L.: Components of care models that influence functionality in people over 65 in the context of long-term care: integrative literature review. In: García-Alonso, J., Fonseca, C. (eds.) IWoG 2020. LNB, pp. 324–335. Springer, Cham (2021). https://doi.org/10.1007/978-3-030-72567-9_30

Electrolyte Imbalances in the Elderly

Eugénia Sardinha[1], Rogério Ferreira[2](✉), João Vieira[2], Teresa Mestre[2], and Ana Clara Nunes[2]

[1] Algarve University Hospital Center, Portimão Hospital, Portimão, Portugal
[2] Polytechnic Institute of Beja, Beja, Portugal
ferrinho.ferreira@ipbeja.pt

Abstract. As human beings age, the percentage of water and electrolytes present in the body decreases, making them more vulnerable to changes in electrolyte balance. Since this balance is crucial for maintaining the human body's homeostasis, the threat of imbalances in this area may have a major impact on the morbidity and mortality of the elderly. Objective: Identify nursing interventions for the control and prevention of Electrolyte Imbalances in the elderly. Methodology: This Integrative Literature Review was based on the PI[C]OD methodology to formulate the following guiding question: "Which nursing interventions (intervention) allow controlling and preventing Electrolyte Imbalances (outcomes) in the elderly (population)?. To answer the research question, we used the EBSCOhost platform to search all databases, namely Academic Search Complete, MEDLINE Complete, CINAHL Complete and MedicLatina, with the respective descriptors. Results: After the organized reading of the studies and the application of the inclusion and exclusion criteria, 5 scientific studies were used to perform the Integrative Literature Review. All of them show, in general, nursing interventions that allow controlling and preventing Electrolyte Imbalances, especially in the elderly. Only 2 of the 5 studies truly specified interventions targeted at the elderly population. Conclusion: Nursing interventions inherent to the control of Electrolyte Imbalances focus on the screening and treatment of symptoms associated with the different imbalances, the administration and control of drug therapy, always paying attention to intercurrences or complications that may occur and, whenever possible, teaching the elderly person and their relatives about Electrolyte Imbalances and how to prevent them.

Keywords: Electrolyte imbalances · Elderly · Nursing interventions · Control · Prevention

1 Introduction

The electrolyte balance is essential for maintaining homeostasis in the human body. Electrolytes are compounds that in solution emit positively charged ions (cations) and negatively charged ions (anions) and are distributed throughout the intracellular and extracellular compartments of fluids of our organism. The main electrolytes are sodium (Na+), potassium (K+), chloride (Cl−), calcium (Ca^{2+}), magnesium (Mg^2+) and phosphate (PO_4^3−) [13, 14]. The most reported imbalances are those involving sodium and

J. García-Alonso and C. Fonseca (Eds.): IWoG 2021, LNBE, pp. 378–387, 2022.
https://doi.org/10.1007/978-3-030-97524-1_35

potassium, and these are the electrolytes that will be specified and addressed in the present work.

An electrolyte imbalance occurs when the level of these electrolytes' changes, increasing or decreasing in number. Regardless of the imbalance, the variation in electrolyte levels interrupts the regular functioning of the body, disrupting homeostasis, and leading to potentially life-threatening complications [11, 13, 14].

In a healthy adult, the electrolyte balance is maintained with regular health care, i.e., correct diet, oral hydration, and physical exercise, among others. However, as one ages, morphological, physiological, biochemical, and psychological changes occur, which facilitate the development of electrolyte imbalances (EIs) in the elderly. In addition, the aging process causes the amount of water present in the body to decrease, and muscle mass is gradually replaced by adipose tissue, which is virtually free of water and electrolytes [6, 7, 10]. Not only the aging process, but also pathological processes and frequent hospitalizations are situations that easily trigger the onset of EIs, due to the vulnerability they cause in the elderly population, increasing mortality and morbidity rates [8].

Considering this, the nursing team plays a key role in this population, as it monitors the elderly's needs and plans a specific and personalized care to identify potential problems [6, 9]. In this sense, nursing interventions are also essential to raise awareness and empower the elderly and their families, as well as to treat the imbalances, prevent complications, promote health, and avoid frequent hospitalizations.

2 Objective

Identify nursing interventions, in the control and prevention of EIs in the elderly.

3 Methods

Type of Study

The Integrative Literature Review is a research method used in Evidence-Based Practice and it allows nurses to incorporate evidence into clinical practice. The methodological procedures used involved the following steps: 1) Identification of a topic and formulation of a clear research question; 2) Use of databases and definition of key words to carry out the search for scientific literature/scientific studies; 3) Establishing criteria for inclusion and exclusion from the scientific literature/scientific studies; 4) Analyzing the data and evaluating the quality of evidence for the integrative review; 5) Interpretation and presentation of the results obtained; 6) Synthesis of the evidence presented [3, 12].

Methodological Procedures

We used the PI[C]OD methodology, whose acronym stands for was used: population (P), type of intervention (I), comparisons (C), result - outcomes (O) and type of study - design (D). To answer the previously established objective and begin the search for scientific evidence, the following research question was defined: "Which nursing interventions (intervention) allow controlling and preventing EIs (outcomes) in the elderly (population)?".

The inclusion criteria focused on scientific studies published in full-text format, with a qualitative or quantitative approach or integrative literature reviews, in Portuguese or English, which showed interventions in the Nursing area concerning EIs control, with available references and publication date between January 2010 and December 2020. Regarding the exclusion criteria, we considered scientific studies that were not within the established date of publication and that did not present Nursing interventions that answered the established research question.

From May 12 to June 12, 2021, 2 searches of scientific literature were performed to support the research question, using the EBSCOhost platform, with the selection of all databases, namely Academic Search Complete, MEDLINE Complete, CINAHL Complete, and MedicLatina. The descriptors used in the first search were the following: "electrolyte imbalance", "nursing care" or "nursing interventions", "elderly" or "aged" or "older" or "elder" or "geriatric", "prevention" or "intervention" or "treatment" or "program"; "water-electrolyte imbalance"; "fluid imbalance". In the second search the following descriptors were used: "hypokalemia"; "hyperkalemia"; "hypernatremia"; "hyponatremia"; "nursing care" or "nursing interventions". They were used in the following order in the first and second search:

First Search:

- [(Nursing interventions) or (Nursing care)] AND
- [(Elderly) or (Aged) or (Older) or (Elder) or (Geriatric)] AND
- [(Fluid and electrolyte balance)] AND
- [(Electrolyte Imbalance] AND
- [(Water-Electrolyte Imbalance)] AND
- [(Prevention) or (Intervention) or (Treatment) or (Program)] AND
- [(Fluid Imbalance)].

Second Search:

- [(Hypokalemia)] AND
- [(Hyperkalemia)] AND
- [(Hypernatremia)] AND
- [(Hyponatremia)] AND
- [(Nursing Care) or (Nursing Interventions)].

The selection of studies involved the evaluation of the title and analysis of the abstract to verify if the articles met the inclusion and exclusion criteria. When these did not prove to be enlightening, the article was read in its entirety to minimize the loss of important studies.

A total of 28 studies were identified on the EBSCOHost platform, with the selection of all databases, namely MEDLINE Complete, CINAHL Complete, MedicLatina, MEDLINE and Academic Search Complete, within the established time limit, and after checking for duplicate or removed studies. After applying the exclusion criteria, 14 studies were analyzed by reading the abstract, and 8 studies were selected to be read in full. Of these, 5 studies were considered to have the quality to be included in the Integrative Literature Review and to answer the guiding question. To synthesize the search, the Preferred Reporting Items for Systematic Reviews and Meta-Analyses (PRISMA) method was applied. It is presented as a flow chart, and it specifies all the steps of the search phase, selection, and inclusion of scientific studies (Flowchart 1).

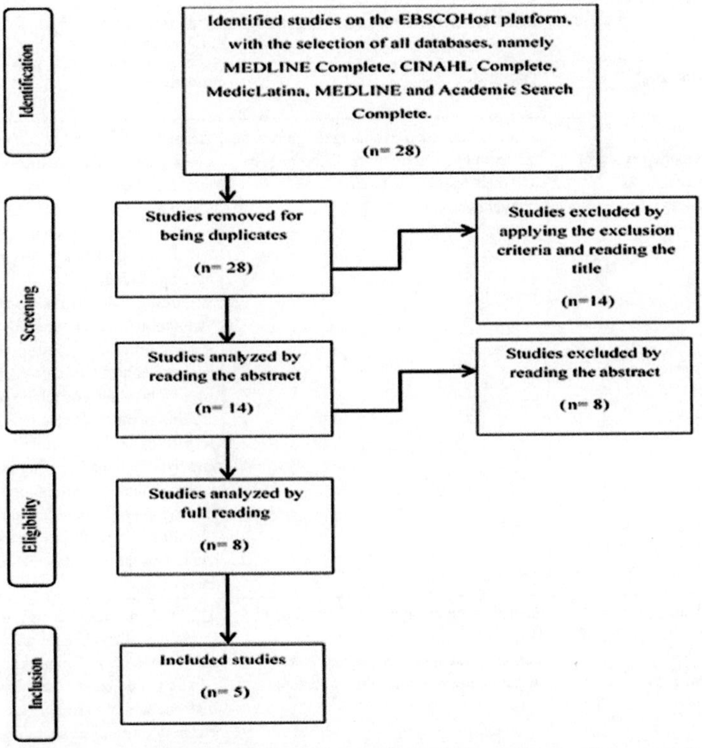

Adapted from: Liberati *et al.* (2009). The PRISMA statement for reporting systematic reviews and meta-analyses of studies that evaluate healthcare interventions: explanation and elaboration. BMJ. Doi: https://doi.org/10.1136/bmj.b2700

Flowchart 1. Flow diagram of the integrative literature review research phase.

For the analysis and assessment of the quality of the selected studies, we used the method of The Joanna Briggs Institute [15], which assigns levels and sublevels of scientific evidence to each study, to identify its degree of methodological quality and understand what type of knowledge it produces.

- Level I - Experimental Designs;
- Level II - Quasi-experimental Designs;
- Level III - Observational – Analytic Designs;

– Level IV - Observational –Descriptive Studies;
– Level V - Expert Opinion and Bench Research.

4 Results

The results come from the analysis and reading of the 5 selected studies and will be exposed in a table format to facilitate interpretation (Table 1).

Table 1. Results obtained for integrative literature review

Authors/Method/Level of evidence	Objective	Results
Fernandes [4] **Method:** Systematic review of descriptive studies **Level of evidence:** IV **Sublevel:** 4a	Aims to indicate the nursing diagnoses for the main hydroelectrolyte disturbances and their respective nursing implementations	According to the study, the most common EIs are those involving sodium and potassium The nursing implementations inherent to each electrolyte imbalance are different, but all aim at a safer and more assertive nursing practice Regarding sodium imbalances (hyper and hyponatremia), the study states that it is important that nurses rigorously evaluate abnormal water losses or low water intake and encourage correct feeding to maintain regular sodium levels Regarding potassium imbalances (hyper and hypokalemia), nursing interventions include monitoring fluid intake, observing electrocardiographic changes, monitoring signs of imbalance, as well as vital signs and capillary blood glucose levels
Crawford and Harris [2] **Method:** Systematic review of descriptive studies **Level of evidence:** IV **Sublevel:** 4a	Aims to review the normal functions of two key electrolytes, sodium, and potassium, and discuss assessment and nursing interventions when imbalances occur	The study reveals that the nursing implementations in case of sodium imbalances involve monitoring the person's fluid balance and assessing his/her state of consciousness For potassium imbalances, the study states that nursing interventions will include checking the signs and symptoms of the imbalance, monitoring vital signs regularly, monitoring the heart, monitoring fluid inflow and outflow, and checking the state of consciousness regularly The study notes that whatever the imbalance in question, it is important to educate the family and the person about the imbalance and its signs and symptoms, about how to avoid the imbalances, and instruct them to inform health professionals or health services if any complications occur

(*continued*)

Table 1. (*continued*)

Authors/Method/Level of evidence	Objective	Results
Kear [5] **Method:** Systematic review of descriptive studies **Level of evidence:** IV **Sublevel:** 4a	Focuses on the role that total body water content, plasma proteins, renal function, and drug metabolism play in age-related human physiology, impacting electrolyte and fluid balance	This study mentions that nurses should employ various strategies to optimize fluid and electrolyte balance in individuals entrusted to their care. Strategies include assessment of fluid and electrolyte status, prevention strategies, and fluid and electrolyte replacement. administration of medications or fluids to decrease electrolyte concentration Careful surveillance for changes in hydro-electrolyte balance, education about EIs, promoting comfort, monitoring fluid balance and vital signs, and frequent physical assessment are essential priorities of nursing care, especially in the elderly person
Bertschi [1] **Method:** Systematic review of descriptive studies **Level of evidence:** IV **Sublevel:** 4a	Improve nursing interventions by explaining how electrolyte changes in potassium and chloride, influence renal function and homeostasis. It also presents are clinical manifestations, etiological and treatment notions	The study stresses that nurses must understand how each treatment works and the importance of patient safety considerations associated with the administration of therapy. In general, people treated for hyperkalemia and hypokalemia should have cardiac monitoring and adequate intravenous access
Pickenhan, Rungg and Schiefermeier-Mach [8] **Method:** Systematic review of descriptive studies **Level of evidence:** IV **Sublevel:** 4a	Discuss the prevalence and management of EIs in long-term care facilities, with a focus on nursing homes	The study mentions that published research studies have reported a higher prevalence of EIs and related mortality rate in nursing homes when compared to older adults in the community. Serum sodium imbalances, hyponatremia, and hypernatremia were the most identified. Risk factors strongly associated with EIs included the dietary/hydration status of nursing home residents, presence of comorbidities, and type of medications prescribed. In this review they also summarize the early signs of EIs and assessments that can be performed locally by nurses. Strengthening awareness of EIs is an important quality improvement effort from the perspective of nursing home residents and their families that can reduce unnecessary hospital transfers, EIs complication rates, and resident mortality

5 Discussion

Overall, in all studies, nursing interventions were identified. However, despite these positive observations, some gaps can be noted. For example, the study by [1] aims to improve nursing interventions in the elderly with EIs, however, it is very little exploratory in the specific interventions.

In terms of the most common imbalances, the studies by [4, 8] are the only ones that identify sodium and potassium imbalances as the most prevalent. The study by [9], further reinforces that sodium imbalances are the most common in the elderly population.

Regarding EIs control and prevention interventions, the studies by [2, 4, 5] refers that the nurse should rigorously assess abnormal water losses or low water intake, i.e., water balance, as this is one of the most important preventive measures. In addition, studies by [2, 4] emphasize that nurses should also encourage a correct diet to maintain regular levels of sodium and potassium to avoid imbalances. Surveillance during the administration of intravenous therapy was considered by all studies as the most important intervention in the screening for complications. The nurse must be cautious and slow in administering components containing sodium and potassium, since these carry risks that affect the morbidity and mortality of the elderly person.

When faced with potassium imbalances, all studies mention the importance of observing electrocardiographic changes through cardiac monitoring. Regarding sodium imbalances, the studies mention the relevance of assessing the person's state of consciousness. Similarly, all studies mention that monitoring vital signs and checking for signs and symptoms of imbalances are key nursing interventions for the prevention of complications.

The studies by [1, 8] are the only ones that mention that nursing considerations in EIs management and control include responsible decision making. When it comes to performing their nursing interventions, nurses must possess a broad knowledge depending on the area where they are intervening. In agreement with this, the study by [8] reinforces that insufficient geriatric knowledge results in difficulties in the early interpretation of signs and symptoms, as well as delays in recognizing them. These authors mention that nurses should be empowered through trainings that include information about EIs, such as signs and symptoms, risk factors and possible complications, and counseling in the screening of these imbalances. The study also argues that the responsibility involved in decision making and the tools used to support it, as well as the presence of strong interprofessional communication skills in nurses, make them capable of preventing complications in the elderly population.

According to the studies of [2, 5], teaching about the signs and symptoms of imbalances in older people, as well as educating them and their relatives about the role of electrolyte excess or deficit and the meaning of imbalances, allows for an early detection of any change suggestive of imbalance. By instructing the person and their family members to go to the emergency services or notify health professionals if any severe symptoms appear, nurses can provide early treatment at discharge, especially when there are changes in the state of consciousness or cardiovascular changes.

Still on the topic of health education, the study by [8], mentions that awareness of EIs allows improving the quality of the elderly and their families, avoiding unnecessary hospitalization, as well as decreasing the rates of EIs complications and mortality in the elderly.

The studies by [1, 2, 8], reflect that at the stage of hospital discharge, the nurse should inform the person and their family members about the principles of proper nutrition, especially if the person has experienced an imbalance such as hypokalemia or hyponatremia, thus it is important to encourage the person to consume foods rich in potassium or sodium, depending on the imbalance experienced. Teaching about fluid intake management and therapeutic regimen management are crucial, particularly in the elderly, as they enable the prevention of EIs at home. Another aspect that should be emphasized in the elderly person is the fact that discontinuation of the current medication regimen on their own may lead to serious health complications and possibly further hospitalization.

6 Study Limitations

Regarding the limitations highlighted during the completion of the Integrative Literature Review, the first limitation was that only 2 [5, 8] out of 5 studies focused on the elderly person with EIs. To circumvent this limitation, we found studies that were similar and completed the information described, to strengthen the interventions directed to the older person. Another limitation was the lack of Portuguese studies, with most studies being of American origin. Thus, it is difficult to understand if all the interventions presented would fit, in their entirety, the reality in Portugal.

The limitation verified right at the beginning of the review was the fact that there was little recent literature on the subject. The only bibliographies found that reported findings on the elderly population had publication dates of two decades prior to the year 2020. However, although relatively recent scientific evidence was found on the topic itself, there is very little evidence on nursing practice in the control and prevention of EIs, especially involving the elderly population. In this sense, there was a need to extend the temporal limits (publication date between 2010 and 2020).

Finally, I consider as a last limitation, the lack of studies involving participants. The studies found are classified as systematic reviews of described studies, with no participants and only describe and synthesize the chosen theme. It would be beneficial to have studies with participants to understand the results of nursing interventions in the elderly person with EIs.

7 Conclusion

When it comes to understanding EIs in the elderly, considering the aging process, with all the changes it entails, and paying special attention to their personal history and existing comorbidities, relating them to the current drug therapy, are the most fundamental tasks for the nursing team. The psychological situation of the elderly also compromises their fluid intake, so nurses should be aware of this aspect to overcome this obstacle.

In general, the nursing interventions explained above allow us to understand that the control of EIs is very much centered on the strict monitoring of signs and symptoms of each imbalance, as well as on caution when administering therapy. These intervention strategies correlate with common nursing interventions, such as monitoring capillary blood glucose and vital signs, physical examination, and assessment of consciousness, and with interventions specific to a client with an EIs, such as fluid balance monitoring and fluid intake management.

In addition, the promotion of health education not only enables the elderly person and their family members or caregivers to manage their health situation autonomously but provides them with tools to prevent future complications and identify symptoms early, as well as to seek health care early.

It is important to emphasize that scientific evidence indicates that the nursing professional should be able to identify the symptoms associated with electrolyte imbalances and understand the positive results of their interventions, as well as, fundamentally, have a thorough knowledge of the geriatric population, to act in accordance with this age group.

References

1. Bertschi, L.: Abnormal basic metabolic panel findings: implications for nursing. Am. J. Nurs. **120**(6), 58–66 (2020). http://dx.doi.org/10.1097/01.NAJ.0000668764.99872.89
2. Crawford, A., Harris, H.: Balancing act: Na+ sodium K+ potassium. Nursing **41**(7), 44–50 (2011). https://doi.org/10.1097/01.NURSE.0000397838.20260.12
3. Donato, H., Donato, M.: Etapas na condução de uma revisão sistemática. Acta Med. Portuguesa **32**(3), 227–235 (2019). https://doi.org/10.20344/amp.11923
4. Fernandes, J.: Assistência de enfermagem ao paciente com distúrbios hidroeletrolíticos. Rev. Científica Semana Acad. **1**(000130), 1–21 (2018). https://semanaacademica.com.br/artigo/assistencia-de-enfermagem-ao-paciente-com-disturbios-hidroeletroliticos
5. Kear, M.T.: Fluid and electrolyte management across the age continuum. Nephrol. Nurs. J. **44**(6), 491–496 (2017). https://s1106788.stacksdiscovery.com/sites/default/files/fluid%20electrolyte%20management.pdf
6. Meneguin, S., Banja, P.F., Ferreira, M.L.: Cuidado ao paciente idoso hospitalizado: implicações para a equipe de enfermagem. Rev. Enfermagem UERJ **25**, 1–6 (2017). http://dx.doi.org/10.12957/reuerj.2017.16107
7. Milovanovic, Z., Adeleye, A.: Making Sense of Fluids and Electrolytes: A Hands-on Guide. Taylor & Francis Group, CRC (2017)
8. Pickenhan, L., Rungg, C., Schiefermeier-Mach, N.: Electrolyte imbalances nursing home residents: a review of prevalence, management, and considerations. J. Nurs. Home Res. Sci. **6**, 14–19 (2020). http://dx.doi.org/10.14283/jnhrs.2020.3
9. Sanguino, G.Z., Previato, G.F., Silva, A.F., Meireles, V.C., Góes, H.L., Baldissera, V.D.: O trabalho de enfermagem no cuidado ao idoso hospitalizado: limites e particularidades. Rev. Pesquisa Cuidado Fundam. Online **10**(1), 160–166 (2018). http://dx.doi.org/10.9789/2175-5361.2018.v10i1.160-166
10. Shlanger, L.E., Bailey, J.L., Sands, J.M.: Electrolytes in the aging. Adv. Chronic Kidney Dis. **17**(4), 308–319 (2010). https://doi.org/10.1053/j.ackd.2010.03.008
11. Shrimanker, I., Bhattarai, S.: Electrolytes. StatPearls Publishing (2020). https://www.ncbi.nlm.nih.gov/books/NBK541123/
12. Sousa, L.M., Marques-Vieira, C.M., Severino, S.S., Antunes, A.V.: Metodologia de revisão integrativa da literatura em enfermagem. Rev. Invest. Enfermagem **21**(2), 17–26 (2017). http://www.sinaisvitais.pt/images/stories/Rie/RIE21.pdf

13. Souza, A.L., et al.: Revisão da literatura sobre os principais distúrbios hidroeletrolíticos. Rev. Saberes **14**(1) (2020). https://facsaopaulo.edu.br/wp-content/uploads/sites/16/2020/09/REVISÃO-DA-LITERATURA-SOBRE-OS-PRINCIPAIS-DISTÚRBIOS-HIDROELETROLÍTICOS.pdf
14. Stivanin, S.C.: Desequilíbrio eletrolítico: sódio, potássio e cloro [master's thesis on the Internet]. Universidade Federal do Rio Grande do Sul (2014). https://www.ufrgs.br/lacvet/site/wp-content/uploads/2014/11/eletrolitico.pdf
15. The Joanna Briggs Institute: JBI Levels of Evidence (2013). https://joannabriggs.org/sites/default/files/2019-05/JBI-Levels-of-evidence_2014_0.pdf

Dehydration Control in Hospitalized Elderly: An Integrative Review

Ana Rita Franco Rodrigues[1], Raquel de Almeida Coelho[1], Luís Sousa[2], Óscar Ramos Ferreira[1,3], and Cristina Lavareda Baixinho[1,3,4(✉)]

[1] Nursing School of Lisbon, Lisbon, Portugal
crbaixinho@esel.pt
[2] Comprehensive Health Research Center, University of Évora, Évora, Portugal
[3] Nursing Research, Innovation and Development Centre of Lisbon (CIDNUR), Lisbon, Portugal
[4] Center for Innovative Care and Health Technology (ciTechcare), Leiria, Portugal

Abstract. Dehydration has a high prevalence in the elder population. 40% of people above 65 years old are dehydrated at hospital admission. This problem becomes worse during hospitalization, due to the therapy, the comorbidities, and the lack of interventions targeted at controlling this malady. The objective of this study was to identify nursing interventions to control dehydration in hospitalized elders. An integrative review was carried out that followed a predefined protocol, with 9 stages, to answer the research question "What nursing interventions are used to control the dehydration of hospitalized elders?" The 7 studies which respected the eligibility criteria allowed to identify interventions to prevent dehydration and intervene for the control of this diagnosis. Stood out: risk evaluation, signal monitoring, and liquid intake. These interventions mostly involved the monitoring of liquid intake during the provision of beverages that are adequate to the preference of the client and to keeping drinks at their disposal, in addition to educating the population, their relatives, and health workers. The results indicate that the problem could be solved with the aid of technological solutions and e-health interventions.

Keywords: Dehydration · Prevention · Hospitalization · Aged

1 Introduction

There is a high prevalence of dehydration in hospitalized elders. Studies have found that 40% of people above 65 years old who are hospitalized are dehydrated at the moment of admission [1, 2]. This prevalence varies from 10% to 44% during hospitalization [2]. It has been estimated that 50% of the elders hospitalized due to chronic or acute dehydration die within a year, and their mortality rates are seven times higher than that of elders with no dehydration [3].

Although the recommended amount of water for daily ingestion varies from 1.5 L to 2 L, these values must be tailored to each individual, considering factors such as food

J. García-Alonso and C. Fonseca (Eds.): IWoG 2021, LNBE, pp. 388–398, 2022.
https://doi.org/10.1007/978-3-030-97524-1_36

ingestion, cognitive function, renal alterations, and liquid restrictions [3]. It has been found that dehydration, in most situations, becomes more severe during hospitalization due to failed interventions, allied to pathophysiological changes caused by the health-disease processes [3–7].

If, on one hand, a broad spectrum of physiological changes related to age increases the risk for dehydration, including low liquid reserves, diminution in the thirst reflex, and diuretic and laxative medication, these are worsened by factors related to memory changes, social isolation, and difficulties to access beverages [4]. On the other hand, the symptoms of some geriatric syndromes, such as vomits, hemorrhages, and diarrhea, lead to the loss of sodium and water through the gastrointestinal system, and are the most common cause of dehydration [4, 5]. There are also other factors that can change the hydroelectrolytic balance, such as medications, hyperventilation, hyperthermia, burns, and diabetes mellitus [4].

Although this is a common diagnosis at admission, whose complications are well known and increase hospitalization time, incapacities, and mortality [1, 2, 8], there is not always a systematized evaluation of the risk for dehydration or the presence of signs of it [8], nor is it commonly verified whether the cause is low liquid intake or excessive loss of liquid [4].

Identifying the elders who are dehydrated or risk dehydration is also a cost-effective measure to prevent other complications, such as falls, fractures, pressure wounds, constipation, urinary infection and other renal issues, coronary events, pneumonias, and thromboembolism [1–4, 9], in addition to cognitive alterations, confusion, and delirium [9]. Dehydration often increases the risk of disabilities in elders in the first four years after its diagnosis [8], and these disabilities may even be permanent.

Considering this issue, some authors report the need to raise the awareness of nurses about how important an issue dehydration is for hospitalized elders, especially the frailest ones, justifying this alert by calling attention to the prevalence of dehydration at admission and due to the fact that nearly half the diseased continue to be dehydrated afterwards [2].

Face the above, the objective of this study is to identify the nursing interventions targeted at controlling dehydration in hospitalized elders.

2 Methodology

This Integrative Review (IR) was guided by the following research question: "What nursing interventions are used to control the dehydration of hospitalized elders?" This question was elaborated using the mnemonic tool PICo (population, phenomenon of interest, and context) [9, 10]. The protocol used to operationalize the research had 9 stages: (1) Formulate a research question; (2) Produce an investigation protocol; (3) Define inclusion and exclusion criteria; (4) Develop a research strategy and research data banks; (5) Select articles; (6) Evaluate the quality of the articles; (7) Extract relevant data from the articles; (8) Summarize the results and evaluate the quality of evidences; and (9) Publish the results [11].

After the research question was determined, the eligibility criteria for the bibliography were established (Table 1). This methodological choice made it possible to narrow confidence intervals, facilitating the comparison between papers, data interpretation, and increasing the precision of the results.

Table 1. Eligibility criteria for the bibliographic sample. Lisbon, 2021.

	Inclusion criteria	Exclusion criteria
Participants	Elders	Children; adolescents; adults
Intervention/Phenomenon of interest	Oral hydration measures; Measures to prevent and/or control dehydration	
Context	Hospitalization	Admission in nursing homes/Emergency Services or home hospitalization units

Studies that described interventions in different contexts could be included, as long as they allowed for the identification of the interventions that control dehydration in a hospital environment.

The research was carried out from March to April 2021, and the descriptors Mesh/DeCS used in it, associated using the Boolean operators AND and OR, were: ("Dehydration" OR "Oral Hydration") AND ("Aged" OR "Elderly" OR "Older person") AND ("Hospitalization") and nurs*.

The research was carried out in the databases available through search engines and in those available in the platforms PubMed, EBSCO (Medline, CINAHL), B-On, ISI (Web of Science), SCOPUS, and JBO, considering the inclusion and exclusion criteria explained above.

The time frame selected was of 5 years (articles published from 2016 to 2021. This criterion was chosen due to the fact that it guarantees the most updated information and recent evidences. In addition to the time frame, the following filters were also used: Full Text; Languages: Portuguese, Spanish, and English.

Data selection and extraction was carried out by two independent investigators, who resorted to a third one when there was no consensus in the different stages of selection of a bibliographic sample. The Rayyan® platform was used for this process.

The flowchart of the extraction of the articles (Fig. 1) allows us to observe that 298 articles were found. 75 of them were excluded for being duplicates. We were able to eliminate 201 articles through an analysis of their titles, after what 22 documents were left. From them, 13 articles were excluded after a reading of their abstract, and 9 were left to be read in full. After a full reading, 2 articles were excluded because they were not in accordance with the objectives of the study, and 7 were left that respected the eligibility criteria.

An Excel spreadsheet was created to extract the title of the paper/work; its authors; year of publication; type of paper; objective(s), method, and techniques; level of evidence; and main results/conclusions.

To systematize the information found, the results of the articles that allowed us to answer the research question were extracted and analyzed. A content analysis of the

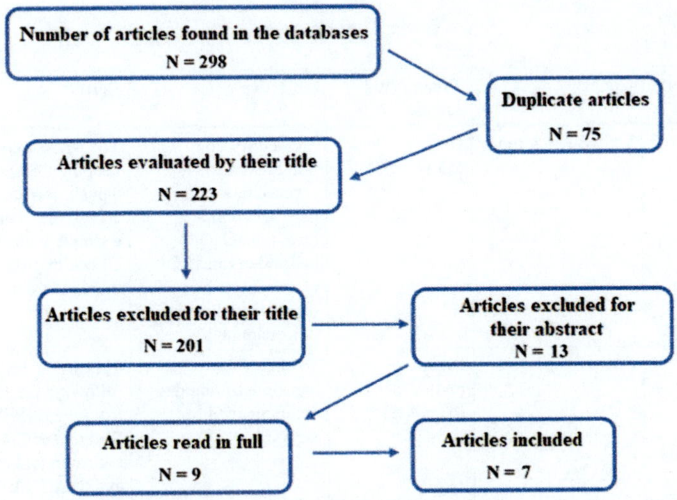

Fig. 1. Flowchart of the triage of the articles for the literature review. Lisbon, 2021.

qualitative findings, considering Bardin's definition [12], was carried out. Two investigators coded the results, which were then assessed by two members of the research team to increase reliability.

3 Results

From the studies (E) that form the bibliographic sample (Table 2), two were published in 2016 [2, 16], two in 2017 [13, 15], one in 2018 [4], and two in 2020 [3, 13]. Three of them are primary studies [2, 14, 15].

Table 2. Studies that form the bibliographic sample. Lisbon, 2021.

Reference (year)	Country	Type of study sample	Objective	Results
E1 Oates and Price (2017) [13]	United Kingdom	Systematic review (23 studies)	To describe clinical evaluation tools that identify people who are under the risk of insufficient liquid intake To describe the impact of interventions to promote oral hydration in hospitals and retirement homes	The authors presented the following interventions as a way to promote hydration in the hospitals: Promoting education for elders; Promoting more opportunities to provide them with beverages; Using visual elements to remind them of this need; Making more liquid available at the time of medication intake; Including the family

(*continued*)

Table 2. (*continued*)

Reference (year)	Country	Type of study sample	Objective	Results
E2 Davidson et al. (2020) [14]	United Kingdom	Observational (559 elders)	To identify up to what point hydration is accessible for the diseased who are hospitalized and bedridden (incapable of moving in bed with no aid from health professionals)	The authors consider that keeping the bedside table in a position where it is easily accessible to the diseased is a simple intervention that all health professionals must consider
E3 Masot et al. (2020) [3]	Spain	Literature review (8 studies)	To clarify the ingestion of liquids recommended for elders	This article recommends following the guidance from the ESPEN (European Society for Clinical Nutrition and Metabolism) and the EFSA (European Food Safety Authority)
E4 Picetti et al. (2017) [15]	2017 United States	Observational (170 elders)	To determine the amount of liquid elders ingest per day To evaluate the knowledge of elders about the ideal state of hydration, signs and symptoms of dehydration and of excessive hydration, as well as some medical conditions associated	The authors recommend carrying out public campaigns to raise awareness about these topics and implementing programs to educate and train health workers According to this article, the standard recommendation for liquid intake is of 8 glasses a day, with a lower amount for those with cardiac diseases or reduced renal function The authors also state that the liquids that must be taken should be individualized, considering their appearance or there should be a promotion of social interaction to make liquid ingestion a more pleasant experience
E5 Hooper et al. (2016) [16]	United Kingdom	Literature review	Systematization of knowledge about the dehydration of elders in several different contexts (including hospitals)	The authors: Individual evaluation of hydration barriers; Education; Monitoring; Encouragement of water intake; Presenting a greater variety of beverages more often; Addressing incontinence and medications that can be needed Health workers must also support the consumption of liquids, even in those with cognitive deterioration, supporting social relations, a routine, and the pleasure of drinking

(*continued*)

Table 2. (*continued*)

Reference (year)	Country	Type of study sample	Objective	Results
E6 McCrow et al. (2016) [2]	Australia	Observational (44 elders)	To evaluate the prevalence of dehydration in hospitalized elders, with or without cognitive impairments To examine the association between dehydration, cognitive impairment, and fragility in the elders	The authors recommend monitoring liquid intake
E7 Volkert et al. (2018) [4]	Scotland	Guideline	To provide evidence-based recommendations for clinical nutrition and hydration in elders, to prevent and/or treat malnutrition and dehydration	This study states that the elders must be consider as a risk group for dehydration and encouraged to ingest the adequate amount of liquids, also adding that all of them should be examined in regard to their hydration status It further states that standard procedures must be determined, and interventions must be adapted and tailored to each patient. Several recommendations are presented to this end, such as: Encouraging the dehydrated and asymptomatic elders to increase their liquid intake by drinking beverages they prefer; Administration of hypotonic fluids to treat dehydration caused by low liquid intake; Monitoring of the state of hydration and liquid intake until they are corrected, and then, monitoring them periodically; Administering intravenous and subcutaneous fluids in parallel to oral liquid intake in dehydrated elders who present symptoms and in elders who cannot ingest liquid orally; Elders with dysphagia must be evaluated, treated, and monitored by a specialist

The articles have a high geographic disparity: three come from the United Kingdom [13, 14, 16], one from Scotland [4], one from Spain [3], one from Australia [2], and one from the United States [15].

The content analysis of the articles made it possible to group the results in two categories: treatment interventions and preventive interventions.

Regarding treatment interventions, their main goal is to deal with a diagnostic that is present, in this case, dehydration. They involve mainly the monitoring of liquid intake during hospitalization [2–4, 15, 16], the provision of beverages that are adequate to the preferences of the diseased [4, 15, 16], the more frequent provision of beverages [3, 4, 13, 15, 16], and the keeping liquids where the client can reach them [4, 13–16], so they can easily have access to beverages independently. To do so, professionals must be educated [4, 13].

The guideline included in the sample still refers to the importance of the administration of hypotonic fluids to correct the deficit of fluids and reduce plasm osmolality [4]. Some studies emphasize the individualization and comprehension of the hydric care in elders to ensure, maintain, or improve the hydric state of the client, as well as their quality of life [4, 15, 16]. The authors also mention the importance of identifying the causes of dehydration and eliminating them as soon as possible, alerting for elders with dysphagia and problems swallowing, as well as their increased risk for dehydration [4].

The use of instruments to evaluate signs of dehydration and monitor hospitalization is important [2, 13], as well as to monitor the quantity and quality of liquid ingested [13].

In regard to preventive interventions, they are addressed by three of the seven articles included. They recommend the ingestion of a minimum of 1.6 L of daily liquid intake for elder women, while elder men should ingest a minimum of 2 L per day [3, 4].

One of the studies recommends, for prevention, the use of clinical assessment tools to identify the elders who are at risk of ingesting insufficient liquid, such as: checklists regarding the health history and physical observations; glycemic and urine tests; checklists with specific or general interventions; identification through characteristics of the urine; promotion of liquid intake; and others [13].

One of the authors warns about the importance of establishing standard procedures to guarantee the implementation of interventions that can ensure all elders are adequately hydrated [4]. These procedures should also be formulated by a multidisciplinary team, including physicians, nurses, and nutritionists. The authors state that all elders must be considered as part of a risk group for dehydration due to low liquid intake. As such, they must be encouraged to consume an adequate amount of liquid, according to their preferences. The article also recommends that an assessment of the hydric state must be carried out for all elders in contact with the health system, to diagnose dehydration early and implement timely interventions [4].

Another measure is an adequate education regarding hydration, that could improve the quality of life of the elders, reducing hospitalization and the economic load associated with mortality and morbidity. This could be carried out through campaigns to disseminate information, aimed at increasing the knowledge of this vulnerable population and their caregivers, relatives, and friends [15].

4 Discussion

Dehydration is a geriatric problem that can be completely avoided through the adoption of a set of simple and cost-effective measures that lead to a daily intake from 1.5 L to 2 L of liquid [3, 4], including the adequate prescription from health workers to individualize intake to the clinical state of the elder [4].

Some authors indicate that simple measures may be enough to increase liquid intake and prevent or control dehydration in hospitalized elderly, including making available more liquid at times of medication intake [13] or keeping the side table in a position where it is accessible to the bedridden person [14]. It is important to mention that the intake of liquid should be fractioned, with small quantities provided several times a day, since a large amount at a single moment may decrease the feeling of thirst due to gastric distention, also interfering on appetite and increasing the risk of malnutrition [17].

Another important measure to avoid accidents, such as falls, is limiting the intake of liquid after 17 p.m., so elders do not get up several times at night to go to the bathroom and/or urinate, risking falls as they get up from the bed or go to the bathroom [18, 19]. It should also be reiterated that coffee, tea, and soft drinks with caffeine have a diuretic effect and, in excess, can increase the risk of falls, especially in elders with cognitive deterioration [19].

One of the studies in the sample shows that 60% of the elder population they studied presented gaps in their knowledge about liquid intake, from the medical conditions that can cause dehydration to the importance of hydration and the need to ingest liquids, or even regarding the need to seek medical help when in situations of risk [15] or the adequate amount of liquid that should be ingested daily [13].

Education in health is a noble priority of nurses, and if we consider the process of disease prevention as a pyramid, its base would indeed be the type of prevention carried out by informing the population [20]. This is why there must be an immediate investment on educating the elders about adequate liquid intake [13].

This educational element can also include health workers and caregivers [21]. In this regard, we believe that it is extremely important to increase the knowledge of the multidisciplinary team in regard to dehydration, risk factors, and interventions for prevention, so everyone is attentive and aware of how important it is to prevent dehydration in elders and monitor the risk and intake [2].

Monitoring can take advantage of technological resources that enable self-monitoring or the recording of one's own liquid intake, such as records in telephone applications, or making available visual and/or sound elements that remind one of the need for hydration [13]. Among risk factors, after all, there are memory problems that lead this population to forget to ingest liquids or the need to hydrate [4].

Resorting to technology can also be a solution to mass disseminate information about the prevention of dehydration in the elderly population at risk, by sending alerts and information about prevention to their telephones, as well as by monitoring them via teleconsultations.

A study with dependent elders and those confined to bed states that 13% of the 138 participants cannot reach the beverage that is at the bedside [14]. The reasons for this include bedside tables distant from the bed or glasses that, despite being full, were out of the reach of the diseased. Considering these results, the authors concluded that a simple intervention, which should be among the first ones made by health professionals, should be moving the bedside table in such a way that each bedridden client can reach the beverage on it [14].

The administration of intravenous and subcutaneous fluids can be a measure to control dehydration, but not for prevention. It should be carried out simultaneously with oral liquid intake in dehydrated symptomatic elders and in those who cannot ingest liquids orally [4]. In cases of severe/grave dehydration, the intravenous administration should be preferred, since a large volume of fluid is necessary. However, the intravenous reposition of fluids is a more delicate situation for elders, since the changes in the skin make it more difficult to place peripheral access points [17]. There is also the risk for iatrogenesis, since endovenous reposition may cause pulmonary edemas in clients with cardiac arrest and hyponatremia [4].

It should be reiterated that, although dehydration is one of the ten most common diagnoses that lead to the hospitalization of elders, it is still seldom discussed, both in regard to statistics or in the elaboration of scales to evaluate the risk of dehydration in the elders and of protocols for the evaluation, prevention, and treatment of this pathology.

We can also state that part of the family of the client are going through a transitional period, since, considering the deterioration of the health state of their relative, it becomes more necessary to help caring for them, and they can assume the role of caregivers [21]. Therefore, it is necessary to recognize these people as partners in the provision of care, especially when it comes to transmitting knowledge, so they can be trained to continue caring for the patient after hospital discharge. They should also be viewed as people under risk for dehydration, since many of them are also of old age.

No qualitative studies were identified in this IR that explore the choices and concerns of the older persons regarding this issue of hydration. We felt that it would be important to bring the 'voices' of these people into the research because the diversification of knowledge is crucial for the promotion of individual and public health. The relationship of the human being with health and with health professionals is complex, as it involves a multiplicity of factors that are not always easy to identify and control, which is influenced by and influences the multiple relations, and cannot be dissociated from the individual experience [22].

This study was limited due to the heterogeneous nature of the studies in the sample. Furthermore, the restriction of articles to Portuguese, Spanish, and English did not allow for an identification of studies published in other languages and may have led to the loss of more international works about the phenomenon being studied.

5 Conclusions

The seven articles that form the bibliographical sample of this study allowed us to identify two categories related to the dehydration of the hospitalized elder: treatment interventions and preventive interventions.

Considering the high prevalence of hospitalized dehydrated elders and the severity of their complications, we believe that it is extremely important for interventions to prevent dehydration to be implemented in the future. These interventions include raising the awareness of health workers, so they can be more alert in regard to this issue, which must be avoided.

Future researches should explore the development of e-health interventions that make it possible to prevent the dehydration of the elderly in the community and in the hospital. We also recommend a Massive Open Online Course (MOOC) to educate health workers about the monitoring and the interventions to prevent and control dehydration.

References

1. El-sharkawy, A.M., et al.: Hydration and outcome in older patients admitted to hospital (the HOOP prospective cohort study). Age Ageing **44**(6), 1–5 (2015). https://doi.org/10.1093/ageing/afv119
2. McCrow, J., Morton, M., Travers, C., Harvey, K., Eeles, E.: Associations between dehydration, cognitive impairment, and frailty in older hospitalized patients: an exploratory study. J. Geront. Nurs. **42**(5), 19–27 (2016). https://doi.org/10.3928/00989134-20160201-01
3. Masot, O., Miranda, J., Santamaría, A.L., Paraiso Pueyo, E., Pascual, A., Botigué, T.: Fluid intake recommendation considering the physiological adaptations of adults over 65 years: a critical review. Nutrients **12**(11), 3383 (2020). https://doi.org/10.3390/nu12113383
4. Volkert, D., et al.: (ESPEN guideline on clinical nutrition and hydration in geriatrics. Clin. Nutr. **38**(1), 10–47 (2019). https://doi.org/10.1016/j.clnu.2018.05.024
5. Hooper, L., Bunn, D., Jimoh, F.O., Fairweather-Tait, S.J.: Water-loss dehydration and aging. Mech. Ageing Dev. **136–137**, 50–58 (2014). https://doi.org/10.1016/j.mad.2013.11.009
6. Anjo, I., et al.: Are hypohydrated older adults at increased risk of exhaustion? J. Hum. Nutr. Diet. **33**, 23–30 (2020). https://doi.org/10.1111/jhn.12702
7. Begg, D.P.: Disturbances of thirst and fluid balance associated with aging. Physiol. Behav. **178**, 28–34 (2017). https://doi.org/10.1016/j.physbeh.2017.03.003
8. Hooper, L., Bunn, D.: Detecting dehydration in older people: useful tests. Nurs. Times **111**(32/33), 12–16 (2015). PMID: 26455128
9. Souza, M.T., Silva, M.D., Carvalho, R.: Integrative review: what is it? How to do it? Einstein **8**(1), 102–106 (2010). https://doi.org/10.1590/s1679-45082010rw1134
10. Sousa, L.M.M., Marques-Vieira, C.M.A., Severino, S.S.P., Antunes, A.V.: A metodologia de revisão integrativa da literatura em enfermagem. Rev. Invest. Enfermagem **2**(21), 17–26 (2017). https://www.researchgate.net/publication/321319742_Metodologia_de_Revisao_Integrativa_da_Literatura_em_Enfermagem
11. Donato, H., Donato, M.: Etapas na Condução de uma Revisão Sistemática. Acta Med. Port. **32**(3), 227–235 (2019). http://dx.doi.org/10.20344/amp.11923
12. Bardin, L.: Análise de Conteúdo. 6ª edn. Edições 70, Lisboa (2016)
13. Oates, L.L., Price, C.I.: Clinical assessments and care interventions to promote oral hydration amongst older patients: a narrative systematic review. BMC Nurs. **16**, 4 (2017). https://doi.org/10.1186/s12912-016-0195-x
14. Davidson, J., et al.: A multicentre prospective audit of bedside hydration in hospital. Br. J. Nurs. **29**(1), 50–54 (2020). https://doi.org/10.12968/bjon.2020.29.1.50
15. Picetti, D., et al.: Hydration health literacy in the elderly. Nutr. Healthy Aging **4**(3), 227–237 (2017). https://doi.org/10.3233/NHA-170026
16. Hooper, L.: Why, oh why, are so many older adults not drinking enough fluid? J. Acad. Nutr. Diet. **116**(5), 774–778 (2016). https://doi.org/10.1016/j.jand.2016.01.006
17. Jimoh, O.F., Brown, T.J., Bunn, D., Hooper, L.: Beverage intake and drinking patterns-clues to support older people living in long-term care to drink well: DRIE and FISE studies. Nutrients **11**(2), 447 (2019). https://doi.org/10.3390/nu11020447

18. Lavareda Baixinho, C., Dixe, M.A.: ¿Cuáles son las prácticas y comportamientos de los mayores institucionalizados para prevenir las caídas?. Index Enferm **26**, 255–259 (2017). https://scielo.isciii.es/scielo.php?script=sci_arttext&pid=S1132-12962017000300004&lng=es&nrm=iso
19. Baixinho, C.L., Dixe, M.A., Madeira, C., Alves, S., Henriques, M.A.: Falls in institutionalized elderly with and without cognitive decline: a study of some factors. Dement. Neuropsychol. **13**(1), 116–121 (2019). https://doi.org/10.1590/1980-57642018dn13-01001
20. Denehy, J.: Health education: an important role for school nurses. J. Sch. Nurs. **17**(5), 233–238 (2001). https://doi.org/10.1177/10598405010170050101
21. Ferreira, B.A.l.S., Gomes, T.J.B., Baixinho, C.R.S.L., Ferreira, O.M.R.: Transitional care to caregivers of dependent older people: an integrative literature review. Rev. Bras. Enferm. **73**(Suppl 3),e20200394 (2020). http://dx.doi.org/10.1590/0034-7167-2020-0394
22. Baixinho, C.L., Presado, M.H., Ribeiro, J.: Qualitative research and the transformation of public health. Cien Saude Colet. **24**(5),1583–1583 (2019). http://dx.doi.org/10.1590/1413-81232018245.05962019

Innovative Educational Approach in Healthcare-Associated Infection Prevention and Control. Results of a European Study

Maria do Rosário Pinto[1](✉), Joaquim Simões[2], Alcinda Reis[2], Fátima Cunha[2], Helena Caseiro[2], Amelia Patrzała[3], Grazina Bączyk[3,4], Aleksandra Jankowiak-Bernaciak[3], Anna Basa[3], Eva Valverde[5], Amaia Yurrebaso-Macho[5], Raquel Guzman-Ordaz[5], Juan Méndez[5], Alexander Ward Mayens[5], Jose Perez Iglesias[5], Jose Miron Canelo[5], Marja Silén-Lipponen[6], Ulla Korhonen[6], Leena Koponen[6], Mikko Myllymäki[6], Paulo S. Costa[7], Beatriz Serambeque[7,8], Eva Fernandes[7], João Pardal[7], Anabela S. Oliveira[7], João Graveto[7], and Pedro Parreira[7]

[1] Higher School of Nursing Lisbon, Lisbon, Portugal
mrosario.pinto@esel.pt
[2] Politechnic Institute of Santarém, Santarém, Portugal
[3] PWSZ University, Gniezno, Poland
[4] Poznan University of Medical Sciences, Poznan, Poland
[5] University of Salamanca, Salamanca, Spain
[6] SAVONIA University of Applied Sciences, Kuopio, Finland
[7] Nursing School of Coimbra | Health Sciences Research Unit: Nursing, Nursing School of Coimbra (ESEnfC), Coimbra, Portugal
[8] Centre for Innovative Biomedicine and Biotechnology (CIBB), Faculty of Medicine, Coimbra, Portugal

Abstract. Prevent and control healthcare-associated infections (HAIs) is a priority in healthcare assistance, not only due to present COVID-19 pandemic. Annually, around 3.2 million patients are affected by one of these infections and it is estimated that without controlling them, by 2050, 10 million more people could die every year, with especial relevance among elderly with infectious situations representing a third of mortality in people over 65 years old. Higher Education Institutions (HEI) in healthcare area have an important role in this panorama, by preparing students to be future professionals, stimulating them to have an innovative and entrepreneurial approach to today's real-life challenges. A mixed-methods research was conducted, at European level (in Portugal, Finland, Poland and Spain), to facilitate learning of good practices on HAIs prevention and control while developing innovative solutions. 1475 participants were enrolled, from all partner HEI: 79 professors and mentors were interviewed (individual or focus group), 1326 final year nursing students made a self-report inventory (application of InovSafeCare Scale) and 70 students participated on focus group (agile piloting of the Model). The result of this research is a pedagogical model that mixes dimensions and methods that take nursing students closer to the demands of HAIs prevention and control and capacitates them to transfer knowledge to work settings with an innovative and entrepreneurial perspective – the InovSafeCare Model.

J. García-Alonso and C. Fonseca (Eds.): IWoG 2021, LNBE, pp. 399–407, 2022.
https://doi.org/10.1007/978-3-030-97524-1_37

Keywords: Healthcare Associated Infections (HAIs) · Elderly · Nursing education · InovSafeCare Model · Entrepreneurship

1 Introduction

One of the 21st Century's most defying challenges is to prevent and control healthcare-associated infections (HAIs), known by its rapid spread and high morbidity and mortality, especially in advanced ages. Approximately 3.2 million patients in Europe suffer every year from HAIs, from which 20 to 30% are considered preventable [1–3].

Current age evolution of the world population increases the concern in this area: 566 million people are at least 65 years old, with estimates of nearly 1.5 billion by 2050. Lengthening life spans correlate with increased time in hospitals or long-term care facilities and exposure to drug-resistant pathogens, although evidence shows that the risk of HAIs increases with age, independent of duration spent in healthcare facilities. Nevertheless, infections constitute a third of mortality in people over 65 years old [4].

Scientific evidence shows these infections can be prevented by adopting measures which are proven to be effective to reduce the risk of transmission during healthcare assistance. Furthermore, guidelines have been published with preventive measures which should be adopted to reduce the risk, but not always healthcare professionals demonstrate excellent knowledge and compliance with these recommendations [5–7].

A situation that obliges all areas related to healthcare, aware of it, to contribute with clear proposals that seek to improve the effectiveness of care, especially focused on populations at higher risk. And the pathway to achieve quality of care begins within the academic context, where students are prepared to be future professionals. Conscious of this and of its implications in healthcare education, a Consortium of five Nursing Higher Education Institutions (HEI) from Portugal, Finland, Poland and Spain developed a European wide mixed-methods research focused on understanding how to promote students' knowledge and competencies in this area, simultaneously with the promotion of entrepreneurial skills.

It is known that healthcare education, specifically in the nursing area, is focused on a dynamic acquisition of knowledge both in theoretical and practical learning environments, allowing the acquisition of theoretical and practical knowledge, promoting its application in practice and the reflection upon action, with the inherent development of critical thinking abilities in real-life contexts. This gains special meaning in HAIs prevention and control area, with the importance of making care safer, free from avoidable infections, of high quality and people centered [8, 9], especially if elderly are the focus of care.

Of high importance in this process is the development of pedagogical models, as structured representations of reality based on different theoretical references or formulated from the combination of previously existing ones [10] which contribute to the synergy between educational approach and the evolution of the health/disease process and the reality of the healthcare assistance, potentiating the articulation between theory and practice, focused on acquiring skills and competences along with an investigative attitude that enables its theorization and allows the combination of the vision(s) for learning and teaching.

Pedagogical models may adopt different orientations, but the constructivist perspective undertakes as consensual that education must promote students' competency(s) to manage their learning process, assume increasing autonomy in their academic path, along with intellectual and social tools that enable them to continue lifelong learning [11]. Based on this premise of student-centered learning is possible to propose basic structures, processes and methods [12], that enable the integration of cognitive and operative strategies as part of the learning process [13], along with the stimulation of students' sense of innovation and entrepreneurship.

From this point of view is possible to produce innovative educational approaches, developing students' competencies along with the learning of good practices, raising their awareness and encouraging them to critically reflect upon the field of HAIs prevention and control, with the aim of proposing innovative solutions that contribute to increase quality of care [14].

Including innovate pedagogical practices for nursing students, that can be used by the different actors involved in the process of developing students' competencies, InovSafeCare Model is the result of this European research, intending to be a reference to inspire and guide the educational pedagogical process in HAIs prevention and control, namely while caring for older people, as evidence suggests that advanced age is the most important predictor for fatal outcomes in current healthcare practice [15].

2 Methods

Mixed-method research was developed guarantying all ethics principles (approved by UICISA: E Ethics' Committee - Opinion nº 635/11-2019), supported on a literature review about pedagogical methods, HAIs protocols and procedures recommended for prevention and control (from Portugal, Spain, Finland and Poland).

Empirical study was performed to understand how learning of these competencies can be integrated in nursing courses, in an innovative perspective. With the objective of getting to know the reality in this area, qualitative and quantitative studies were developed.

Interviews and focus groups were conducted to identify the perspective of teachers and tutors involved in the learning and teaching process of nursing students on HAIs prevention and control. According to previously defined criteria, 79 participants were enrolled - nursing course Coordinators and Presidents of HEI Boards were interviewed while invited assistants and clinical mentors participated in focus groups [61 females and 18 males, medium age of 51 years; with a general work experience in the profession of 28.8 years (min. 17/max. 40) and an experience in didatics applied to the healthcare sciences of 16.5 years (min 3/max. 35)].

The convenience sample composed of 1326 students from Portugal, Finland, Poland and Spain, enrolled in the quantitative study, allowed the characterization of students' point of view about learning/teaching methods usually applied, namely contents and its organization in the syllabus, along with the identification of personal dimensions that interfere in the process [16].

The triangulation of all data obtained constituted the empirical structure of the model, permitting the design of the InovSafeCare Model, which, through Focus group method, was piloted in all academic realities of the five HEIs, involving a total of seventy students that analyzed the proposal, giving their perspective and specific suggestions to improve its design and implementation perspective.

3 Results and Discussion

Results of studies are aligned with a constructivist perspective, that places students in the center of the process, identifying a vectorial relation between theoretical approach (result of teachers' intervention), motivation and students' attitude, as can be seen in Fig. 1.

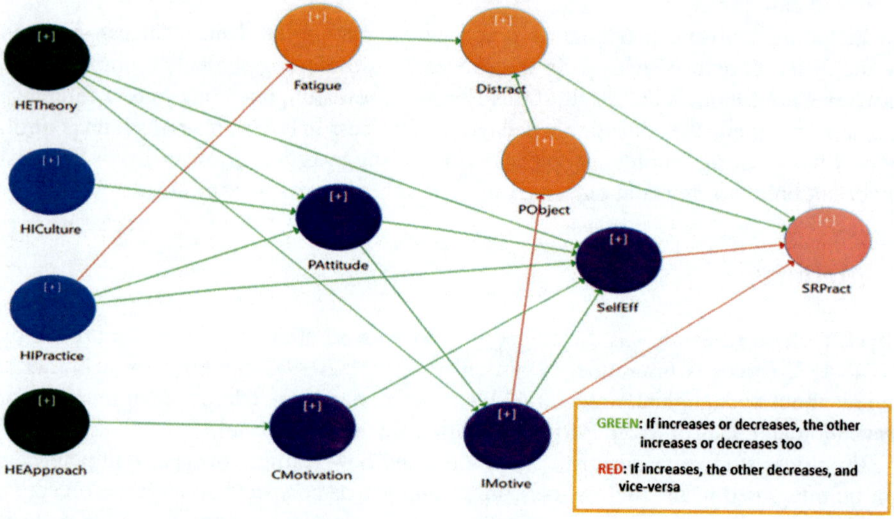

Fig. 1. InovSafeCare Ecosystem Model (Source: adapted from Yurrebaso-Macho et al. 2021)

The importance of an active learning environment is highlighted, pointing out that this can stimulate and inspire engaged, reflexive and critical thinking with the implementation of methods that take students closer to the real world of care, capacitating them to transfer knowledge to work settings [17].

Another dimension, that arises from the qualitative study, is self-directed learning, in which students have the initiative to identify their learning needs [18] while they develop skills to increase active citizenship and work HAIs prevention and control issues with a creative perspective, making decisions applicable to nursing care [19] at the same time they increment their creativity and innovative skills.

The results of qualitative study highlight students "*…have this characteristic (…) have creativity…*" and make "*…suggestions for intervention (…) innovative things…*" that can "*…contribute to the behaviour change within the [healthcare] team*", in the line of thought of Alves and his partners [20], that defend the importance of creativity, opportunity identification, decision-making for innovation, idea generation, autonomy and networking, in order to develop an entrepreneurial spirit and explore opportunities in healthcare and technological areas that will promote quality of care. Consequently, this generates more assertiveness on prevention and control of HAIs, reducing morbidity and mortality rates. As one of the participants in qualitative study mention, "*Entrepreneurship contributes to development [of practices and educational strategies]*".

Empirical outcomes also point out the pedagogical strategies and methods to encourage reflexive thinking and entrepreneurial potential, suggesting a perspective of acquisition and development of skills that allow students to become entrepreneurs in the field of HAIs, a very specialized area, with objective, specific and constantly updated information, periodically worldwide regulated as new evidence is produced, leading to the need for regular acquisition or actualization of information (see Table 1).

Table 1. Excerpts from the speech about the utilization of technological and non-technological strategies to approach HAIs prevention and control

Non technological strategies	Technological strategies
"… giving information to students in an **active lecture**, (…) with examples…" FT2 L 260–262 "…provide a **clinical case** that (…) already has (…) data that we want (…) to mobilize…" FT5 L807–809 "**situations of the observation**…" FT2 L 566 "There should also be a greater integration of the contents, (…) for example **problem solving**" FT5 L 212–213 "Move from what is theoretical content, to problem solving, in different circumstances" FT5 L 214–215 "… it seems to me that perhaps **theoretical-practical classes** were necessary, even if truly theoretical-practical, where one could actually exemplify the area that is sterilized, what is sterilization…" B5 "…**laboratories** are equipped, (…) for demonstration and explanation (…) I am thinking of very practical things, which are the taps, the way they are handled (...) it is adequate and adapted…" E3 "In a **laboratory practice**, different adjustments can be made throughout the process…" FT5 L 843–844 "…[students] come to [clinical] **practice** and the real models are [nurses]…" FC3 L160–163 "… during the **clinical** teaching (…) there is always a relationship with the institution's teacher, and there is proximity." A3 "when students go to my ward, they are guided and focused on hand hygiene…" A3. "… we [University and Hospital] can make some materials together..." SE	"as an **online course**, …" S1 "[It was important to have] the possibility to **record the procedures** that they [the students] did in these laboratories" FC2 L 390–391 "[It was a facilitator to have conditions like the] **mannequins** [that interact with the students] and that we see and that there is a teacher out there who visualizes and records everything" FC1 L393 "… simulation processes should cover more than one domain" FT5 L 827-829 "The simulation processes are also part of a good strategy to acquire knowledge" FT5 L 834–835 "I think that it would be, in fact, a very important [simulation] context to integrate these aspects [infection prevention and control]" IPPC L 301–302 "We are trying to create several scenarios (…) from the patient's history to the situation… all the equipment, what is going to be done and what the student is expected to answer… later, at the end, there is debriefing" B8

This European research substantiated the design of InovSafeCare Model, whose structure is delineated on Fig. 2, encouraging the mobilization of non-technological and technological strategies [21], consistently organized within an active learning environment that enables students to be engaged in self-learning, critical and reflexive thinking, with an entrepreneurial attitude. Consequently, its main objectives are:

- to provide a student-centered learning environment that capacitates to intervention in HAIs control and prevention process;
- to enhance learners' awareness and involvement in the process of HAIs prevention and control;
- to develop creative and critical thinking in clinical decision making, evidence-based supported, to prevent and control HAIs;
- to encourage learners' entrepreneurship towards innovative approach perspectives in HAIs prevention and control.

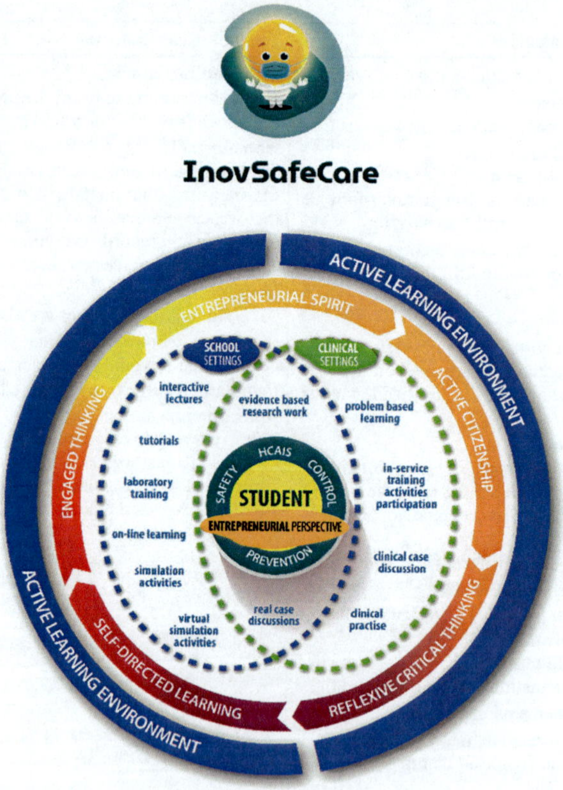

Fig. 2. Explicative diagram of the InovSafeCare Model

This innovative educational proposal understands learning and teaching process in which all components support each other, specifically methods, strategies and the curricula, ensuring that the learning outcomes agreed are achievable and levels or standards expected at different stages are clear [22]. Basically, it consists of the integration of dimensions and methods to make students closer to the demands of expertise related to HAIs prevention and control, simultaneously seeking to integrate the discussion about learning and cognition, with an innovative and entrepreneurial glance.

4 Final Considerations

Currently, HAIs prevention and control are a worldwide healthcare concern and priority, not only due to the present COVID-19 pandemic situation, but directly related to its global prevalence, especially in the situation of people over 65 years, due to what appears to be a network of factors in the aging body, including degenerative alterations along with the decrease of immune response, that interact and lead each other to distinctly increase vulnerability to infection.

This defies the pedagogical capacity to innovate and improve practices focused on achieving higher quality in all its dimensions, enabling healthcare students to acquire and develop cognitive, technical and interpersonal competencies, proposing innovative solutions that can contribute to the prevention and/or minimization of HAIs.

The results of the studies developed allowed the design of a specific educational proposal, essentially directed to nursing education, that can be applied transversally to other healthcare areas. Supported upon the perspective of all the actors involved in the learning and teaching process (students, professors and nurses), with deep knowledge about HAIs prevention and control area, about general and specific competencies to be achieved/developed, as well as about the syllabus of nursing courses and teaching academic reality (qualitative and quantitative studies), InovSafeCare Model was accomplished.

The uniqueness of this proposal consists of its dynamic and interactive system developed to encourage a student-centered pedagogical methodology that promotes an entrepreneurial perspective focused on generating innovative projects that can contribute positively to the quality and security in healthcare practice, potentiating the interaction between scholars and clinical contributes.

Specifically in HAIs area, this approach has already produced suggestions about personal protection equipment namely to protect the face, solving the issue of decreased vision due to blurring, and about disinfection of common spaces. These devices, by contributing to the security of caring process, are an asset in HAIs prevention and control, as they contribute to the safety of assistance and therefore do decrease the risk of exposure of the care receivers, especially in the case of the elderly.

Further research is in development, concerning the assessment procedures, fundamental to provide feedback about the process and needs for future improvement.

Acknowledgments. We acknowledge professor **Cassilda Vaz Sarroeira** for her contribution to the design of *InovSafeCare Model*, essential to this final achievement.

Funding. ERASMUS+ Programme (InovSafeCare Project: 2018-1-PT01-KA203-047453).

References

1. Harbarth, S., Sax, H., Gastmeier, P.: The preventable proportion of nosocomial infections: an overview of published reports. J. Hosp. Infect. **54**, 258–66 (2003). https://doi.org/10.1016/s0195-6701(03)00150-6
2. Council of the European Union: Council conclusions on patient safety and quality of care, including the prevention and control of healthcare-associated infections and antimicrobial resistance (2014/C 438/05). Official Journal of the European Union (2014)
3. ECDC: European Centre for Disease Prevention and Control. An agency of the European Union (2019)
4. Kline, K.A., Bowdish, D.M.: Infection in an aging population. Curr. Opin. Microbiol. **29**, 63–67 (2016). https://doi.org/10.1016/j.mib.2015.11.003
5. Castella, A., et al.: Surgical site infection surveillance: analysis of adherence to recommendations for routine infection control practices. Infect. Control Hosp. Epidemiol. **27**, 835–40 (2006). https://doi.org/10.1086/506396
6. Zhou, Y., et al.: Healthcare-associated infections and shanghai clinicians: a multicenter cross-sectional study. PLoS One **9**(8), e105838 (2014). https://doi.org/10.1371/journal.pone.0105838
7. Kołpa, M., Grochowsk, A., Gniadek, A., Jurkiewicz, B.: Level of knowledge among medical personnel about infections transferred through direct contact – results of questionnaire survey. Przegl. Epidemiol. **69**, 503–6 (2015)
8. WHO: Health care without avoidable infections. The critical role of infection prevention and control. WHO, Geneve (2016)
9. WHO: Global infection prevention and control priorities 2018–22: a call for action, Lanc, vol. 5, December 2017, pp. e1178–80 (2017)
10. da Silva, M.I.L.: Prática Educativa, Teoria e Investigação. Rev Interações **27**, 283–304 (2013)
11. Simão, A.: Integrar os princípios da aprendizagem estratégica no processo formativo dos professores. In: Silva, A., Duarte, A., Sá, I., Simão, A. (eds.) Aprendizagem Auto-Regulada pelo Estudante. Perspectivas psicológicas e educacionais, pp. 95–106. Porto Editora, Porto (2004)
12. Campbell, A., Gutierrez, M., Lancelott, M.: Operating Model Canvas. Aligning Operations and Organization with Strategy. Van Haren Publishing (2017). ISBN 978 94 018 0071 6
13. Laureano-Cruces, A.L., Ramírez-Rodríguez, J., Mora-Torres, M., Arriaga, F., Escarela-Pérez, R.: Cognitive-operative model of intelligent learning systems behavior. Interact. Learn. Environ. **18**(1), 11–38 (2010). https://doi.org/10.1080/10494820802160872
14. Pinto, M.R., et al.: Educating nursing students for innovative infection prevention and control practices: the InovSafeCare model. In: Proceedings of 1st CIEQV International Congress, Santarém, 18–19 February 2021, pp. 101–2 (2021)
15. Perrotta, F., et al.: COVID-19 and the elderly: insights into pathogenesis and clinical decision-making. Aging Clin. Exp. Res. **32**(8), 1599–1608 (2020). https://doi.org/10.1007/s40520-020-01631-y
16. Yurrebaso-Macho, A., et al.: Nursing students' perceptions on healthcare-associated infection control and prevention teaching and learning experience: development and validation of a scale in four European countries. Front. Psychol. **12**, 701208 (2021). https://doi.org/10.3389/fpsyg.2021.701208
17. Adkins, J.: Active learning and formative assessment in a user-centred design course. Inf. Syst. Educ. J. **16**(4), 34–40 (2018). ISSN 1545-679X

18. Laureano-Cruces, A., Terán-Gilmore, A., de Arriaga, F., El Alami, M.: La importancia de las estrategias cognitivas en el disseño del curricula didáctico. In: Sossa Azuela, H., Sánchez Guerrero, H., Polito Olvera, J., Fuenlabrada Velásquez, S. (eds.) Proceedings XVI Congreso Nacional y II Congreso Internacional de Informática y Computación de la ANIEI, vol. I, pp. 35–41. Zacatecas, México (2003)
19. Ku, Y.-L.: Evaluating creative thinking of RN-BSN students in the course of clinical case study and practicum. Innov. Educ. Teach. Int. **52**(3), 290–299 (2015). https://doi.org/10.1080/14703297.2013.838144
20. Alves, C., Felgueira, T., Paiva, T.: Competências empreendedoras. In: Parreira, P.M., Alves, L., Mónico, L., Sampaio, J., Paiva, T.: Competências empreendedoras no Ensino Superior Politécnico: Motivos, influências, serviços de apoio e educação, pp. 65–76. Instituto Politécnico da Guarda, Guarda (2018)
21. Dearnly, C., McClelland, G., Irving, D.: Innovation in Teaching and Learning in Health Higher Education: Literature Review. Council of Deans of Health and the Higher Education Academy, Bradford (2013)
22. Stefani, L.: Planning teaching and learning. Curriculum design and development. In: Fry, H., Ketteridge, S., Marshall, S. (eds.) A Handbook for Teaching and Learning in Higher Education: Enhancing Academic Practice, 3rd edn., pp. 40–57. Routledge, New York (2009). ISBN 1

Author Index

J. García-Alonso and C. Fonseca (Eds.): IWoG 2021, LNBE, pp. 409–411, 2022.
https://doi.org/10.1007/978-3-030-97524-1